National Health Policy

National Health Policy

What Role for Government?

Proceedings of a
Conference on National Health Policy
held at the Hoover Institution,
Stanford University, on March 28 and 29, 1980

Editor
Isaac Ehrlich

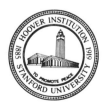

Hoover Institution Press
Stanford University, Stanford, California

ACKNOWLEDGMENTS

Table 1.10: Courtesy of McKinsey & Company, Inc.,
New York, N.Y.

Tables 3.3, 3.4, and 3.6: Courtesy Institute of Applied
and Economic Social Research, University of Melbourne.

Table 3.7 and Figures 3.1, 3.2, and 3.3: Courtesy
of the Australian Consumers' Association, publishers
of CHOICE magazine.

Hoover Press Publication 265

Contents

Foreword
A Market-Side Approach to Health Care

Isaac Ehrlich

Much of the material included in this conference volume differs from what is typically found in similar publications dealing with health policy issues in that it exhibits willingness to re-examine and question the all-too-frequent assertion by many specialists that the transformation of the American health system from a private to a public enterprise is inevitable. It is commonly argued that the American health care system is imperfect: health levels of the population are not the highest in the world; access to health care services is incomplete, especially for the poor and the chronically ill; there are no complete health insurance plans against all medical and related contingencies; and some segments of the population lack any insurance coverage. Moreover, there is medical cost inflation; and despite an apparent unchecked trend to commit a growing share of the national pie to health care services, the system still fails to eliminate various inequities in the distribution of services across different areas or population groups. Thus everyone knows, goes the argument, that it is the government which must intervene and shoulder a major responsibility for alleviating these problems. Indeed, if one looks at the developments in some other Western countries in recent decades, the inevitable solution seems to be in the direction of establishing at the very least a national health insurance plan, if not a national health system modeled after the British or Canadian examples.

Yet many of the papers included in this volume express skepticism regarding both the diagnosis of the American health system as fundamentally ailing and the prescription of greater public intervention in the financing and delivery of medical services as the remedy and sure path to recovery.

Authors in this volume question the standard literature because it has not systematically considered the evidence from other countries that have experimented in various degrees with a national system of health insurance or health care. While no comprehensive examination of these experiences is offered in this volume, the papers in Section I nevertheless point at the various distortions that are bound to emerge with the replacement of a voluntary, market-oriented system by a government-controlled setup in which bureaucratic predispositions replace consumer preferences for health care services and wasteful means of rationing replace the more flexible and efficient method of rationing by fees or prenegotiated insurance contracts. Matt Lindsay, for example, argues on the basis of the recent experience in Great Britain that the circumvention of the private market in determining what services to produce or how to produce them is likely to generate predictable consequences that undermine individual welfare, such as: a bureaucratic bias in favor of "visible" services instead of the proper mix of "visible" and "invisible" services that patients truly seek; a developing tendency among highly trained native physicians and surgeons to migrate to countries maintaining a higher degree of consumer and market sovereignty; and a resulting deterioration in the quality of medical care through arbitrary rationing of services, forced reliance on foreign-trained medical personnel, and reduced efficiency in the management of hospital and ambulatory services. John Pierce's and Uwe Reinhardt's papers also indicate that, contrary to popular beliefs, the current trends in other Western countries in terms of a shift toward greater reliance on the government for the provision or financing of medical services are not as clear-cut as proponents of a socialized system of medicine have been suggesting. In Australia, according to John Pierce, different political camps are pulling in different directions, with the recent Frazer government reversing the previous policy of the labor government by reintroducing a major role for private health insurers and rejecting a uniform national health insurance option. In Germany, where the idea of a limited national health insurance system was born in the 1880s, the actual system has not progressed, according to Reinhardt's account, in the direction of a British-type national health service. Instead, it has continued to rely on an essentially voluntary system of numerous competing and largely self-sufficient "sickness funds" with the role of the government limited to a modest degree of subsidization of the bulk of these funds.

Some conference papers also question the standard theoretical arguments made in favor of government intervention in the health services sector because of an alleged failure of private markets to deliver the range and quantity of services U.S. patients (or some population groups in the United States) need by some academic standards, and in order to control the apparent explosion in health care costs in recent decades. One aspect of the alleged market failure argument—the unequal access to medical services—is eloquently expressed and documented in Lu Ann Aday's paper and Diana Dutton's comments. Representing a general sociological perspective, the latter author also expresses doubts concerning the validity and practical relevance of an economic approach to medicine.

The objections raised by many of the economists in the conference to allegations that the private system of medicine in the United States has failed to achieve maximum potential benefits to consumers and providers stem partly from these economists' different assessment of the empirical evidence bearing on the performance of the private system and partly from a different perception concerning the relationship between genuine shortcomings of the present system and public intervention. There often seems to be a general confusion in the literature regarding the relation between imperfections in the type and level of medical services rendered and the economic system producing them. Medical care in the United States, as well as in other countries, is indeed imperfect, incomplete, and frequently perhaps even inadequate, not because the private voluntary system has failed but because resources are scarce. We do not have the "right" amounts of hospital and ambulatory services, nursing homes, dental and psychiatric care, or full insurance against all the related financial contingencies—especially in specific geographical locations—in the same way that we can't produce unlimited food, clothing and shelter, perfectly safe or fuel-efficient cars, or full life insurance benefits for all. Yet most critics would not espouse the socialization of the industries producing these services because no one expects the government to produce more of these goods at similar or lower costs. The distinction between the scarcity of resources, or the "limited size of the markets," underlying specific medical services and market failure is particularly important in this era of rapid technological and scientific breakthroughs in medicine, which create the potential for superior treatment of the medical problems of all groups at all ages—a potential which cannot be fully realized because resources are limited and must serve competing personal needs. In the same vein, the "failure" of the private health insurance system to provide full coverage of all medical and related personal services at zero deductibles and zero coinsurance rate, as advocated in the Kennedy Plan (the Health Care for All Americans Act) summarized in the article by Stanley Jones, cannot be interpreted as indicative of market failure that must be remedied through some form of a governmental takeover. The fact is that no governmental takeover can eliminate the resource limitations, technological constraints, monitoring and management requirements, and other true sources of the cost of doing business in the health services and health insurance sectors. There is no evidence to suggest that government officials can produce more efficiently than private entrepreneurs any type of medical care or health insurance services, especially when decisions pertaining to allocation of resources are to be made with no regard to resource costs and implicit prices. As my analysis of the Health Care for all Americans Act reveals, the provision of "full" and "free" financial coverage of most medical care contingencies and the guarantee of unlimited access to the markets providing these services are illusionary under any realistic assumptions regarding budget constraints, and even the present level of medical services would be achieved under the proposed guidelines at a dramatically higher social price tag because of the plan's inevitable reliance on nonprice methods of rationing. My analysis shows that the original estimates of the true social costs required to implement the new Kennedy Plan have been severely understated.

As for the evident increase in the share of national income going to health care services, the increase can be attributed to a number of important factors, none of which is linked to the private and voluntary aspects of the present medical care system. These factors include (1) the growth in per capita real income in the United States in the post–World War II period raising the general demand for health care; (2) the significant advances in medical technology raising the quality and effectiveness of a variety of new and old treatment procedures; (3) the general aging of the population (itself, in part, a derivative of advances in health care); and (4) innovations in the system of financing medical care expenditures through hospital, physician, and dental insurance plans. Undoubtedly, the growth of health insurance has been one of the important factors behind the increased expenditures on health care services in the United States; but the extent to which the latter increase has been "excessive" in a welfare-theoretic sense can be attributed in large measure to the artificial public subsidization of the private cost of insurance premiums through a variety of direct subsidies, exemptions from taxation, and the combined effects of medicare and medicaid, rather than to the market failure of private health insurance plans. The fact is that most of the growth of *private* hospital and physician insurance in the United States has taken place from the early 1950s to the mid-1960s—a period which has not been characterized by the stepped-up rate of growth of medical expenditures and medical costs, as has been the situation since the late 1960s following the increased public subsidization of the private consumption of medical care services.

Much of the apparent "failure" of the private system thus may be the result of inefficient government intervention. As the figures presented in my own paper and that of Laurence Seidman indicate, in 1980 the share of the national health bill financed by the government may have already exceeded the 50 percent mark; in this sense, the U.S. medical sector has already been "socialized." While the extent to which the apparent medical cost inflation is the product of distortive subsidies is yet to be determined through careful research, the article by Patricia Munch-Danzon in Section III of the volume clearly demonstrates, at the very least, how well the standard predictions of economic analysis concerning the effects of implicit subsidies and explicit regulation of the pricing system hold against the empirical evidence concerning our experience with medicare and medicaid. Her analysis demonstrates the potential distortive effects inherent in the latest Carter administration's National Health Plan.

Of course, beyond the question of the quality and efficiency of the health care system, there is also the issue of achieving a fair distribution of medical services in the population. Few persons would deny the existence of a strong sentiment in society for guaranteeing indigent persons and those persons suffering from medical conditions requiring enormous financial expenditures access to the medical care system. As many participants have pointed out, however, if it is care for people in extreme medical and financial conditions that is being sought, why not attack this problem directly through a genuinely progressive system of guaranteed premium subsidies or other transfer payments? Why should the solution involve a mandatory comprehensive package for all people and all types of medical expenses, which, coupled with direct supply controls to contain costs, would decrease the choices available to patients, providers, and insurers and increase the real costs of providing services only because of the desire to extend medical assistance to a small segment of the population unable to afford coverage. Indeed, a frontal attack on this problem need not cost more to finance than the implicit rational health insurance system of inefficient and regressive public subsidies that is presently used to support private outlays on insurance and health care.

The solution to the present ills of the health services sector in the United States outlined by several participants in the second and third sections of this volume rejects a continuing shift toward the socialization of medicine as the remedy and relies instead on the power of voluntary private markets, unadulterated by regulatory constraints and inefficient subsidies, to synchronize the wants of consumers and providers and ensure the provision of a socially optimal level of services at the lowest social cost. This market orientation to health care, which is generally adopted in other sectors of the economy, has never been tried to the same degree in the health services sector due to (1) the existence of strict licensure arrangements and other supply controls; (2) the unusual degree of authority granted to physicians and other providers in determining entrance into the medical profession and other aspects of the practice of medicine in the United States; (3) the stringent regulation of the drug industry; (4) the direct intervention by government through regulation and planning of hospital and specific ambulatory services; and (5) the unselective and largely regressive subsidization of health insurance premiums.

The detailed proposals included in the paper by Clark Havighurst generally call for the identification of all areas of health care and health insurance services in which competitive forces have been thwarted, governmental and legal controls have been excessive, and the public subsidization unfocused and distortive. His proposals also call for the replacement of the current set-up in those areas by increased private competition and use of the market mechanism to regulate the flow of medical inputs and services and to determine optimal financing arrangements. A genuine market orientation would also require that subsidization of health care services would be made directly to consumers on the basis of financial need, rather than to individual providers or specific types of organizations of health care services such as health maintenance organizations (HMOs). A truly competitive structure of the health services sector should also result in the most efficient organization of the health care delivery and financing system in terms of the variety of options and practices available to consumers: preventive as well as remedial care; home care as well as hospitalization; solo practices as well as HMOs; fee-for-service as well as physician and dental insurance coverages; and indemnity as well as reimbursement provisions in health insurance contracts. The relative mix of all of these options should thus be determined by consumers' relative preferences for the options and the true costs of producing each one rather than by use of artificial subsidization and public planning.

Although it appears under my name alone, the editorial work on this book would not have been possible without the dedicated assistance of a number of individuals. My greatest debt is to Chaya Ehrlich for her superb assistance in editing the material included in this volume and for taking care of various editorial tasks during the summer of 1981. Fred Floss, Jr., has also participated enthusiastically in the editorial work with the transcripts of the conference proceedings and in the administration of the project. I have also benefitted from the careful review of the manuscript and the many suggestions given by Mr. Richard Osborne, copy editor for Hoover Institution Press, and by Phyllis Cairns, publications manager. Finally, I wish to thank Dr. Rita Ricardo-Campbell, a senior fellow of the Hoover Institution, and Dr. Thomas Moore, the director of the institution's Domestic Studies Program, both of whom organized the conference itself and have been mainly responsible for its outcome.

Preface

Rita Ricardo-Campbell

This conference was called because I could see no clear direction in national health policy that would result in containing the extraordinary increases in the costs of health care. Countries worldwide have not been successful in containing costs, and new approaches were sought. The conference was thus organized to find out what can be learned from the experiences of other countries. Australia, for example, has in part reversed its national health insurance program. Western Germany has found that the costs of a national program are extraordinarily high. The United Kingdom, by contrast, has contained its costs by deliberate limitations of government budget amounts, thus forcing into public view the problem of deciding who gets what type of health care.

To me it has been clear for a long time that national health insurance is not inevitable in the United States because of the unique, rapid growth of private health insurance coverage. In recent years, this has become recognized by increasing numbers of policymakers and economists. Ironically, it is the growth in private health insurance, subsidized by the federal government's policy to permit expensing of the premiums by business, that also primarily accounts for the runaway rise in the costs of medical care in the United States. This policy is responsible for the fact that out-of-pocket costs remained constant despite the growth of inflation. Rapid increases in medical costs are worldwide and result in part from the driving factor of rapid technological changes that supports longer life expectancy. Expansive and supportive, not curative, medicine has been increasing, and populations of the industrialized nations are aging.

The health sector, which absorbs one-tenth of the gross national product in the United States, has for a long period been considered part of the government sector, not of business. Although private businesses, profit and nonprofit alike, are still providing most of our health care services, in professional meetings of economists and physicians it has been assumed that the United States would follow in the footsteps of all the other industrialized nations by eventually adopting a comprehensive government health insurance program.

With the election of President Reagan (an event that took place after this conference), it is now quite clear that at least for a period of four years the health sector will be viewed and analyzed as a business. There will be a strong attempt to increase competition in the health sector by decreasing the regulations that are protective of established firms and encouraging the provision of information to allow informative choices as an alternative to national health insurance and more regulation. The range of available choices will greatly expand. The conference, after a review of the successes and failures of U.S. policy, sought innovative, nongovernment solutions and methods that promise lesser government participation in the future. Several of the papers speak to these issues.

The early evolvement of private health insurance in the United States and subsequent government subsidies of health insurance premiums have structured the existing forms of organization of delivery of medical care and the financial underwriting of them. Means will evolve to divert part of the premiums from underwriting first-dollar coverage of comprehensive care of workers to catastrophic expense coverage of workers and their dependents.

To require employers to provide catastrophic health expense coverage is, for those employers who do not already provide this benefit, equivalent to a new payroll tax levy. This, like similar increases in social security taxes, would depress the economy. In most instances, employers will in the short run adjust to higher payroll taxes by reducing their number of employees and possibly increasing unemployment. My preference is to induce diversion of some part of the existing premiums to support catastrophic expense coverage. This proposal is supplemental to Laurence Seidman's recommendations made in his paper

to increase consumer cost sharing and, coupled with my voucher proposal, fits well with Clark Havighurst's proposal to make "employed
people pay their way without the help of government subsidies beyond
some minimum point."

The federal government has put both money and sustained effort
into the development of prepaid group practices, or health maintenance organizations (HMOs), as the only counteractive, competitive
form of medical organization. Policymakers have not faced up to the
fact that this has narrowed competition to one form rather than permitting the evolution of the variety of forms that a competitive market
would sustain. Freeing the market of restraints imposed by the medical
profession and in conjunction with others, which has begun under the
Federal Trade Commission (FTC), is also needed to foster competitive forces. National health policy will hopefully reverse itself away
from government subsidization and regulation towards greater freedom of choice. Industry is beginning to realize its power as a large
purchaser in negotiating the price of health insurance.

My personal preference is to strengthen the market aspects of the
health sector by developing, or permitting to develop by removal of
hampering government rules, a variety of suppliers while simultaneously improving consumers' knowledge about various choices open
to them and their anticipated costs and benefits. With this end in
mind, I propose a voucher system. Medicare and Medicaid limit reimbursement of a consumer's choice to only a qualified health-care plan
with community-rating set by actuarial category. The choice open to
consumers should encompass all types of plans: those of commercial
insurers and the "Blues" that have experience-rating, group plans with
less comprehensive benefits and lesser charges, and also plans of solo
practitioners who are willing to risk a prepaid, per capita arrangement.

The latter arrangement might be especially suitable for pediatricians who are being squeezed out of the market where HMOs are
strong.* The solo pediatrician could, under prepayment arrangements,
cover ambulatory care of children including well-baby care, immu-

---

*This suggestion evolved during discussions with Mary Lee Ingbar, Ph.D.,
M.P.H., Professor of Family and Community Medicine, University of Massachusetts Medical Center.

nization shots, and checkups. Although HMOs do cover these items, most private health insurance plans do not. Pediatricians could compete with HMOs by offering their own per capita arrangements and also by holding office hours during some evenings and Saturday mornings. A major group of children who receive lesser amounts of medical care are those whose mothers work. The pediatrician could self-insure against the rate expenses of hospitalization among children. Further, the solo general practitioner could explore the same route and possibly work out with a hospital and an insurer a similar plan for adult patients.

My proposal for more competition via vouchers recognizes that some employees are receiving well over $2,000 annually in tax-free health insurance premiums. Under my proposal, the employer would be required to pay the voucher and Medicare could also issue a voucher. The consumer may spend the voucher for health services from any provider and/or insurer that he or she chooses. Employees would not have to use only employer-approved or government-approved arrangements. The voucher system would permit wider competition. If both husband and wife work and have health insurance protection, arrangements to eliminate duplicate benefits would be worked out.

This too-briefly outlined proposal could combine a competitive approach with catastrophic expense coverage. Fifty-five percent of the uninsured are dependents; they are not in the labor force. This proposal could give them catastrophic expense coverage by permitting employees to use the voucher to purchase only catastrophic expense coverage, rather than first-dollar coverage, for themselves and all dependents. Thus, persons with different family obligations could make different choices and competition would be encouraged.

National Health Policy Conference Participants

Lu Ann Aday
Senior Research Associate and
Associate Director for Research
Center for Health Administration
  Studies
University of Chicago
5720 S. Woodlawn Avenue
Chicago, IL 60737

Martin Anderson
Assistant to the President for
  Policy Development
Senior Fellow
Hoover Institution
Stanford University
Stanford, CA 94305

Diana Dutton
Assistant Professor
Stanford University Medical
  School and Department of So-
  ciology
Stanford, CA 94305

Richard Egdahl
Director, Boston University
  Medical Center

53 Bay State Road
Boston, MA 02215

Isaac Ehrlich
Melvin H. Baker Professor of
  American Enterprise and
  Professor of Economics
State University of New York at
  Buffalo
611 O'Brian Hall
Buffalo, NY 14260

Paul Feldstein
Professor, Department of Econom-
  ics and School of Public Health
University of Michigan
Ann Arbor, MI 48109

Scott Fleming
Senior Vice-President
Kaiser-Permanente Medical Care
  Program
One Kaiser Plaza
Oakland, CA 94612

Victor Fuchs
Professor of Economics

Stanford University
Stanford, CA 94305

Willis B. Goldbeck
Washington Business Group on
    Health
922 Pennsylvania Avenue, S.E.
Washington, D.C. 20003

John Goodman
Professor of Economics
University of Dallas
Irving, TX 75061

Clark C. Havighurst
Professor, School of Law
Duke University
Durham, NC 27706

Mary Lee Ingbar
Director, Department of
    Institutional Studies
University of Massachusetts
    Medical Center
Amherst, MA 01002

Stanley B. Jones
Consultant, Blue Cross/Blue
    Shield Association
1700 Pennsylvania Ave., NW
Washington, D.C. 20006

Cotton M. Lindsay
Professor of Economics
Emory University
Atlanta, GA 30322

Harold S. Luft
Associate Professor of Health
    Economics
Institute for Health Policy Studies
School of Medicine
University of California, San
    Francisco
1326 Third Ave.
San Francisco, CA 94143

Thomas Moore
Senior Fellow
Hoover Institution

Stanford University
Stanford, CA 94305

Patricia Munch-Danzon
Senior Research Fellow
Stanford University
Stanford, CA 94305 and
The Rand Corporation
1700 Main Street
Santa Monica, CA 90406

Mark Perlman
University Professor
Department of Economics
University of Pittsburgh
Pittsburgh, PA 15217

Charles Phelps
Director, Regulatory Policies and
    Institutions Program
The Rand Corporation
1700 Main Street
Santa Monica, CA 90406

John P. Pierce
National Health and Medical Re-
    search Council of Australia and
    Research Fellow
Stanford Heart Disease Prevention
    Program
Cypress Hall, Stanford University
Stanford, CA 94305

Uwe E. Reinhardt
Professor of Economics
    and Public Affairs
Department of Economics
Princeton University
Princeton, NJ 08540

Rita Ricardo-Campbell
Senior Fellow
Hoover Institution
Stanford University
Stanford, CA 94305

Dorothy P. Rice
Director, National Center for
    Health Statistics

Department of Health and Human
  Services
Center Building-2 Rm. 2-19
3700 East-West Highway
Hyattsville, MD 20782

Stuart O. Schweitzer
Professor, School of Public Health
Center for Health Science
University of California
Los Angeles, CA 90024

Laurence S. Seidman
Assistant Professor of Economics
Swarthmore College
Swarthmore, PA 19081

Caspar Weinberger
Secretary of Defense
Former Secretary of Health, Education, and Welfare in the Ford
  and Nixon Administrations

Michael Zubkoff
Professor and Chairman, Depart-
  ment of Community and Family
  Medicine
Dartmouth Medical School and
  Professor of Health Economics
Amos Tuck School of Business
  Administration
Dartmouth College
Hanover, NH 03755

Abbreviations

AFDC Aid to Families with Dependent Children
AGSP Australian Government Printing Office
AHA American Hospital Association
AJPH American Journal of Public Health
AMA American Medical Association
CAT Computerized Axial Tomography
CBO Congressional Budget Office
CHAMPUS Civilian Health and Medical Program of the Uniform Service
CHAS Center for Health Administration Studies
CPI Consumer Price Index
DM Deutsche Mark
DO Doctor of Osteopathy
DOL Department of Labor
ER Emergency Room
ESP Economic Stabilization Plan
FICA Federal Insurance Contribution Act

GB Great Britain
GE General Electric
GM General Motors
GNP Gross National Product
GP General Practice
HCFA Health Care Financing Administration
HEW (Department of) Health, Education, and Welfare
HHS (Department of) Health and Human Services
HIAA Health Insurance Association of America
HMO Health Maintenance Organization
HMSO Her Majesty's Stationery Office
HSA Health Systems Agencies
HUD Housing and Urban Development
IBM International Business Machines
ICDA International Statistical Classification of Diseases
IPA Individual Practice Association
IRS Internal Revenue Service

ISR Institute for Social Research
ISSUS Studies in Surgical Services in the United States
JAHA Journal of American Hospital Association
JAMA Journal of the American Medical Association
KVs Kassenaerztlichen Vereinigungen (Associations of Sickness-Fund Physicians)
MCA Multiple Classification Analysis
MD Doctor of Medicine
NAMCS National Ambulatory Medical Care Service
NCHSR National Center for Health Services Research
NCHS National Center for Health Statistics
NHI National Health Insurance
NHP National Health Plan (U.S.)
NHS National Health Service (G.B.)

NORC National Opinion Research Center
OB/GYN Obstetrics and Gynecology
OLS Ordinary least squares
OPD Out-patient Department
PSRO Professional Standards Review Organization
PUB Public
RCCAC Ratio-of-charges-applied-to-costs
RVs Reimbursement visits
SMSA Standard Metropolitan Statistical Areas
SSI Social Security Income
UAW United Auto Workers
UCR "usual, customary, and reasonable" (fees)
U.K. United Kingdom
UR Utilization Review
USA United States of America
VA Veterans Administration
VE Voluntary Effort

Section I

Worldwide Experience
with National Health Insurance

The British National Health Service as a Government Enterprise

*Cotton M. Lindsay**

This paper seeks to test features of a theory of government enterprise using the experience of the British National Health Service (NHS). It is hoped that in so doing a somewhat larger picture of results under such arrangements may be drawn than can be developed by actual description. A well-developed theory that has been confirmed by empirical testing can inform us about aspects of this behavior that have not been statistically analyzed. This procedure, if successful, can prove a much richer source of understanding than a piece-by-piece comparison of the NHS with other health systems. The method followed, therefore, involves presenting a model of bureaucratic government supply in which the implied behavior for these institutions differs from that predicted for similar private institutions. These implications are then tested by reference to the actual experience of NHS and Ameri-

*Department of Economics, Emory University. This paper draws on results reported in a larger study of resource allocation under the British National Health Service which I authored: *National Health Issues: The British Experience* (Nutley, N.J.: Roche Laboratories, 1980). I gratefully acknowledge the careful assistance in this research by Thomas Hall, Steven Honda, and Kenneth Tamor. The research was financed by a grant from Hoffman-La Roche, Inc.

can (largely private) institutions concerning remuneration and qualifications of physicians, hospital resource use, and other data on the
operations of these contrasting forms of medical industry organization.

Bureaucratic Supply and Visible Output

When we consider the behavior of government enterprises, we often
take for granted that they will behave as private firms do when confronted with similar choices. We assume, for example, that private
firms which produce attractive, convenient, low-cost products will
continue to do so when they are nationalized. We tend to think of such
changes as purely administrative; hence, the internal decision making
of the organization will continue unaffected. This assumption is incorrect. When government ownership replaces private ownership, pro-
found changes are made in the incentive structure of the entire
organization, which have implications for both the quality of the product and the efficiency of the production process.

In an earlier paper[1] I developed a model of some aspects of decision
making within a government organization in connection with a study
of Veterans Administration hospitals and pointed out that there are
two principal differences in the economic environments of private
firms and government agencies. First, the private firm gets its direction on what to produce from the customer alone. A private firm
watches the market performance of its product in competition with
others and adopts features which the market will buy and drops those
which do not sell. Government agencies like the NHS typically offer
their product at zero price; hence, they get no information from this
source. Their products always "sell"; they are free. Government agencies depend on the governmental process, the legislative and executive
branches of government, to determine what should be produced and
how much. If, of course, the governmental process transmits the same
information which consumers themselves communicate to producers
through markets then the information source can make no difference.
The extensive theoretical literature on the democratic process suggests that information transmitted via these channels will not be un-
biased. Even if a bureaucracy perfectly executes the instructions it
receives from the legislature, these results will be different and possibly inferior to the results of market organization of production.

In this paper, we focus on a second difference between market and government agency organization of activity. It concerns the movement of information in the opposite direction. It is unfortunate but nevertheless true that giving the correct instructions is only part of the task of ensuring that things get done. This is a particularly complicated problem for producing organizations because the tasks we set for them are at cross-purposes. On the one hand, we want economical production. On the other hand, we want a high-quality product, and more quality can in general be obtained only at greater cost. These are balanced for us nicely by competitive private firms, which use information provided by profit signals. If the manager of such an enterprise is excessively zealous in his pursuit of economy, the quality of the product will fall as will price. This poor management will be reflected in the profit statement of the firm. If excessive quality is embodied in the product (at too great a cost), the cost increase will more than offset the increased revenue for the better product, and profits will also fall.

Needless to say, the profit picture of the government enterprise does not provide similar information. Government output is given away, and the agency invariably operates at losses, which depend only on the level of output and expenditure per unit. The balance between the two offsetting influences on producer decisions is therefore lost. Managers who are able to reduce unit cost by increasing the efficiency of their enterprises are, of course, influenced to do so. Those with executive authority must be rewarded for efficient management or they will not manage. Those who reduce costs by decreasing the quality of the product produced (and therefore give the appearance of greater efficiency) will not be restrained by lost sales. Zero-priced output sells, regardless of quality.

Government administrators acknowledge this problem by engaging in quality control efforts far beyond the scope observed in the private sector. The mountainous paperwork observed in connection with the operation of government agencies clearly represents an attempt to monitor the products of these agencies to prevent them from cutting costs at the expense of quality. To the extent that all aspects of government output can be monitored at reasonable cost, this tendency will be vitiated. For many government products (and services are particularly troublesome in this regard), certain features of the output cannot be monitored at almost any cost.

Those aspects that cannot be economically monitored are referred to as "invisible." Cost-conscious government administrators will invest less resources in these invisible aspects of the products they supply than will private producers. Consider some examples where the operation of this principle is at least hypothetically at work. Government may easily collect data on the volume of mail that passes through a particular postal region. It obtains information on the speed with which mail is delivered only with great difficulty. Speed is thus an invisible characteristic of mail service. It is not therefore surprising that private messenger services offering rapid delivery of letters and parcels between stations successfully compete with the subsidized U.S. Postal Service. The testing of reading and quantitative skills can be accomplished at low cost, while measuring the extent to which public schools impart a genuine appreciation of literature and analytical skills is very costly. These latter characteristics of the educational process are therefore invisible and receive inadequate attention in many public school classrooms keenly attuned to trends in standardized testing results.

Invisible Characteristics of Health

This model of government enterprise was originally developed to study the supply behavior of American Veterans Administration (VA) hospitals. It has already proven its usefulness in predicting deficiencies in certain output characteristics of the hospital and medical sector. Several implications for the model for VA hospitals may be applied directly to the care provided for the whole of the British population. We shall consider each of these implications in turn.

One of the most important implications for any health system is that government will tend to spend less on medical care than people would spend on themselves. Medical attention is demanded for many reasons, and many characteristics of the demanded care are predicted to be invisible. Medical customers demand pleasant surroundings and prompt attention by their physicians. They demand privacy in their hospital accommodations and answers to their questions about their health. Even when well, they seek reassurance about troubling symptoms and ailing relations. Because it is not observed, provision for this aspect of service will be given less attention in the budget. Bureaucratic managers will devote fewer resources to providing this type of care because it cannot be counted and does not therefore reflect favorably on their recorded performance as managers.

Because it does not spend on such invisible output, the NHS finds it possible to operate at a much lower per capita expenditure level than does the health care sector in the United States. Thus it is not surprising that the Health Service consumes only about 5.3 percent of the British gross national product (GNP), while total expenditure in the United States on health consumes about 10 percent of our GNP. This does not imply that Britain's organization is more technically efficient in producing health care than ours. Lower cost is an *implication* of organization of health under a bureaucratic system. Medical care in the United States is more costly because it is a more varied, higher quality product.

It would be incorrect to infer that a McDonald's dinner is more efficient than one at a gourmet restaurant even though they were equally nutritious. It is similarly incorrect to infer that the British Health Service is more efficient than the American system simply because it spends less per capita and achieves the same record with respect to health statistics.[2] Indeed, health indicators are one of the few sets of visible characteristics available with which Parliament may assess the performance of the NHS. It is not surprising that such indicators do not fail to show that health under the NHS is maintained at levels equivalent to those in other countries. If the aim is to give the *appearance* of a high level of health produced with minimum resources,[3] then resource use has been quite intelligent in the United Kingdom. It is important to keep in mind in reading such reports that it is precisely those areas where statistics are unavailable that NHS care is likely to be found deficient.

The Economic Experience of Physicians

Let us consider the case of physician care. Our theory of government enterprise predicts that government managers will find it uneconomical to reward such invisible characteristics of physician care as providing information not related to the patient's health, pleasant surroundings for outpatient visits, and similar features likely to be associated by patients with higher quality care. They will therefore inadequately reimburse doctors for providing such niceties. Physicians will have an incentive to spend less time with each patient since attendance to the patient's health needs is the only monitored characteristic. We would therefore predict that health service may get along with fewer physicians since each is providing a narrower range of services and doctor time is not devoted to providing these invisible characteristics. We are not surprised to find therefore that since 1960 there have been consistently between 21 and 27 percent more doctors per capita in the United States than in England and Wales.

Because of its monopsony power in the market for doctors, government will be able to pay doctors less than the competitive wage. The economic position of doctors will decline. How is this to be measured? The first task was to find a control group with which to compare the doctor's economic position. There is a distressing paucity of earnings data categorized by occupation and/or schooling in the United Kingdom. The British census collects and reports virtually no earnings information. The Review Body, established by Parliament to determine appropriate physician pay levels, found it necessary to generate its own survey data on incomes of other occupations. Ideally, the control group should possess qualifications and credentials similar to doctors. However, adequate time series data were available only for the general category of manual workers. Physician pay was taken to be the target incomes for general practitioners (GPs) that were set by the Review Body.

We compared the economic status of these occupations by calculating the net present values of earnings in each occupation. This method compensates appropriately for the differing life-cycle patterns in the earnings of different occupations and recognizes the large investments required to enter medicine. The rationale here is to view the decision to become a doctor as an investment and to analyze the economic attractiveness of this decision. In doing this it is necessary to make adjustments in these calculations for various characteristics of the two cohorts, which are probably dissimilar. One of these is native ability.

It is typically assumed that the group of people who ultimately succeed in completing all of the education required for medicine have higher than average ability. Manual workers probably have lower than average ability. An ability adjustment factor is therefore applied to manual workers' incomes. In the early literature on education as an investment, an adjustment was made directly to income differentials reflecting the portion due to education. In the mid–1960s, it was thought that approximately two-thirds of observed differentials were attributable to education. More recent evidence suggests that this percentage is around 80 or 90. The present analysis therefore adjusts manual worker earnings upward by 20 percent, reflecting the assumption that people with the ability to become doctors will have higher productivity in this alternative occupation.

This mode of comparison also requires that a discount rate be chosen to use in the present value (PV) calculations. General education is an alternative investment open to an individual, so this was used as a basis to determine the appropriate discount rate. Rates of return to education have yielded various estimates, as shown in table 1.1 Because physicians' earnings are delayed, the lower the discount rate employed, the better will doctors' economic positions appear relative to others. A rate of return of 12 percent was chosen for analysis, which is on the lower side of these estimates.

Present values for manual workers are calculated by discounting their income streams.[4] Data limitations make it possible to analyze only the earnings of GPs. For these physicians, the present values are

TABLE 1.1
Private rates of return

	Secondary education	Higher education
1. Henderson-Stewart	13.0	14.0
2. Richardson	–	15.3
3. Layard, et al.	–	12.0
4. Ziderman	8.5	20.0

1. D. Henderson-Stewart, appendix in M. Blaug, "The Rate of Return on Investment in Education in Great Britain." *The Manchester School* (September 1965). $\alpha = .60$ used.[a]

2. V. A. Richardson, "The Problems of Manpower and Educational Planning: Analysis and Appraisal of Alternative Techniques, Illustrated by Some Empirical Models" (Ph.D. diss. University of Manchester, 1969).

3. P. R. G. Layard et al., *Qualified Manpower and Economic Performance* (London: Allen Lane, The Penguin Press: 1971). $\alpha = .66$ used.

4. A. Ziderman, "Incremental Rates of Return on Investment in Education: Recent Results for Britain," Mimeographed. (Queen Mary College, University of London, 1971).

a. The symbol α used in these citations refers to the percentage of observed earnings differences attributed to education.

calculated by discounting their maintenance grants received while attending school and their career income stream. The earned income streams used are net of taxes. These present value calculations are done for each year from 1948 to 1978. To facilitate comparisons over the time period, the pound sterling values were translated into constant 1978 pounds using the retail price index for consumer goods and services.

The results of the present value calculations are presented in table 1.2. The differences in the present value of a doctor minus the present value of a manual worker are shown in the third column of table 1.2 and in figure 1.1. This difference shows the economic attractiveness of becoming a doctor over a manual worker as measured in 1978 pounds. The use of a higher discount rate would decrease this attractiveness in each year. Looking closer at these results, one can see that the attractiveness of becoming a doctor in the early years was fairly high, but deteriorated until the mid–1960s. For a few years from 1967 to 1971, the attractiveness of becoming a doctor rose again, but after that period started a severe downturn that has not yet abated. One can see that except for a short period from the late 1960s to the early 1970s, the economic attractiveness of becoming a doctor has deteriorated dramatically. This decline is also apparent in rate of return calculations on physician training reported in column 4 of table 1.2.

This evidence suggests that the attractiveness of a medical career has lost much ground since the inception of the NHS, and doctors now are being severely underpaid. We may estimate the extent of this over- and underpayment by determining what level of earnings would make medicine and manual worker careers equally attractive economically in each year. The average remuneration of GPs that would make such an investment economically attractive has therefore been calculated. The percentage of an over- or underpayment has been calculated by taking the difference of the actual and this "equilibrium" pay level and dividing by the equilibrium pay level. These results are included in the last column of table 1.2 and in figure 1.2.

Although all of this analysis concerns only the earnings of GPs, the same pattern should be observed in an analysis of specialists' incomes. The decline noted for GPs in the last decade should be even more dramatic for the case of specialists' incomes, which were affected more severely by the Incomes Policy applied during this period.

TABLE 1.2
Results of present value (PV) calculations

Year	1[a] Manual workers' PVs at 12%	2[a] Physicians' PVs at 12%	3[a] 2 − 1	4 Rate of return	5 Percentage over- or underpaid
1948	16870.	26174.	9305.	22.649	98
1949	16914.	25502.	8588.	21.841	86
1950	17216.	24825.	7610.	20.561	76
1951	18248.	24221.	5974.	18.510	54
1952	18436.	24832.	6396.	18.826	55
1953	19324.	24565.	5241.	17.437	45
1954	20405.	24350.	3946.	15.911	31
1955	21349.	23998.	2650.	14.607	19
1956	21637.	23120.	1483.	13.440	10
1957	22259.	23483.	1224.	13.147	8
1958	22058.	23350.	1291.	13.258	8
1959	23039.	25961.	2923.	14.560	19
1960	24210.	25732.	1521.	13.278	10
1961	24643.	25103.	460.	12.383	4
1962	24274.	24607.	333.	12.292	3
1963	25220.	26913.	1693.	13.362	9
1964	26128.	26083.	−45.	11.965	0
1965	26424.	26513.	88.	12.069	1
1966	26048.	26501.	453.	12.350	2
1967	26479.	25701.	− 778.	11.395	−4
1968	26749.	29399.	2649.	13.867	14
1969	27052.	28912.	1860.	13.296	9
1970	28505.	30797.	2292.	13.484	11
1971	28820.	31051.	2231.	13.444	10
1972	30700.	30852.	152.	12.094	0
1973	32025.	29485.	−2540.	10.415	−9
1974	31974.	27553.	−4421.	9.189	−18
1975	30653.	28320.	−2333.	10.523	−12
1976	30077.	25207.	−4870.	8.693	−23
1977	27966.	22508.	−5458.	7.882	−26
1978	30196.	22583.	−7613.	6.547	−32

a. Calculations reflect present values in 1978 £ sterling.

FIGURE 1.1

Net attractiveness of general practice by year (1948–1978) in
constant 1978 £ Sterling

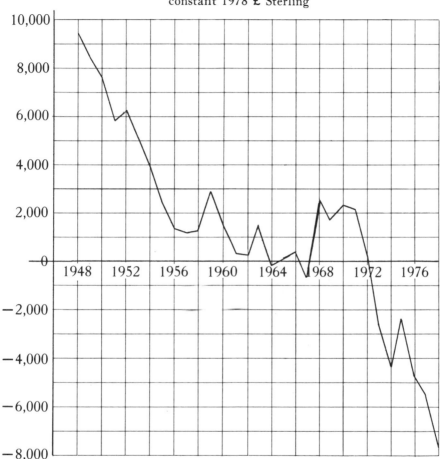

Economic Status and Physician Emigration

The evidence presented indicates a decline in the economic position of
doctors in the United Kingdom under the NHS. It is useful to look at
this finding in the light of other phenomena observed during this period. We may, for example, validate our estimates of the attractiveness
of a medical career by observing the rate of emigration of doctors. If
our measure of the economic position of doctors is accurate, we should

FIGURE 1.2

Over- and underpayment relative to the earnings of manual
workers (1948–1978)

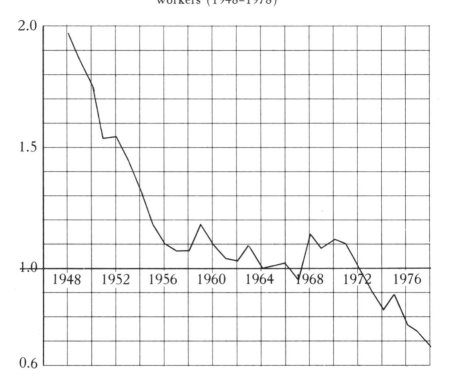

find it negatively correlated with the rate at which physicians leave
the United Kingdom permanently to practice elsewhere.

Unfortunately, data on emigration of physicians was not collected
or fully reported until recently. We have data for the ten-year period
from 1965 to 1975 on physicians fully or provisionally registered in
Great Britain who were born in the United Kingdom or the Irish Republic and who emigrated. As there are a certain number of physicians
each year returning to the United Kingdom who had previously emigrated, the number we chose to employ in our estimates is net emigrations, i.e., total leaving less the number returning in each year. This
total is presented in table 1.3.

The decision to leave one's native country is not taken lightly and
probably involves considerable delay between the decision to emigrate
and the departure. One must find a new practice, obtain the necessary

TABLE 1.3
Net physician emigration from the United Kingdom
(1965–1975)

Year	Net emigrations
1965	520
1966	380
1967	450
1968	480
1969	320
1970	290
1971	330
1972	110
1973	370
1974	450
1975	470

visas and licenses, settle one's affairs, and arrange transportation. In other words, we expect to find lags between deterioration in the economic situation of doctors and changes in the rate of emigration. As we cannot specify these lags on a priori grounds, we employed several specifications using both single and distributed lags. These results are reported in table 1.4.

Although one cannot place great reliance on time series observations over a period of only ten years, these results do support the hypothesis that migration of physicians is influenced by economic welfare of doctors. The dependent variable in each regression is the number of net emigrations in each year. This is regressed on a constant term C and the rate of return from our earlier calculations given various lags. These results suggest a robust and strong effect of rate of return on the emigration rate with a one-year lag. In each of the specifications, it is statistically significant at the 10 percent level or better, and the coefficient is remarkably stable. Durban-Watson statistics indicate the absence of first order autocorrelation.

These results lend credence to our estimates of rates of return as accurate indicators of the economic welfare of physicians. As our measured rates of return decline, the rate at which physicians leave the United Kingdom for practice elsewhere increases. Our estimated coefficient for this relationship suggests that for each unit decline in the rate of return, 54 doctors depart each year. Expressing this in elasticity, a 1 percent decline in the rate of return produced a 1.74 percent increase in the rate of emigration. In view of the extremely low rates of return calculated for the later 1970s, the outlook for emigration of physicians over the next few years may be a source of serious concern.

Foreign-Trained Doctors and the Quality of Care

Our model of bureaucratic production implies that government enterprises will inadequately reward production of invisible characteristics of medical care provision, leading to their undersupply relative to a market-organized industry. They will therefore undersupply physician services so long as these services are used to produce the invisible aspects of treatment discussed above. The deterioration of the economic position of doctors described in the previous section is consistent with this interpretation only so long as the rate of emigration of physicians, which it produces, does not in turn produce a visible deterioration in the health of the public. This will be far easier to achieve if there is an offsetting immigration of foreign-trained physicians to take the place of those who leave.

It was observed in the study of Veterans Administration hospitals mentioned earlier that government-organized medical care facilities hire disproportionate numbers of foreign-trained physicians, since these doctors will supply medical attention at lower prices than will locally-trained doctors. In the market-organized medical industry of

TABLE 1.4

Physician emigration related to rates of return
to physician training (1965–1975)

C	964.3	961.2	1040.3
	(2.39)	(3.55)	(4.19)
RR_t	21.18	21.23	–
	(0.76)	(0.83)	
RR_{t-1}	−68.73	−68.94	−54.46
	(−1.99)	(−2.55)	(−2.69)
RR_{t-2}	−0.41	–	–
	(−0.01)		
r^2	.49	.49	.44
F	2.22	3.81	7.17
D.W.	1.96	1.96	1.59

the United States, American-trained physicians command higher earnings because they are more valued by the patients whom they serve. These patients are willing to pay more to American-trained physicians for a number of reasons. They feel they communicate better—there is no language barrier—with native Americans, and they have greater confidence in the skills imparted in American schools.

A similar process may be predicted to have occurred in the United Kingdom. Locally-trained physicians in the United Kingdom have higher priced alternatives than do the foreign-trained physicians who take their places. At the earnings level adopted by the government, locally-trained physicians are influenced to emigrate while foreign-trained physicians find NHS positions attractive. The Health Service is thus able to hold the cost of physician care down by supplying a physician force which contains a larger representation of lower cost, foreign-trained physicians.

How important have overseas doctors been to the NHS? In the early years, data were not kept on the training or birthplaces of doctors; hence there is little one can say concerning overseas-born doctors before the 1960s. We report the available data in table 1.5. Data for all hospital doctors are available from 1967 to 1977 and, by 1967, the proportion is surprisingly high. Throughout that time period, about 30 to 33 percent of all hospital doctors were born outside of the United Kingdom or the Irish Republic. There was an overall growth of about 3.5 percent per annum in hospital medical staff, so although the proportion of overseas-born doctors was not increasing, their absolute numbers have been increasing.

Of doctors that held positions of registrar or below, data are also available for the years 1963 and 1966. These numbers suggest that the proportion of foreign-born doctors increased steadily from 1963 to 1969 where it leveled out at about 50 percent. Since that time, the share has diminished somewhat but remains in the neighborhood of 50 percent. Roughly half of those engaged in delivering primary care in NHS hospitals are foreign-born doctors.

The scenario for general practice has been slightly different. Overseas-born doctors are not as heavily represented here as in hospital appointments. However, there has been a steady upward trend from 1965 to 1977 in the numbers and proportion of general medical practitioners (unrestricted principles) who were born overseas.

Comment on the clinical performance of medical practitioners is out

TABLE 1.5
Percent of physicians born outside the United Kingdom and
the Irish Republic

	All hospital staff (Great Britain)	Registrar and below (Great Britain)	GPs (England and Wales)
1963	–	39.4	–
1964	–	–	–
1965	–	–	11.3
1966	–	45.7	11.6
1967	29.7	47.5	12.1
1968	30.5	48.6	12.6
1969	31.4	49.8	13.4
1970	31.2	49.0	14.2
1971	30.8	47.6	–
1972	31.4	48.0	15.5
1973	32.5	49.6	16.3
1974	33.1	50.1	17.1
1975	33.3	49.7	17.7
1976	32.7	48.1	18.4
1977	31.8	45.8	–

of place in an economic analysis. We shall therefore restrict our discussion to a brief survey of the findings of a recent inquiry conducted by physicians themselves. In the *Report of the Committee of Inquiry into the Regulation of the Medical Profession* in 1975 (published by HMSO), the competence of overseas doctors was investigated. Evidence was submitted by the Royal College of Psychiatrists and the Royal College of General Practitioners regarding the performance of foreign-born doctors in tests administered for membership.

From the Royal College of Psychiatrists came results of 1,031 candidates who took their examinations. Pass rates were compared for the candidates who came from the United Kingdom, Australia, and South Africa and the candidates who came from the United Arab Republic and the Indian subcontinent. The results in table 1.6 suggest that qualifications for overseas doctors from the second group are significantly lower than for the doctors from the first group.

In other evidence submitted by the Royal College of General Practitioners, results of examination from spring 1972 to autumn 1974 of practitioners who desired to become members were reported. Of the

869 doctors who came from the United Kingdom and the Republic of Ireland, 82 percent passed, while only 21 percent of the 141 candidates who were from other areas passed.

The report draws "the inescapable conclusion . . . from the evidence we have received . . . that there are substantial numbers of overseas doctors whose skill and the care they offer to patients fall below that generally acceptable in this country, and it is at least possible that there are some who should not have been registered" (p. 60). Furthermore, the report states the belief that "this unsatisfactory situation is principally to be attributed to a willingness on the part of the General Medical Council (GMC) to allow its duty as the protector of medical standards to be compromised by the manpower requirements of the NHS" (p. 61).

Hospital Spending and Beds per Capita

Managers of government hospitals are particularly difficult to monitor in the performance of their jobs. As long as patients do not die in disproportionate numbers, there is little else that Parliament or any other

TABLE 1.6

Pass rates for home-trained and foreign-trained candidates for
Royal College of Psychiatrists (1972)

	Percent passing examinations			
	I	II	III	All
U.K., Australia, South Africa	80	84	79	81
U.A.R., Indian Subcontinent	47	44	48	47

Pass rates for home-trained and foreign-trained
candidates for Royal College of General Practitioners (1972–1974)

	Number	Percent passing examinations
U.K. and Republic of Ireland	869	82
Elsewhere	141	21

Source: *Report of the Committee of Inquiry into the Regulation of the Medical Profession.* (London: HMSO, 1975).

overseeing agency can do to distinguish high quality treatment from low. This is not to say, of course, that patients themselves cannot be made more comfortable, more confident, or in general more satisfied with the quality of their care. The point is that, without some way (such as a price signal) for patients to convey this information to the appropriate level of government, this information will not be transmitted. Characteristics of hospital care affecting patient satisfaction in these dimensions will be invisible; hence, less resources will be devoted to their production.

The hospital manager who succeeds in producing hospitalization at the lowest cost per patient-day will appear the most successful, in spite of the fact that other managers who spend more making their hospitals more comfortable may be producing a more valuable product in the eyes of their individual customers. One way to economize on such invisible characteristics is to reduce the man-hours devoted to nonessential activities which affect merely patient comfort. Much nursing and domestic labor is devoted by American hospitals to this type of activity (as well as to treating and curing disease). We therefore expect government-operated systems such as the NHS to devote fewer resources to these activities than a system like that in the United States, which is more sensitive to market forces. This inference is supported by table 1.7 and figure 1.3, which compare personnel inputs per available bed in the two systems. Although staff per bed ratios in the United States exceeded those in the NHS hospitals at the advent of the system, the difference in the figures has widened over the following 30 years.

In 1950, for example, the staff per bed ratio in the United States exceeded that of the NHS by 39.5 percent. By 1960 this difference had grown to 47.1 percent. Finally, by 1971 this excess of personnel in U.S. hospitals compared to the NHS had grown to nearly 110 percent. Some part of this growth in personnel spending may be attributable to the cost-plus hospital reimbursement policy adopted by the federal government for Medicare and Medicaid. Indeed, the dramatic upward kink in the U.S. curve in 1965 is consistent with such an explanation. The entire difference cannot be attributed to declining cost-consciousness on the part of U.S. hospitals associated with federal government reimbursement practices, however. By 1965 the difference in the personnel to staff ratio had already grown to 58.5 percent.

One would expect a similar economy in capital spending devoted to invisible characteristics of hospital output. That is, government man-

TABLE 1.7
Total staff per available hospital bed in the United States and
NHS (various years)

Year	Total personnel per available bed	
	NHS	U.S.
1948	–	.665
1949	–	.671
1950	.521	.727
1951	.524	.706
1952	.532	.716
1953	.539	.739
1954	.534	.790
1955	.534	.811
1956	.595	.855
1957	.606	.899
1958	.629	.932
1959	.647	.942
1960	.655	.964
1961	.674	1.016
1962	.697	1.044
1963	.702	1.099
1964	.710	1.113
1965	.723	1.146
1966	.745	1.254
1967	.761	1.318
1968	.756	1.388
1969	.758	1.470
1970	.767	1.570
1971	.793	1.664
1972	–	1.723
1973	–	1.804
1974	–	1.929
1975	–	2.062

agers are predicted to eschew investment in capital which merely increases the comfort and convenience of patients. As those who must
monitor the productivity of hospital managers cannot economically determine how much comfort and convenience is actually produced,
managers will devote less capital resources to these activities, as well.
Measuring the capital stock is a difficult task, however. Merely

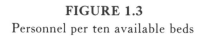

FIGURE 1.3

Personnel per ten available beds

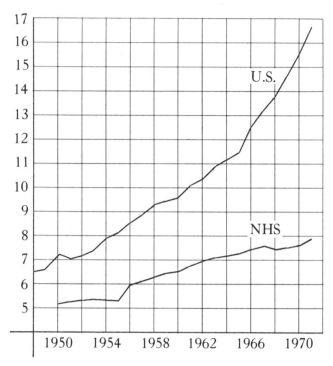

counting available beds is a crude measure, for beds themselves are visible outputs. Bureaucratic managers will cut back first on carpets, drapes, televisions, and privacy before reducing beds. We would like to compute some standardized unit of capital, which might be compared per bed as was done for expenditure on personnel. Expenditure itself is deceptive too, since hospital capital is likely to vary in cost among countries. Furthermore, investment itself should depend on the existing level of capital; and at the inception of the NHS, the United Kingdom was more heavily endowed with hospital beds than was the United States. Bearing this in mind, evidence that we are able to gather is not inconsistent with the hypothesis that capital, too, has been subject to the law of "visible production."

Consider capital expenditures on hospitals. These are presented in table 1.8 and in figure 1.4. From 1950 to 1960, hospital investment in the United States exceeded that under the NHS by 200 to 600 percent.

FIGURE 1.4

Capital expenditures
per capita in real U.S. dollars (1970-71)

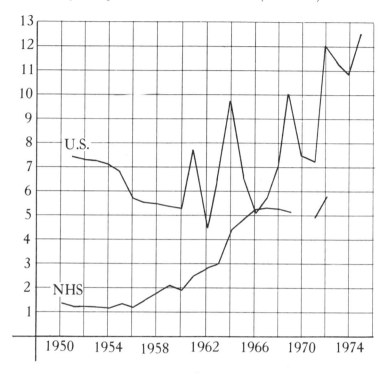

In the mid–1960s, during the heyday of the Powell-led hospital build-ing program, there was a brief period of catching up. As our data on the NHS investment levels run out, however, the United States pulls ahead on hospital investment again. Such comparisons can be mislead-ing, as was mentioned, for hospital capital may be less costly in the United Kingdom than in the United States. Lower levels of invest-ment need not imply less capital. For this reason, we also include hos-pital investment as a percentage of GNP. As GNP per capita is much smaller in the United Kingdom than in the United States, this predict-ably improves the picture for the United Kingdom, particularly in more recent years. Unfortunately, data beyond 1971 were unavailable from published sources to complete this picture.

Complete data on hospital beds were also unavailable from pub-lished sources. We were able to construct a series on total beds, but

TABLE 1.8

Hospital investments: NHS versus the United States (1948–1976), in U.S. dollars

Year	Capital expenditures per capita[a]		Capital expenditures per GNP		Capital expenditures per total revenue expenditures		Beds per thousand persons	
	NHS	U.S.	NHS	U.S.	NHS	U.S.	NHS	U.S.
1948	–	–	–	–	–	–	–	9.59
1949	–	–	–	–	–	–	10.34	9.58
1950	1.26	–	.0008	–	.041	–	10.73	9.56
1951	1.20	7.42	.0007	.0025	.038	.184	10.93	9.82
1952	1.20	7.29	.0007	.0024	.038	.164	11.02	9.92
1953	1.12	7.17	.0006	.0023	.034	.155	11.11	9.87
1954	1.04	7.05	.0006	.0023	.031	.144	11.13	9.68
1955	1.28	6.92	.0007	.0021	.038	.137	11.06	9.67
1956	1.23	5.76	.0006	.0023	.036	.111	10.80	9.52
1957	1.45	5.66	.0007	.0022	.040	.107	10.75	9.06
1958	1.80	5.56	.0009	.0022	.050	.099	10.71	8.99
1959	2.02	5.47	.0010	.0020	.053	.092	10.63	9.07
1960	1.97	5.39	.0009	.0019	.049	.087	10.47	9.18
1961	2.41	7.81	.0011	.0021	.058	.116	10.35	9.09
1962	2.89	4.37	.0013	.0011	.070	.062	10.14	9.05
1963	2.94	6.68	.0013	.0016	.069	.090	10.03	8.99
1964	4.44	9.75	.0019	.0023	.102	.124	9.96	8.83
1965	4.88	6.69	.0021	.0015	.111	.082	9.84	8.77
1966	5.22	5.03	.0022	.0011	.114	.059	9.74	8.54
1967	5.47	5.76	.0023	.0012	.115	.060	9.66	8.41
1968	5.40	7.16	.0026	.0015	.130	.068	9.63	8.29

1969	–	10.13	–	.0021	–	.088	9.51	8.14
1970	4.97	7.39	.0024	.0015	.123	.059	9.37	7.89
1971	5.58	7.36	.0024	.0015	.122	.056	9.22	7.15
1972	–	12.57	–	.0025	–	.088	9.03	7.42
1973	–	11.75	–	.0022	–	.079	8.89	7.30
1974	–	11.35	–	.0022	–	.074	8.68	7.14
1975	–	12.61	–	.0025	–	.076	8.52	6.86
1976	–	–	–	–	–	–	8.38	–
% change	1951–1971	1951–1971	1951–1971	1951–1971	1951–1971	1951–1971	1949–1975	1949–1975
	+365.0	–0.8	+200.0	–40.0	+221.1	–69.9	–17.6	–28.4

a. Data for NHS measure real capital expenditures in U.S. dollars (1970 = 1) divided by the population of England and Wales. Data for the United States measure the change in real plant assets from the previous year, in U.S. dollars (1970 = 1).

this series contains long-term as well as short-term general hospital beds. As these two categories are quite imperfect substitutes and the proportions of each represented in the totals differed substantially over the period of our study, these aggregate data are of limited usefulness. They are presented in table 1.9 and in figure 1.5. After a brief rise in the early 1950s, beds per capita declined secularly for more than two decades. Throughout this period, however, the NHS had more total beds per capita than did the United States. The smaller level of investment in hospital capital in the NHS might appear to be reasonable in light of these data. Lower levels of investment might be thought consistent with a higher initial capital stock, which the NHS wishes to reduce. This parallel movement in total beds conceals significant compositional changes, however, which are inconsistent with the explanation of rational reductions in the stock of beds.

Disaggregated data on hospital beds per capita are available for certain years. When we examine these data, we find that the parallel movement in total beds does not carry over to the short-term general hospital capacity, which is more important to measured national health.

In table 1.10 we report data on disaggregated hospital beds in the United States and Great Britain. Here the differing trends in hospital

FIGURE 1.5
Beds per thousand persons

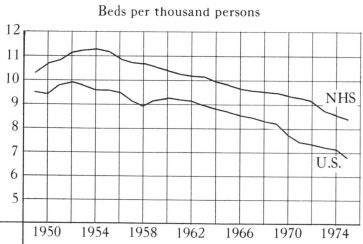

priorities are immediately apparent. While total beds in the two countries declined at roughly parallel rates, the number of short-term general hospital beds per capita actually increased in the United States by 12 percent, at least during the eleven-year period covered by these statistics. During the same period, short-term general hospital beds declined in England and Wales by almost exactly the same rate. It will be remembered, too, that the period covered here represents the peak of hospital investment by the NHS. The reason for the similar paths followed by total beds in the two countries is not that experience was similar. The real explanation is that, coincident with the relative growth of general hospitals in the United States, there was a far greater decline there in the number of psychiatric beds.

Of course, these figures are open to many interpretations. It could be argued that health spending in general has been assigned a low priority by political leaders, who have discovered that it is politically expedient to spend less on health than people would spend for themselves. Another interpretation is that Americans have constructed an excessive number of general hospital beds in the past decade and that the NHS has achieved a budgetary coup by cutting back on the resources devoted to such expensive institutions. We can shed some light on these two competing hypotheses by examining data on lengths of stay. According to the American surplus hypothesis, the NHS is able to get along with fewer hospital beds by using their smaller endowment more efficiently. We should therefore expect inpatient cases per available bed to be higher in the NHS than in the United States. We find the opposite to be true. Figure 1.6 depicts the inpatient case rate per available bed in the two countries. Although the case rates per bed have increased in both countries, the United States has consistently used its hospital stock to treat more patients than has the NHS. Although far from conclusive, this finding does raise doubts about the hypothesis that the NHS uses its hospital stock more efficiently and therefore is able to get along with less.

Hospital Inpatient Lengths of Stay

In my earlier study of Veterans Administration hospitals in the United States, it was argued that government-operated hospitals would be observed to use hospital capacity less efficiently than hospitals operated

TABLE 1.9

Hospital capacity: NHS versus the United States (1948–1976)

Year	Hospitals[a]		Beds[b] (thousands)		Beds per thousand population[c]		Total personnel[d] (thousands)	
	NHS	U.S.	NHS	U.S.	NHS	U.S.	NHS	U.S.
1948	–	6160	–	1411	–	9.59	–	939
1949	–	6277	453	1435	10.34	9.58	227	963
1950	–	6788	472	1456	10.73	9.56	236	1058
1951	–	6832	479	1522	10.93	9.82	242	1075
1952	–	6903	484	1563	11.02	9.92	249	1119
1953	–	6978	490	1581	11.11	9.87	254	1169
1954	–	6970	492	1578	11.13	9.68	254	1246
1955	–	6956	491	1604	11.06	9.67	254	1301
1956	–	6966	482	1608	10.80	9.52	284	1375
1957	–	6818	482	1559	10.75	9.06	289	1401
1958	–	6786	483	1572	10.71	8.99	300	1465
1959	3027	6845	482	1613	10.63	9.07	308	1520
1960	–	6876	479	1658	10.47	9.18	311	1598
1961	2989	6923	478	1670	10.35	9.09	316	1696
1962	2975	7028	473	1689	10.14	9.05	326	1763
1963	2953	7138	472	1702	10.03	8.99	327	1840
1964	2935	7127	472	1696	9.96	8.83	331	1887
1965	2938	7123	469	1704	9.84	8.77	336	1952
1966	2921	7160	468	1679	9.74	8.54	344	2106
1967	2885	7172	467	1671	9.66	8.41	351	2203
1968	2890	7137	465	1663	9.63	8.29	347	2309

Year								
1969	2857	7144	461	1650	9.51	8.14	345	2426
1970	2808	7123	456	1616	9.37	7.89	345	2537
1971	2760	7097	450	1556	9.22	7.51	353	2589
1972	2748	7061	443	1550	9.03	7.42	–	2671
1973	2724	7123	437	1535	8.89	7.30	–	2769
1974	2736	7174	427	1513	8.68	7.14	–	2919
1975	2684	7156	419	1466	8.52	6.86	–	3023
1976	2657	–	412	–	8.38	–	–	–
	1961–1975		1949–1975		1949–1975		1949–1971	
Percent change	−10.20	+3.37	−9.05	+2.16	−18.96	−28.39	+55.51	+168.85

a. Data are for hospitals of all types (for the United States, American Hospital Association [AHA] accredited hospitals only).

b. Data for NHS measure fully staffed beds.

c. Data for NHS measure fully staffed beds per 1000 population in England and Wales.

d. Data for NHS measure whole-time nurses and midwives plus domestic staff. For the United States, data measure all personnel as reported annually in the *Journal of the American Hospital Association* (JAHA) Hospital Statistics.

TABLE 1.10

Disaggregated data on hospital beds in the United States and
England and Wales (various years)

	England and Wales	United States
Total beds		
1960	104.7	91.8
1971	92.4	75.1
percent change	−11.7	−18.2
Short-term general		
1960	46.0	41.4
1971	40.7	46.7
percent change	−11.5	12.8
Psychiatric		
1960	46.5	43.7
1971	35.9	27.7[a]
percent change	−22.8	−36.6

a. 1970
Source: R. Maxwell, *Health Care: The Growing Dilemma,* 2nd ed. (New York: McKinsey and Co., Inc., 1975).

for profit.[5] Data on lengths of stay in VA and private hospitals strongly supported this implication of bureaucratic behavior. The argument presented there is that government managers seek to produce the visible characteristic of their product (i.e., hospital days of care) as cheaply as possible. A patient who is gravely ill requires a great deal of costly care, while a patient who has fully recovered or was never very ill requires little. Thus, if a patient who has already recovered is replaced by one who is seriously ill, costs per patient-day will rise, and such a report will reflect unfavorably on the productivity of the hospital manager—regardless of whether management had anything to do with the cost rise or not. This phenomenon will bias hospital administrators to seek to influence physicians to retain patients after they might have been discharged. Longer lengths of stay imply lower costs per patient-day, and a patient-day of care is virtually the only useful measure of hospital output with which productivity may be gauged.

The results presented in figure 1.6 are consistent with the hypoth-

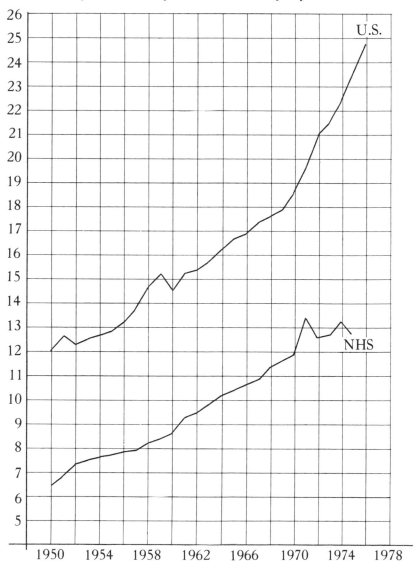

FIGURE 1.6

Inpatient cases per available bed per year

TABLE 1.11

Mean length of stay by diagnosis in the United States and
Great Britain (1973)[a]
Diseases

ICDA category	Diagnostic category	Mean stay (days) U.S.	Mean stay (days) G.B.
174	Malignant neoplasms—breast	12.2	12.1
185	Malignant neoplasms—prostate	12.4	20.7
210–239	Benign neoplasms and neoplasms of unspecified nature	6.7	7.4
218, 219	Benign neoplasm of uterus	8.1	8.8
240–279	Endocrine, nutritional, and metabolic diseases	10.0	20.4
250	Diabetes mellitus	11.1	24.6
230–289	Diseases of the blood and blood-forming organs	8.1	16.1
290–315	Mental disorders	11.6	47.6
374	Cataract	6.4	11.3
380–389	Diseases of the ear and mastoid process	3.5	4.6
390–458	Diseases of the circulatory system	11.4	35.2
390–398	Rheumatic fever and rheumatic heart disease	11.6	17.4
400–404	Hypertensive disease	8.3	20.9
410	Acute myocardial infarction	15.6	19.9
411–414	Ischemic heart disease	10.8	24.2
454	Varicose veins of the lower extremities	8.5	10.3
455	Hemorrhoids	6.8	7.8
460–519	Diseases of the respiratory system	6.0	11.0
480–486	Pneumonia (all kinds)	9.0	17.9
490–492	Bronchitis and emphysema	8.2	23.4
493	Asthma	6.8	10.0
500	Hypertrophy of tonsils and adenoids	2.1	3.9
520–577	Diseases of the digestive system	7.9	9.7
540–543	Appendicitis	6.4	7.9
550–553	Hernia (with or without obstruction)	6.7	8.1
560	Intestinal obstruction without mention of hernia	11.3	14.0
574, 575	Cholelithiasis and cholecystitis	10.2	13.0
580–629	Diseases of the genito-urinary system	6.3	7.5
580–584	Nephritis and nephrosis	6.6	20.8
590	Infections of kidney	8.6	21.4
600	Hyperplasia of prostate	11.4	16.4

610–611	Diseases of breast	3.4	4.0
623	Uterovaginal prolapse	9.3	13.6
650	Delivery without mention of complications	3.8	6.8
680–686	Infections of skin and subcutaneous tissue	7.5	10.6
690–709	Other diseases of skin and subcutaneous tissue	7.4	13.3
710–738	Diseases of the musculoskeletal system and connective tissue	9.6	23.6
713	Osteoarthritis and allied conditions	12.2	37.8
725	Displacement of intervertebral disc	11.7	18.7
740–759	Congenital anomalies	6.6	11.9

a. British data are for England and Wales and include all disease groups of comparable levels of aggregation.

Sources: United States: U.S. Department of HEW. *Vital and Health Statistics,* series 13, no. 25, "Inpatient Utilization of Short-Stay Hospitals—United States 1973." (Washington, D.C.: Government Printing Office, 1976).

Great Britain: Department of Health and Social Security. *Report on Hospital Inpatient Enquiry for the Year 1973.* (HMSO, 1977).

esis that hospital managers in NHS hospitals, like their American VA counterparts, influence the retention of patients longer than they would be retained in private hospitals. Those results reflect excessive aggregation, however. As case loads clearly vary between countries, these case rates may reflect the differing lengths of stay associated with case mixes between countries. What we require are length-of-stay comparisons for individual hospital case categories. We have assembled this information in tables 1.11, 1.12, and 1.13.

Tables 1.11, 1.12, and 1.13 present figures for mean length of stay in NHS and U.S. proprietary hospitals for several categories of disease, injury, and surgical procedure. Since both countries use adaptations of the same international classification scheme, correspondence for diseases and injuries should be very good (though mental disorders, congenital anomalies, and the skin disease residual are questionable). All categories for which the level of aggregation are comparable are included in these tables. Since some of the categories are part of other listed categories, the information content is less than the apparent 40 pairs. The NHS does not use the international categories for operations, so only those with obviously similar names are listed.

TABLE 1.12

Mean length of stay by diagnosis in the United States and
Great Britain (1973)
Injury

ICDA category	Injury	Mean stay (days) U.S.	G.B.
800–804	Fracture of skull and face bones	6.3	6.8
810–819	Fracture of upper limb	5.8	7.8
820	Fracture of neck or femur	21.0	42.7
821–829	Other fracture of lower limbs	12.1	28.8
805–809	Fracture of other and multiple sites	13.2	20.4
830–839	Dislocation without fracture	6.3	12.1
846, 847	Sprains and strains of back (including neck)	7.8	10.5
850–854	Intracranial injury (excluding those with skull fracture)	5.4	4.1
860–869	Internal injury of chest, abdomen, and pelvis	11.9	10.8
870–873	Laceration and open wound of eye, ear, and head	4.7	5.3
874–907	Laceration and open wound of other and multiple locations	5.9	6.7
940–949	Burns	14.5	17.5

Sources: Same as table 1.11.

The results tend to support the hypothesis. Of the 40 diseases compared, 39 involved longer mean lengths of stay in NHS hospitals. Ten of the twelve injuries and twelve of the fourteen surgical procedures also involved longer mean stays in NHS hospitals. In most cases NHS stays are substantially longer. Where they are shorter, the difference is always quite small. Approximated standard errors for various categories suggest that, while some cases receive significantly longer treatment in Britain, the reverse is never the case.

Conclusion

In this paper we have considered the influence of government organization of the health industry on the supply of these services. We developed a model of government bureaucratic supply in which those

TABLE 1.13

Mean length of stay by procedure in the United States and
Great Britain (1973)
Surgery[a]

| | Mean stay (days) | |
	U.S.	G.B.
Thyroidectomy	6.8	8.9
Inguinal hernia	6.2	7.2
Vagotomy	16.2	15.6
Hemorrhoidectomy	7.3	9.6
Nephrectomy	17.7	20.1
Dilation of urethra	6.5	4.3
Prostatectomy	13.9	19.5
Orchidopexy	5.1	5.7
Oophorectomy	9.4	12.0
Hysterectomy	9.5	14.2
Golporrhaphy	7.4	14.1
Caesarean section	7.2	15.5
Anthorclesis	9.0	17.8
Plastic surgery	7.8	17.1

a. Definitions may not always be precisely comparable.
Sources: United States: U.S. Department of HEW. *Vital and Health Statistics,* series 13, no. 24, "Surgical Operations in Short-Stay Hospitals—United States 1973." (Washington, D.C.: Government Printing Office, 1976).
Great Britain: Department of Health and Social Security, Hospital In-Patient Enquiry, (1973).

who must gauge the performance of these suppliers are denied the information supplied by the accounting statements of competitive firms. This monitoring process must inevitably result in reliance of the monitors on statistical indicators of the quantity and quality of output. As many of the characteristics of health output may not be economically monitored, and thus are invisible, the incentives of these organizations influence the diversion of resources from such invisible characteristics of output as patient comfort, information, and convenience toward visible aspects such as patient-days (i.e., "hotel" services).

We have examined many phenomena from the point of view of this hypothesized behavior and find much evidence that supports it. We observe that the NHS spends less per capita than Americans do on themselves, even allowing for the possible influence of the higher income in the United States on spending. As it does not pay for NHS doctors to devote time to invisible characteristics of patient care either, the NHS may get along with fewer doctors. We find that they have in fact done so. In this connection, we observe that under the NHS the economic position of physicians has plummeted. We also find a statistically significant relation between this economic problem of physicians and their rate of emigration from the United Kingdom. Thus we observe declining earnings of physicians driving out home-trained physicians whose places are taken by foreign-trained doctors with lower qualifications.

Personal attention and comfort are very difficult for Parliament to monitor, and we therefore predict that factors useful in producing these invisible aspects of hospital care will not be as extensively employed by the NHS as by American proprietary hospitals. This implication is confirmed by the observation of fewer personnel per available bed in NHS hospitals and in the lower levels of capital spending. While hospital beds themselves are visible and therefore should be less susceptible to governmental economies of this type, we also note a relative deprivation of short-term acute hospital beds in the United Kingdom relative to the United States. Finally, we note that hospital managers may improve their performance (in the important statistical sense) by retaining patients in hospital beds beyond the point when it is medically advisable. Evidence suggests that U.S. VA hospitals use this ploy to improve their reported productivity. Such an inference finds additional support in the data on in-patient hospitalization for U.S. and NHS hospitals.

Chapter 1 Notes

1. Cotton M. Lindsay, *Veterans Administration Hospitals: An Economic Analysis of Government Enterprise* (Washington, D.C.: American Enterprise Institute, 1975). Also see, Cotton M. Lindsay, "A Theory of Government Enterprise," *Journal of Political Economy,* 84 (October 1976): 1061–77.

2. In Lindsay, *National Health Issues,* health indicators are analyzed and are found to be insensitive to the introduction of government health plans.

3. The British have taken considerable pride in their performance in de-

tailed international comparisons such as Robert Maxwell, *Health Care: The Growing Dilemma* (New York: McKinsey and Company, 1974).

4. Lifetime income streams were assumed to follow cross-sectional age income profiles.

5. Lindsay, "A Theory of Government Enterprise."

Health Insurance and Health Policy in the Federal Republic of Germany

*Uwe E. Reinhardt**

Introduction

Modern societies, without exception, view certain basic health care services as commodities to which every member of society should be guaranteed access, regardless of their ability to pay. This general proposition seems widely shared among nations, whatever their cultural and political complexions. Vastly different approaches, however, have been adopted for acting on that precept.

Some nations have proceeded on the assumption that the desired guarantee requires the nationalization of both the production and the financing of health services. This approach has been favored in the United Kingdom and in the socialist nations. The overall capacity of the delivery systems in these nations is determined by a political al-

*Professor of Economics and Public Affairs, Princeton University. Research for this paper was supported by the Health Care Financing Agency of the Department of Health and Human Services under Grant No. 95-P97309/2-01. That support is gratefully acknowledged. The author is indebted to Professor Klaus-Dirk Henke, Technische Universitat, Hannover, West Germany and to Dr. Peter McMenamin of the Health Care Financing Agency of the Department of Health and Human Services for their careful review of the manuscript and their many helpful comments.

gorithm, and available capacity is distributed regionally on the basis of explicit planning. It is rationed among individual consumers on some basis other than monetary charges—usually on the basis of time prices or on the basis of the providers' medical judgement. The time prices faced by individual patients are, of course, also set indirectly by some provider's assessment of the patient's need for health services.

At the other end of the spectrum are nations that seek to provide the desired guarantees with a minimum of public-sector intrusion into the production and financing of health services. These nations would prefer, in principle, to effect the guarantee simply by redistributing appropriate amounts of general purchasing power—for example, through negative-income tax schemes. Upon making the requisite transfers one could once again, in principle, rely on the price mechanism to determine the system's overall capacity and to allocate that capacity among members of society. In practice, however, this ideal approach has typically been found infeasible because the requisite transfers of general purchasing power tend to exceed the political tolerance for such transfers. Consequently, even in these nations one observes varying degrees of public-sector intrustion into at least the financing of health care services. The production of health services, however, has remained more or less completely in the private sector.

From the perspective of health policy in the United States, the second set of approaches is clearly the more interesting. To be sure, the nationalized and centrally planned health systems can, and do, claim for themselves certain advantages. In the United States, however, it is not generally believed that the advantages of centrally planned, publicly owned health systems compensate adequately for the rigidities inherent in them. Should Americans ever wish to copy other nations' approaches to national health insurance, for example, they would more probably look to contexts in which at least the production of health care services remains in the private sector.

Even that confined purview, however, presents one with a remarkable variety of mechanisms used to provide the desired guarantees. Some nations (for example, Canada) have chosen to nationalize the financing of health services completely. Other nations (for example, Australia) seem to view complete nationalization of the financing mechanism as unnecessary and, indeed, undesirable. Still other nations (for example, France) have sought to have the best of both worlds. Although the financing of health services in France is effected through nongovernmental insurance funds (*caisses d'assurance maladie*), these insurance funds operate under close supervision of the central government's ministry of health. So close is this supervision on a day-to-day basis that the insurance funds have, in effect, become the central government's arm in the implementation of national health policy.

In this paper I shall focus almost exclusively on the health insurance system of West Germany. That system is interesting because (1) the delivery system resembles in important respects those systems found on the North American continent; (2) virtually the entire West German population is now covered by the most comprehensive health insurance imaginable; and (3) the public sector's role in the production and financing of health care extends merely to the provision of a statutory framework, to occasional compulsory arbitration, and to the financing of capital expenditures by hospitals (and with it, participation in the planning of inpatient capacity).

The remainder of this paper is organized as follows: presented next is a brief description of the West German health care delivery system, its health insurance system, and recent trends in health care expenditures; the focus then shifts to current issues in West German health policy, notably, the approaches to the control of health care costs and expenditures. The paper concludes with some general remarks on the arbitration of social conflict over the allocation of health care resources.

Health Care Resources and Their Utilization in West Germany

West Germany currently has a population of about 61.5 million. As indicated in table 2.1, this population is served by roughly 1.7 million health workers—a total defined to include any person employed by the health care sector, in whatever capacity. Only about 700,000 of this total are health professionals as that term is used in the United States; of these, roughly 120,000 are physicians.

The labor force in the health care sector is complemented by about thirty-five hundred hospitals with a capacity of about 11.6 beds per 1,000 population. As shown in table 2.2, slightly over 54 percent of all hospital beds are in publicly owned facilities (mainly municipal hospitals); 35 percent are in hospitals founded and administered by private organizations (churches or foundations) on a not-for-profit basis; and 10.5 percent are in other private hospitals, some of which are operated

TABLE 2.1

Employment in the West German health care sector
(1976)

Category	Total number	Number per 100,000 population	
Total employment	1,710,000	2,780	
Physicians			
inpatient	54,648	89	} 182
ambulatory	56,969	93	
other[a]	12,949	21	
Dentists	31,858	51	
Pharmacists	25,885	42	
Other health professionals[b]	487,709	793	
Other persons employed in health care[c]	1,039,982	1,691	

a. Includes physicians in public health departments, administration, and industry.

b. Includes nursing personnel and physicians in training.

c. Includes workers in the industries producing supplies, medical equipment, and drugs.

Source: Bundesverband der Ortskrankenkassen 1978, p. 33.

on a for-profit basis. Only about 7.9 beds per 1,000 population are allocated to general acute care. The remainder serve long-term or special care.

American or Canadian physicians typically treat their patients in their own practices and in the hospitals with which they are affiliated. Hospital privileges following this North American pattern are enjoyed by only about 6 percent of the West German physicians—the *Belegsärzte*. Other West German physicians work full time either in their own private practice or in the hospital. Physicians in private practice (*Niedergelassene Ärzte*) typically treat their patients on a fee-for-service basis, with the bulk of the fees (about 85 percent) coming directly from third-party payers. Physicians in hospitals (*Krankenhausärzte*) are salaried, and only the chiefs of staff enjoy the privilege of treating private patients on the hospital's premises for a fee.

The dichotomy between the ambulatory and inpatient physician practice is statutory and strictly enforced. It has a number of peculiar consequences. First, most hospitals are prohibited from operating out-

TABLE 2.2

Hospitals, hospital beds, and hospital utilization
in West Germany (1974)

Number of hospitals (all types)	3,483	100%
Public	1,309	38%
Private, nonprofit	1,200	34%
Other private	974	28%
Number of hospital beds	716,530	100%
In public hospitals	387,590	54%
In private, nonprofit hospitals	253,949	35%
In other private hospitals	74,991	11%
Number of beds per 100,000 population		
All hospitals	11.56	
Acute-care hospitals	7.85	
Special hospitals	3.71	
Number of admissions per 100,000 population	159	
Acute-care hospitals	140	
Special hospitals	19	
Average length of stay		
Acute-care hospitals	17 days	
Special hospitals	63 days	
Average utilization rate		
Acute-care hospitals	84%	
Special hospitals	89%	
Number of patient days per 1,000 population		
Acute-care hospitals	2,405	
Special hospitals	1,206	

Source: Bundesminister für Jugend 1977, pp. 239–49.

patient departments because the provision of ambulatory care is the preserve of the *Niedergelassene Ärzte* (the physicians in private practice). Hospitals may intrude on this monopoly only if they are affiliated with a medical school and their outpatient clinic serves a teaching function. Second, a private physician sending a patient to a hospital loses both medical and economic control over the patient during his or her hospital stay (although hospitals may and often do report back to the patient's private physician). A corollary is that although West German patients have the right to choose their own physician for ambulatory health services, freedom of choice does not extend to treatment within the hospital unless the patient is treated on a private basis by one of the chiefs of medicine. Finally, the strict division between ambulatory and inpatient care contributes to an excessive application of diagnostic tests, because hospital physicians do not invariably accept the diagnosis determined by the private practitioner and prefer to conduct their own tests, at the risk of repeating some tests. While this practice may enhance the accuracy of the diagnosis, it is expensive.

As is evident from tables 2.2 and 2.3, West Germans rely rather more heavily on the hospital than do Americans. Although the West German admission rate is below the comparable rate in the United States, the average length of stay per admission in West Germany is roughly double the comparable rate in the United States. Case-mix differentials may distort this comparison to some extent; but it is known that the average length of stay for specific illnesses in West Germany tends to be much higher than it is for identical illnesses in the United States. As a result of this differential, the number of patient days per 1,000 population is substantially higher in West Germany than it is in the United States.

Unfortunately, similar data on the utilization of ambulatory services are not publicly available in West Germany as they are in the United States. There is evidence that West German physicians see far more patients per office hour than do their American counterparts and, in particular, that they place heavy emphasis on diagnostic and other technical procedures in the composition of treatment packages. In this respect, West German physicians appear to respond to fee schedules

TABLE 2.3
Hospital utilization in the United States
(1974)

	General and special hospitals	Psychiatric and tuberculosis hospitals
Admissions per 1,000 population	165	4.2
Total days in hospital per 1,000 population	1,432	662
Average length of stay (days)	8.7	NA
Occupancy rate	76%	NA

Source: *Statistical Abstract of the United States 1978*, 1979 table 168, p. 110.

that tend to reward technical procedures relatively more generously than face-to-face contact with patients, at least in comparison with the typical structure of fees in the United States.

The West German Health Insurance System

Institutional and Historical Background

The onset of national health insurance in Germany is usually dated 1883, when low-income industrial workers and their families were compelled by law to become members of sickness funds, many of which had already been in existence throughout the nineteenth century. At that time (1883), the statutory system covered only about one-sixth of the population. The benefit package mainly included sickness cash payments and only a modest range of medical services in kind. In the ensuing decades, the system evolved in predictable directions: coverage was extended across both population groups and medical services. Today the system covers the bulk of the population and offers a remarkably comprehensive benefit package. Expenditures on benefits-in-kind now dwarf sickness cash payments.

During the period of 1883 to the 1930s, the sickness funds negotiated contracts privately with individual physicians and had the right to limit the number of physicians participating in their schemes. In 1931 the statutory basis was laid for collective contracts between regional associations of sickness funds and newly created professional associations of sickness-fund physicians—the *Kassenaerztlichen Vereinigungen* (KVs). These physician associations were originally chartered on a *Land* (state) basis, but they eventually formed national associations as well. Under the 1931 statute the sickness funds collectively transferred an agreed-upon lump sum per each insured patient to the physician associations, which in turn agreed to have their members render the insured patient all medically necessary services and disbursed the lump sum to their members, typically on a capitation basis. The sickness fund associations have always negotiated separate contracts with individual hospitals, usually on the basis of agreed-upon per diem charges.

After World War II, West German physicians won the right to establish themselves as sickness-fund physicians without the funds' prior approval. The distribution of funds from the physician associations to individual physicians began to proceed more and more on a fee-for-service basis, according to fee schedules negotiated between the sickness funds and the professional associations. Until very recently, this system was open-ended. The sickness funds paid for whatever billings were submitted by physicians to their physician associations. Since 1976 there have been attempts to place a cap on overall physician reimbursement, although the success of this approach is not assured. These attempts, culminating in a formal cost-containment act in 1977, are described later in this paper.

Parallel to the compulsory insurance system, there developed the *Ersatzkassen* (literally, "substitute funds"), whose membership primarily includes white-collar workers. For the most part, these funds have not been accessible to blue-collar workers.[1] Individuals not mandated by law to join a sickness fund often enjoy the right to join a fund voluntarily; and in competing with the compulsory sickness funds for voluntary members, these *Ersatzkassen* have frequently sought to attract patients by offering their physicians better financial terms. It is sometimes alleged that the *Ersatzkassen* can do this because of an ability to select among risks. In any event, there is evidence that the role of the *Ersatzkassen* has served to shift the evolution of the West German health insurance system in directions favored by physicians. The shift from capitation to fee-for-service reimbursement is said to be one such instance. That shift was spearheaded by the *Ersatzkassen* during the 1960s.

Administration and Financing of the Current (1980) System

As noted, the West German health insurance system is actually a mosaic of roughly 1,500 autonomous sickness funds organized on the basis of geography (the *Ortskrankenkassen*), of enterprise (the *Betriebskassen*), or of trade (*Innungskassen*). About one-half of the insured population has membership in the *Ortskrankenkassen,* and one-quarter are members of the *Ersatzkassen.* Tables 2.4 and 2.5 provide further details on the insurance status of the West German population and the distribution of insured members across sickness funds. "Member," in this context, means the insured employee or retired person. Membership in a sickness fund automatically extends full coverage to

TABLE 2.4

Percentage breakdown of West German population
by health insurance status (1974)

Insurance status	Percent of the population
1. Insured under the statutory system	90.15
Mandatory members	30.75
Voluntary members	7.53
Retired people who are members	11.82
Dependents of members who are automatically covered	37.04
2. Covered by private health insurance	7.20
3. Covered by special insurance schemes	2.36
Policemen	1.00
People on public assistance	1.07
Students	0.29
4. Not insured	0.29
Total population	100.

Source: Schmidt 1978, table 15, p. 57.

all of the member's dependents. The number of persons insured by a sickness fund thus tends to exceed the number of its members significantly (see table 2.4, item 1).

Depending on the member's economic status, he or she is either a voluntary member of a sickness fund or must join on a mandatory basis. Included in the group of mandatorily insured are: all blue-collar workers, white-collar workers with incomes below a certain level, retired persons, virtually all farmers, students and apprentices, and sundry other groups of modest economic status. Over three-quarters of the persons insured under the statutory system now are mandated to do so. Persons not mandated to seek coverage have the right to join sickness funds on a voluntary basis.

About 7 percent of the population obtains private insurance coverage. This group includes civil servants, who receive a cash supplement from the government in case of illness and obtain private supplemental insurance to handle costs not covered by the government indemnity.

The sickness funds are governed by boards composed of members

TABLE 2.5

Membership in the statutory health insurance system
(1974)

		Percentage of all insured "members"
Local sickness funds (*Ortskrankenkassen*)		48.5
Enterprise funds (*Betriebskrankenkassen*)		12.9
Other funds[a]		11.0
Substitute funds (*Ersatzkassen*)		27.6
Blue-collar workers	1.1	
White-collar workers	26.5	
Total: 31.64 million members		100

a. Funds organized around a trade or craft, e.g., funds for sailors, miners, farmers, and agricultural workers.
Source: Schmidt 1978, table 18, p. 60.

representing employers and employees. The individual funds are members of associations at the level of the *Land* (state), which in turn form the national associations. The *Land* and national associations negotiate with their counterpart associations of health care providers.

In principle, each individual fund is expected to be fiscally autonomous. Its financial affairs are supervised, however, at the level of the *Land*. Overall supervisory authority over the statutory insurance system rests with the federal government's Ministry of Labor and Social Affairs. Since the sickness funds must operate within statutory guidelines that prescribe, inter alia, the benefit package that must be offered the insured under Statutory Health Insurance, the funds are actually fairly similar to one another. Broadly speaking, membership in a sickness fund entitles members and their families to all necessary medical and hospital services in case of illness, to certain types of preventive care, to prescribed drugs, and to cash benefits that cover loss of income due to illness.[2] Also included in the typical benefit package are maternity benefits, the services of health workers in patients' homes, medical appliances, dental care (including dentures), eyeglasses, stays in rest homes, and rehabilitative services. Indeed, it is hard to think of medical services that are not covered by the statutory health insurance scheme.

For the most part, West Germans insured under the statutory system enjoy first-dollar coverage for insured items. There is a modest copayment on prescription drugs (one Deutsche Mark, DM, or about 50 U.S. cents per item in 1980) and a 20 percent coinsurance rate on dentures. A wide range of medical supplies are fully covered, but only for certain basic models. Thus the insurance funds will fully cover the cost of a basic type of eyeglasses, leaving the cost of a more attractive frame entirely to the consumer. A valid generalization, however, would be that cost sharing by patients in West Germany is rare and trivial in both absolute and relative amounts.

Tables 2.6–2.8 provide information on the financing of the Statutory Insurance System. It is seen that the system is almost wholly financed by employers and employees. Contributions for insured members are raised in the form of a flat payroll tax, with employers and employees each paying an equal share. Contributions for members who are retired are made by their respective pension funds. The public sector itself makes only modest contributions to the system, mainly indirectly through pension funds (table 2.6).

Contributions to the sickness funds are made on the "solidarity principle," which is understood to mean that members should contribute in accordance with their ability to pay, regardless of the number of their dependents or their health status. No attempt has ever been made to set contributions for individual members within a fund on actuarial principles. A fund as a whole, however, must set its overall contribution rate strictly on the basis of the actuarial cost of serving the entire membership (and dependents). Because the actuarial cost per member

TABLE 2.6

Direct and indirect sources of finance for the statutory
health insurance system in West Germany
(1974)

Employers	39.0%
Private households (mainly employees)	48.8%
Federal government (*Bund*)	7.2%
States (*Länder*)	1.7%
Municipalities	1.9%
Other	1.4%
Total	DM 51.705 billion

Source: Schmidt 1978, table 20, p. 96.

TABLE 2.7
Secular change in contribution rates to the statutory health
insurance system (1974–1978)—in percentage of gross
earnings[a]

Year	Local sickness funds	Enterprise funds	Other funds	Substitute funds for		All funds in the system
				Blue-collar workers	White-collar workers	
1974	9.35	8.63	8.95	9.38	9.81	9.36
1976	11.34	10.20	11.10	11.09	11.85	11.30
1978	11.51	10.61	11.34	11.47	11.82	NA

a. Shared equally by employers and employees.
Source: Bundesverband der Ortskrankenkassen 1978, table 2.

depends on the demographic mix of members, which can and does vary
among sickness funds, one observes a rather striking variability in the
contribution rates imposed by the various funds (see table 2.8). In recent years, this disparity in contribution rates has quite understandably become an increasingly controversial issue. The disparity has

TABLE 2.8
Variation in contribution rates to the statutory health
insurance system (1975)

Contribution rate (in percent)[a]	No. of local sickness funds	No. of enterprise funds	No. of other funds	No. of substitute funds	All funds
0–6	–	12	–	–	12
6.1–7	–	56	1	–	57
7.1–8	7	155	8	–	170
8.1–9	34	299	30	1	364
9.1–10	84	318	53	2	457
10.1–11	134	113	60	8	315
11.1–12	49	12	12	4	77
12.1–13	6	–	–	–	6
Total	314	965	164	15	1458

a. Percentage of gross earnings shared equally by employer and employee.
Source: Schmidt 1978, table 43, p. 97.

persisted because there is actually little effective competition for members among the numerous funds. By and large, an employee's or retired person's membership is dictated by his or her employment and/or geographic location.

Expenditures

Table 2.9 presents details on the pattern of expenditures under West Germany's Statutory Insurance System. To provide a basis of comparison, data on gross national product are shown as well.

Total expenditures by the statutory system (excluding cash benefits) amounted to about 5.4 percent of West Germany's gross national product in 1978. This figure is, of course, not directly comparable to the national health care expenditure series published in the United States. The West German figure excludes expenditures by private households for nonprescription drugs; public-sector expenditures for capital investments in hospitals, medical schools, and medical research; as well as expenditures made by the private insurance carriers. It is difficult to estimate an exact counterpart of the U.S. figure from

TABLE 2.9

Total expenditures under the statutory health insurance
system by type of service[a] (1978)

Category	Billions of DM	Percent of total
Ambulatory medical services	13.2	19.1
Dental services and dentures	10.6	15.3
Drugs	10.6	15.3
Hospital services	21.8	31.6
All other expenditures (medicinal aids, maternity benefits, preventive care, etc.)	9.6	13.9
Administration	3.3	4.8
Total expenditures, excluding cash benefits and administration	69.1	100.0
Cash Benefits	5.3	7.7
Gross national product	1,278.0	

a. Preliminary data.

Source: Federal Department of Labor and Social Affairs; cited in Geissler 1978, table 4.

the available West German data. A reasonable approximation, however, can be developed from data published by West Germany's Federal Ministry of Labor and Social Affairs (see Bundesminister für Arbeit und Sozialordnung 1978). According to these data, total national expenditures from all sources for inpatient care, ambulatory care, drugs, supplies and dentures, medical research and public health services amounted to DM 97 billion in 1975, a figure that includes DM 6 billion for administrative costs. Gross national product in 1975 amounted to DM 1,030 billion (Geissler 1978, table 4). On the more comprehensive U.S. definition of health expenditures, then, West Germans appeared to spend roughly 9.4 percent of their gross national product on health care proper in 1975. In other words, the total expenditure figure of DM 69.1 billion attributed to the Statutory Health Insurance System in table 2.9 represents only about 71 percent of the total that approximates the American concept of national health expenditures. This ratio should always be kept in mind regarding data strictly on the statutory system.

Table 2.10 presents the distribution of expenditures by the statutory

TABLE 2.10

Distribution of expenditures over categories of sickness funds and expenditures per member by category of sickness funds (1974)

	Percentage of total expenditures paid by funds	Expenditure per "member" (in Deutsche Marks)
Local sickness funds	47.7	1,446
Substitute funds for white-collar workers	26.7	1,467
Enterprise funds	13.3	1,529
Funds for miners	4.2	1,902
Funds for trade guilds	4.1	1,306
Funds for rural workers	2.7	1,368
Substitute funds for blue-collar workers	1.1	1,488
Funds for seamen	0.2	1,396
Total	100.0	1,469[a]

a. Standard deviation of category means about overall mean (1488) is DM 182.
Source: Adapted from Schmidt 1978, tables 34 and 35.

system (including DM 4.2 billion cash-benefits payments) over the various categories of sickness funds in 1974. The table also indicates the variability of expenditures per insured member. This number, incidentally, is not to be confused with expenditures per capita, because membership in a sickness fund automatically extends full coverage also to all of the insured member's dependents. The interfund variability in expenditures per member therefore reflects, to some extent, more differences in the demographic mix of the funds' membership, including differences in the number of dependents per member.

The secular growth in health care expenditures by the statutory system is exhibited in table 2.11. Although all categories of these expenditures increased more rapidly than the gross national product during the 1960s, that differential in growth rates reached remarkable proportions during the first half of the 1970s. Overall expenditures during that period grew at more than twice the rate of growth in gross national product. The pattern received widespread and highly critical comment in the media and eventually triggered public intervention in the form of a federal cost-containment law.

Reimbursement of Providers

Hospitals are reimbursed by the sickness funds on the basis of negotiated per diems. These per diems cover all operating costs incurred in connection with inpatient physician care, including the cost of drugs and supplies. The per diems do not cover capital costs, which since 1972 have been supplied from state and federal sources in conjunction with regional planning. The negotiated per diems are unique to each hospital; but they are subject to approval by a state authority. As already noted, hospital physicians are salaried, and only chief medical officers are permitted to deliver health care to private patients on a fee-for-service basis.

The sickness funds pay pharmacists for drugs and supplies furnished to patients against prescriptions obtained from ambulatory care physicians. Payment is at "market prices," which are the sum of wholesale prices paid by pharmacists to the producers of pharmaceuticals or to wholesalers, plus a markup (*Handelsspanne*) fixed by law and not subject to any influence by the sickness funds. Precisely what countervailing power makes this retail price a market price is an intriguing

TABLE 2.11

Average annual growth rates in selected expenditures
under the Statutory Health Insurance System (1960–1978)

Category	Average annual percentage growth					
	1960–1965	1965–1970	1970–1975	1976	1977	1978[a]
Ambulatory medical care	11.3	11.4	15.6	5.9	4.6	5.7
Dental services and dentures	13.1	13.8	26.8	15.6	3.4	6.2
Drugs	13.1	15.9	16.1	8.3	1.5	8.7
Hospital services	13.5	15.3	23.9	9.8	5.7	7.1
Total expenditures excluding cash benefits for sickness and administration	12.3	13.8	20.1	10.0	4.3	7.2
Gross national product	8.8	8.3	8.5	9.1	6.2	7.1

a. Preliminary

Source: Federal Department of Labor and Social Affairs; cited in Geissler 1978, table 5.

question. In principle, the individual physician is to prescribe the lowest-priced drug within any set of drugs of comparable bio-availability and effectiveness. In practice, this mandate had been widely circumvented for want of information on drug equivalence.

A recently established commission of physicians, pharmacists, and representatives of the pharmaceutical industry has been charged with the task of devising an officially accepted list of bioequivalencies and associated drug prices. That list is expected to contribute toward greater economy in the prescription of drugs. Furthermore, there have been experiments—notably in the state of Bavaria—with reimbursement methods that hold the individual physician fiscally responsible for the excessive prescribing of drugs.

The reimbursement of ambulatory patient physicians and dentists is somewhat complicated as is shown in figure 2.1. Each insured person in Germany receives from his or her sickness fund a sickness voucher every three months. The patient surrenders this quarterly voucher to his or her physician on their first contact of each quarter. Referrals to specialists proceed on a transfer certificate issued by the referring physician, although patients may go directly to a specialist as initial contact with the medical system. The physician notes individual services rendered on the voucher (or transfer certificate) and submits it to the appropriate physician association for reimbursement on a fee-for-service basis. If the association faces an overall cap on distributable funds—as is being attempted now—then individual fees are scaled up or down by the association to meet the budget constraint. Utilization review to control overservicing is, in the first instance, in the hands of the physician associations, although the sickness funds have recently gained the right to participate actively in utilization reviews. The reimbursement system for dentists parallels that for physicians.

The fee schedules used under the statutory system are negotiated periodically between associations of the sickness funds and the professional associations. The overall structure of the fee schedule (that is, relative value points) is negotiated at the national level. The original basis for these negotiations is a federal fee schedule issued by the Ministry of Economics in 1965.[3] The national negotiations take the form of amendments to this schedule.

The money value of the relative value points is negotiated between sickness funds and professional associations at the level of the *Land*

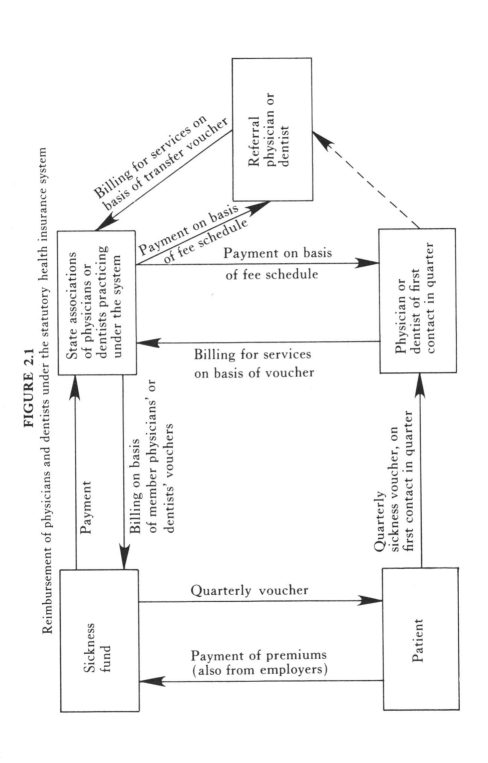

FIGURE 2.1

Reimbursement of physicians and dentists under the statutory health insurance system (state). Although fee levels vary across the states, such variations are small compared to regional variations of fees in the United States. (In 1976, for example, the highest level of fees in West Germany was only 6 percent above the lowest level of fees.) There are also minor variations in fee levels among the various types of sickness funds; but, again, in no way are these comparable to the variations in fees one observes in the United States.

For patients insured under the statutory scheme, physicians and dentists must accept the negotiated fees as payment in full. They may, and invariably do, charge private patients considerably higher fees. Indeed, it is not uncommon for physicians to divide their day into practice hours for statutorily insured and privately insured patients, and to adopt different practice styles for the two types of patients. Table 2.12 presents data from a recent study of practice styles in the city of Munich. These data suggest that practice styles are sensitive to differences in insurance coverage. Patients covered by the *Allgemeine Ortskrankenkasse* (local sickness fund), which offers physicians the relatively least-generous terms, tended to spend considerably more time in the waiting room than private patients (who paid relatively higher fees). Private patients also spent more time per visit with the physician than did patients under the statutory system.

Control of Cost and Expenditures Under the Statutory Health Insurance System

Under the Statutory Health Insurance System of West Germany, providers and patients are mandated to exercise economy in the use of health care resources. That mandate, however, is not really compatible with the financial incentives built into the system. With few exceptions, all insured services and supplies are received by patients free of charge at the point of delivery. Physicians are reimbursed on a fee-for-service basis; hospitals are reimbursed for the number of patient-days they report. Both face a fiscal incentive to service their patients generously. In the wake of a rapid expansion of health care resources—both facilities and manpower—the sharp secular increase in expenditures during the 1970s is not surprising.

To be sure, the system has always been equipped with formal cost-control mechanisms. The prices of drugs, for example, are reviewed and authorized by the Ministry of Economics. The fees for physician

TABLE 2.12

Average wait time in the office and average
length of patient visits by insurance status of patients
Munich, West Germany (1979)

	Patients insured by:		Local sickness fund
	Local sickness fund	Private insurance	Private insurance
Men aged 18–55			
Wait time in the office (minutes)	45.2	28.9	1.56
Length of patient visit (minutes)	10.5	11.9	0.88
Women aged 18–55			
Wait time in the office (minutes)	47.0	28.0	1.68
Length of patient visit (minutes)	10.5	13.5	0.78

Source: Neubauer and Birkner 1980, figures 1 and 2, pp. 155 and 156.

services are negotiated between sickness funds and physician associations. The utilization of physician services, as well as the prescription
of drugs, is monitored by the physician associations themselves and, in
principle, controlled by them. The funds flowing to the hospital sector
are controlled, at least in part, through negotiated per diems on the
basis of approved cost sheets. Finally, since 1972, the physical capacity
of the hospital sector has come under the influence of regional planners, whose approval is required for state and federal financing of capital expenditures by hospitals.

As is clearly evident in table 2.11, these sundry controls either failed
to work during the early 1970s or were not applied at all. Because the
secular growth during this period led to successive increases in the
premium rates (see table 2.7), both organized labor and employers
pressed for more overt forms of cost control. In that climate the federal
government succeeded in enacting its Health Care Cost-Containment
Act of 1977, an act that seems in keeping with West Germany's penchant for policy by consensus.

The overall thrust of the Cost-Containment Act is to constrain the growth of expenditures to the growth of gross national product. The basic mechanism is an annually negotiated agreement of overall health care budgets at the federal and state level. To this end the act mandates the establishment of a National Health Conference (*Konzertierte Aktion*) embracing all major interest groups active in the health care sector, including the sickness funds, the associations of sickness funds' physicians, hospitals, the pharmaceutical industry, unions (representing consumers), associations of employers, the state governments, and the federal government (Geissler 1978). The conference is mandated to develop annually a consensus on guidelines for the economic development of the Statutory Health Insurance System, including, of course, the growth of total expenditures by type of service and, indirectly, increases in fees and prices. To illustrate: during its first sessions in December 1977 and March 1978, chaired by the Federal Minister of Labor, the conference reached a consensus on the following recommendations for the period of July 1, 1978 to June 30, 1979.

1. Expenditures per insured member for ambulatory physician services are to increase by not more than 5.5 percent above the previous fiscal year. Of this total, 2.5 percent is allocated to increases in fees and 3.0 percent is allocated to increases in utilization.
2. Similarly, expenditures per member for dental services (excluding materials and laboratory costs) from July 1, 1978 to June 30, 1979 may exceed the previous year's by only 2.5 percent.
3. Expenditures on drugs per insured member in the second half of 1978 may exceed average expenditures during 1977 by only 3.5 percent.

Physicians, pharmacists, the pharmaceutical industry, and the sickness funds agreed on recommendations 1 and 3. These recommendations, therefore, had force. Because the dental association dissented from recommendation 2, the reimbursement of dentists was left for further negotiations between dentists and the sickness funds. An explicit recommendation for the hospital sector could not be offered because that sector is not covered by the Cost-Containment Act.[4]

To implement the recommended guidelines, the sickness funds and physician associations were mandated under the act to establish Economic Monitoring Committees at the state level, with equal representation of both parties and rotating chairmanship. The committees' monitoring system screens the charge profile of every physician. Physicians whose average number of services or prescriptions per case (voucher) exceeds their class average by 30 percent are selected for further examination. In the absence of justification for the observed deviations, these physicians' reimbursements are cut accordingly. Under this system the individual physician can, therefore, be held fiscally liable for excessive prescribing of drugs.

A remarkable feature of the West German approach to cost containment is that the guidelines recommended by the conference are reached by consensus and that they are not binding upon the negotiating parties. Although the guidelines may thus appear as a toothless tiger, they are nevertheless thought to influence the direction of negotiations and even more so the compulsory arbitration that is triggered whenever negotiations between the sickness funds and providers break down. In effect, the law represents an attempt to replace the vacuum left by the secular erosion of market forces with a new type of market—one in which professional and economic interest groups bargain collectively toward a national consensus within a set of constraints provided by statute.

By contrast, the thrust of public policy in the United States has been, by and large, to replace the eroding market forces in health care by direct and often unilateral regulation of the health care sector. Ironically, then, policymakers in a country that prides itself on its respect for the individual's freedom seem more taken by the potential of bureaucratic management in health care than policymakers in a country with an alleged penchant for bureaucracy.

How successful the West German approach to cost containment will be in the longer run remains to be seen. As is shown in table 2.11, the growth of expenditures under West Germany's statutory health insurance system has abated markedly since 1975, although the most dramatic decline in the growth rate actually preceded the introduction of the Cost-Containment Act of 1977. The explanation generally given for this early decline is that health care providers agreed to a stringent voluntary cost-containment effort in anticipation of federal legislation, to demonstrate its redundancy.

Also, the relative harmony prevailing at the early sessions of the conference has given way to more open dissent in subsequent sessions. Some observers of the West German health system—policymakers among them—appear increasingly disillusioned with the approach.[5] One reaction to this sense of frustration may be stronger government interference in the health sector. A provision in the Cost-Containment Act, for example, mandates the federal executive to report in 1981 to Parliament on the effectiveness of the act and to assess the need for more potent policies.[6]

An alternative reaction might be to subject the delivery and financing of health care more extensively to classical market mechanisms— for example, to significant cost sharing among patients. Some economists (for example, Henke and Metze 1978) have advocated this approach, as has organized medicine in West Germany. On the other hand, neither policymakers nor politicians in West Germany have shown so far any inclination to employ cost sharing by patients as a cost containment strategy.

The economist's case for coinsurance rests on a well-known body of theory. Implicit in that case is the assumption that patients are (1) well informed and (2) capable of acting rationally on accurate information concerning their health status and on alternative approaches to treating given medical conditions. Alternatively, it is assumed that even if patients were not well informed or were incapable of choosing rationally among treatment alternatives, physicians would keep the patient's financial interest in mind when choosing treatment on the patient's behalf.

Why physicians would favor cost sharing by patients is not as clearly evident. When physicians do make the case for cost sharing they typically do so on the argument that it would (1) elicit more responsible conduct on the part of patients, (2) free medical practice from trivial cases, and (3) contribute toward expenditure containment. There may be validity to the first argument and possibly to the second as well. One doubts, however, that physicians seriously believe the third. Organized medicine is not known to favor policies that reduce the aggregate flow of funds to physicians. As Barer et al. (1979) recently argued, a more plausible explanation for the profession's posture is that cost sharing, coupled with third-party coverage, is believed by physicians to draw more fiscal nourishment overall to the physician sector than could otherwise be had from third-party payers under universal first-dollar coverage, because it is usually more difficult to maintain an overview of, and control over, fiscal flows from many spigots than to control a single source.

In West Germany, the discovery of additional sources of fiscal nourishment for physicians has a particular urgency. Current prognoses put the number of active physicians per 100,000 population in the year 2000 at 406 to 485,[7] depending on the assumptions embodied in the forecast. Because the hospital sector is not likely to expand significantly, the bulk of this projected increase in physician density will spill over into the ambulatory-care sector where physicians are free to establish a private practice without the approval of an intervening institution, such as a hospital. Table 2.13 indicates the effect of this expected spillover. In reaction to these projections one should keep in mind that the physicians included in the table will cater solely to the population's need for ambulatory physician services. Just how, in the face of these numbers, West Germany proposes to keep the growth of total physician remuneration roughly in line with the growth of gross national product (the stated goal of cost-containment policy in that country) is an interesting question. From the American vantage point, the resolution of this question may yield instructive lessons.

Concluding Remarks

In the Western democracies, conflicts over the allocation of real resources among members of society are usually arbitrated by private-

TABLE 2.13

Actual and projected number of active physicians in
West Germany (1975–2000)

Category	1975	1980	1990	2000
Total number of active physicians	118,007	136,900	190,400	256,600
In research and administration	11,819	13,100	18,900	24,200
Primarily in the hospital	52,340	57,000	60,000	62,000
In private, ambulatory practice	53,848	66,800	111,500	170,400
Number of physicians in private ambulatory practice, per 100,000 population				
Number	87	110	191	306
Index (1975=100)	(100)	(126)	(220)	(351)

Source: Adapted from Lefelmann and Geissler 1978, tables 2 and 3, pp. 16 and 17.

market forces. Ideally, this process takes the form of competitive bidding with purchasing power that is distributed among individuals on the basis of a mixture of merit, lineage, and luck. In general, the resource-allocative verdicts of this arbitration process tend to be accepted with remarkable equanimity, even by those whom mere misfortune had shunted aside in the original distribution of purchasing power, as long as the bidding process itself has been reasonably fair (competitive). Almost invariably the impersonal, though often harsh, verdicts of private markets are accepted more tranquilly than possibly less harsh verdicts by identifiable individuals, for example, public servants.

For many decades—indeed centuries—this form of arbitration was also accepted in conflicts over the allocation of health care resources. As I have asserted in the introduction, however, one cannot think of a modern society that still favors this process. Many societies (for example, the United States and Australia) wish to guarantee their members access to at least a minimally adequate set of health services, regardless of the distribution of purchasing power, although not necessarily on an equal footing.[8] Other societies (for example, Canada, the United Kingdom, the continental European nations, and the socialist nations) profess as a basic tenet that all members of society ought to have unfettered access to all technically available and medically justifiable health care, and on an equal footing. Although these nations have not so far been able to implement this tenet fully in practice, at the very least they pretend to structure their health care and health insurance systems on this fundamental principle.

Whatever particular ethical principle various societies posit for their health systems, all of them have found it necessary to replace wholly or partially the classical process of free-market arbitration with some alternative, collectivized process of arbitration over resource conflicts in health care. A widely shared belief among American health economists (and some 'European ones as well) is that one ought to move cautiously in this direction and never more than is absolutely necessary for the sake of equity.

Many policymakers in the United States, and apparently most policymakers elsewhere, seem to have despaired long ago of the economist's favored strategy. In particular, little credence is given to the notion that consumers could participate sensibly in resource-allocative decisions in health care, even if they were given the basic information for such decisions—information which health care providers now deliberately withhold from them.[9] Expressing no faith in the consumer's competence, the thrust of public health policy almost everywhere has been to replace market mechanisms altogether with something else, in piecemeal or wholesale fashion.

In the United States this tendency has manifested itself in a penchant for centrally directed planning and direct regulation of individuals' behavior, for example, Professional Standards Review Organizations (PSROs) or Certificates of Needs (CONs) for hospital capacity. In West Germany the thrust of public health policy so far has been neither to move sharply towards planning and direct regulation[10] nor to resurrect the long-moribund play of free market forces. Instead, public policy has attempted to create novel, quasi-economic, quasi-political markets that fall somewhere between the extreme of classical markets and central planning.[11] The ideal decision-making units in these quasi markets are freestanding associations of the individuals and organizations active in these markets (such as, association of providers, of insurers, of the insured, and so on). The atomistic *tatonnement* of classical markets gives way to collective bargaining among these free-standing associations, all within a statutory framework that guards the rights of weaker parties and provides for compulsory arbitration of inconclusive negotiations. The Health Care Conference *(Konzertierte Aktion)* provided for in the Health Care Cost-Containment Act of 1977 can be interpreted as an attempt to refine this type of "market" mechanism.

It can be asked whether, at this time, anyone can seriously claim to know the superior, universally applicable form of arbitration in health care, or even the clearly superior mechanism for the United States.

During the 1960s and early 1970s, when economic growth was rapid everywhere and resources were plentiful, almost any chosen form of conflict arbitration in health care seemed to work, after a fashion. Potential conflicts over real resources were simply smothered in funds and resolved by muddling through with what was thought to be only temporarily fixed physical capacity. In the meantime, the very nature of the allocation problem has changed. There is plenty of physical capacity, but widespread unwillingness to allocate budgets for the use and long-range maintenance of this capacity. All of the Western industrialized nations find themselves in the midst of this new game and all of them are seeking to develop civilized and acceptable rules for it.

Just what set of rules other nations, such as West Germany, will develop and how they will work will be of more than mere academic interest to American observers. After all, in the United States the fabled Yankee ingenuity seems to have taken a long rest sometime before reaching the arena of social policy.

Chapter 2 Notes

1. In 1974 only 3.9 percent of the members of the *Ersatzkassen* were blue-collar workers (see Schmidt 1978, table 17, p. 59).

2. Since 1970, employers have been mandated to provide such cash payments (*Lohnfortzahlung*, i.e., continuation of wages) directly, at least for some weeks. As a result, the percentage of such cash payments in total disbursements by the funds shrank from 21 percent in 1969 to 10.7 percent in 1978.

3. This is the *Gebührenordnung fur Ärzte* (fee schedule for physicians). The annual amendments to the relative value structure in this basic schedule are called *Bundesmantelverträge* (federal envelop contracts).

4. The hospital sector was excluded from the act, because some of the states (notably the city-state of Hamburg) were reluctant to relinquish their control over hospitals to the conference. At the time of this writing, the hospital sector still remains outside the act and has not been subject to any separate cost-containment legislation. In this context see "Kostendämpfung und Strukturverbesserung im Gesundheitswesen" 1978.

5. See, for example, Spivak 1979.

6. Cost-Containment Act, Art. 2, par. 6. In this context see Geissler 1978, p. 13.

7. Lefelmann and Geissler 1979, p. 11.

8. Practically, equal footing in health care could mean that two patients falling victim to the same medical condition in a given locality would receive the same treatment regardless of their socioeconomic position.

9. This asymmetric management of information in health care is often justified by physicians as part of a good therapy. As it happens, however, the asymmetry bestows both medical and market power on the provider. The motives behind it may therefore be questioned.

10. The exception here is the application of planning in the hospital sector as part of the financing of capital expenditures.

11. A clear exposition of this strategy can be found in Herder-Dornreich 1979.

Chapter 2 References

Barer, M. L.; Evans, R. G.; and Stoddart, G. L. 1979. *Controlling Health Care Costs by Direct Charges to Patients: Snare or Delusion?* Occasional paper no. 10. Ontario Economic Council.

Bundesminister für Arbeit und Sozialordnung. 1978. *Die Struktur der Ausgaben im Gesundheitsbereich und ihre Entwicklung seit 1970.* Gesundheitsforschung Series Vol. 7. Bonn. September 1978.

Bundesminster für Jugend, Familie und Gesundheit. 1977. *Daten des Gesundheitswesens—Ausgabe 1977.* Bonn-Bad Godesberg. July 1977.

Bundesverband der Ortskrankenkassen. 1978. Die Ortskrankenkassen im Jahre 1977. Bad-Godesberg. Mimeographed.

Geissler, Ulrich. 1978. Health Care Cost-Containment in the Federal Republic of Germany. Mimeographed. Paper presented at Princeton University, November 1978.

Herder-Dornreich, Philipp. 1977. *Soziale Ordnungspolitik.* Stuttgart: Verlag Bonnaktuel GMBH. 1979.

Henke, Klaus Dirk, and Metze, Ingolf. 1979. "Selbstbeteiligung und Kostenentwicklung." In *Medizin Mensch Gesellschaft* Vol. 4, pp. 34–40.

"Kostendämpfung und Strukturverbesserung im Gesundheitswesen," Part A. III of *Sozialbericht 1978 der Bundesregierung.* BT-Drucksache 8/1805. December 12, 1978, pp. 26–32.

Lefelmann, Gerd, and Geissler, Ulrich. 1979. "Die Entwicklung des Ärzteangebotes bis zum Jahre 2000: Analyse, Bewertungsgesicht-punkte, Massnahmen." In Wissenschaftliches Institut der Ortskrankenkassen, *Gesundheitsökonomische Aspekte der Vergütungspolitik.* Bonn-Bad Godesberg, pp. 9–24.

Neubauer, Grunter, and Birkner, Barbara. 1980. "Beeinflusst die Krankenversicherungsart das Verhalten von Arzt und Patient?" *Sozialer Fortschritt* 29 (July/August 1980): pp. 153–60.

Schmidt, Reinhart. 1978. *Strukturanalyse des Gesundheitswesens in Schleswig-Holstein.* Vol. 8. Kiel.

Spivak, Jonathan. 1979. "Health Cost Controls in Germany." *Wall Street Journal,* December 19, 1979, p. 81.

U.S. Department of Commerce. 1979. *Statistical Abstract of the United States 1978.* Washington, D.C.

Experiments with Government Funding of Health Care in Australia

*John P. Pierce**

Introduction

In 1948 the United Nations declared that every individual had the right to good health. The acceptance of this declaration by a government raises a number of social policy issues; that is, issues concerned with the distribution of resources, opportunities, and life changes between different groups and categories of people (Donnison 1976). The term good health has been variously defined, but governments have tended to operationalize it as "access to medical care." The social policy of a government with respect to health is concerned with reducing gross inequalities and deprivations, especially when they involve people whose capacity to earn income in the market is weakest.

However, general acceptance of the need for a government social policy in the health area does not lead to obvious courses of action that should be followed. Controversial issues center around what constitutes deprivation and how much of the utilization of the health care

*Australian National Health and Medical Research Council Scholar at Stanford Heart Disease Prevention Program and Senior Lecturer (on leave), Department of Community Health Science, Western Australian Institute of Technology.

system can be demonstrated to improve health status. As a minimum, it would seem that social policy should provide an insurance that protects against the huge personal expense that can be incurred by a health catastrophe. At the other end of the scale, there are those who advocate that consultation with any health professional should be covered by a tax-based insurance scheme.

The questions that this conference is addressing today relate not only to what should be covered by public expenditure but also to how this public intervention can best be incorporated into what has traditionally been a private, professional service. At a time when the economy is ailing, the recent vast increases in the total community cost of health services create added tension, as the traditional method of countering inflation has been to reduce government expenditure.

This paper will discuss the evolution of National Health Insurance in Australia from the point of view of what information would be useful to health care policymakers in the United States. This is particularly relevant as Australia has experimented with a number of methods of government funding of health care, ranging from a tax-based system covering total health care to a catastrophe-type tax-based system, all maintaining professional freedom as expressed in fee-for-service practice. Furthermore, Australians are not that different from Americans in their health care experience (see table 3.1), nor is their health care system much different in technology or quality.

For a proper assessment of the implications of the different health schemes, it is important that one have a feeling for Australia. The following part of this paper provides this. Social policy is evolutionary and tends to be a controversial political issue; for these reasons, an understanding of Australian politics since World War II is very important. They are discussed in the third part of this paper.

The balance of the paper deals in chronological order with the different systems of health care funding that Australia has implemented. Each scheme is discussed in terms of the issues of equity, cost, and the respective roles of the public and private sector.

Australia in Perspective

The Land

The continent of Australia has an area of 7,682,300 square kilometers (about 2.9 million square miles), making it nearly as large as main-

TABLE 3.1

Comparative health indicators

	Australia (1977)	Sweden (1976)	United States (1976)
1. Life expectancy at birth			
Male	69.9	72.2	69.0
Female	76.8	78.1	76.7
2. Crude birth rate (per 1000 population)	16.1	11.9	15.3
3. Crude death rate (per 1000 population)	7.7	11.0	8.8
4. Infant mortality rate (per 1000 live births)	12.5	8.3	14.0[a]
5. Alcohol consumption (liters of absolute alcohol per capita)	9.8	6.2	7.6
6. Tobacco consumption (lbs. per year)	4.96[b]		8.33[a]
7. Major causes of death (per 100,000 population)			
a. Ischaemic heart disease	232.1		301.0
b. Malignant neoplasms	151.8		175.8
c. Cerebrovascular disease	103.3		87.9
d. Motor vehicle accidents (15–24 age bracket)	27.2 (58.2)		21.9

a. 1977 figure.
b. 1978 figure.
Sources: Australia: Annual Report of Director General of Health 1978–79.
United States: *Statistical Abstract of the United States 1978.* (U.S. Census Bureau.)

land United States. It is considered the oldest of the land masses and is also the flattest, with a mean elevation of 300 meters (the world mean is 700 meters). The country lies in latitudes of 10°S to 40°S; and it is less subject to extremes of climate than regions of comparable size in other parts of the world because of the moderating effect of the surrounding oceans and the absence of extensive high mountain masses. In January and July, average temperatures vary from 29°C to 24°C in the north, and 18°C to 10°C in the south. Regular winter snowfalls occur only on the highlands and tablelands of the southeast corner of the mainland and Tasmania. Australian soils have been highly leached from their formation in earlier, wetter climatic cycles and are generally low in fertility. However, the use of trace elements and artificial fertilizers has transformed some of these soils into highly productive pastures.

The Population

It is estimated that Australia was first settled some 38,000 years ago by a people now known as the Australian Aboriginal. When European settlement began in 1788 there were thought to be some 300,000 aboriginals living in nomadic families or tribal groups scattered mainly through the better watered country of the coastal fringe, particularly in the south and east. This population had been reduced to 139,800 by June 1978. Half of the population lived on the fringes of towns or in the less well-to-do parts of the cities. By March 1978, there were 14.3 million people in Australia, approximately 20 percent of whom had been born in other countries.

The crude birth rate is approximately 16 babies per 1000 people and is slowly decreasing, as is the population growth rate, which is approximately 1.05 percent. More than 25 percent of the population is under the age of 15 and a further 9 percent of the population is over the age of 65. Eighty-five percent of the population lives in urban centers, the majority in the five major coastal cities: Sydney (three million), Melbourne (three million), Brisbane (one million), Adelaide (one million), and Perth (one million).

The Economy

By any standard, Australia is a wealthy country, and it possesses the resources to ensure continued prosperity. In 1977–78 the gross domestic product per head was $A6,332, of which 10 percent (and declining) came from rural industry, 25 percent from manufacturing, and 65 percent from tertiary industries. Most of the labor force (85 percent) is composed of wage and salary earners who work a 40-hour week over five days and receive between three and four weeks paid annual leave in addition to sick and long-service leave—demonstrating the strength and cohesiveness of the union movement. The seasonally adjusted average weekly earning per employed adult male for the September quarter of 1978 was $A220.40. As in most Western countries, inflation has been a serious problem over recent years even though Australia supplies 70 percent of its own oil requirements. In the three years corresponding to the Whitlam Labor government (1972–75) the consumer price index rose an average of 14.4 percent. In 1978 the rise was 7.7 percent. In December 1978 unemployment was estimated at 6.8 percent of the labor force.

The Nation's Health Indicators

Australia's health indicators are very similar to those of the United States and Canada, as can be seen in table 3.1. The similarity in the causes of death is continued through age-specific breakdowns. The time trend on these data demonstrates a slow increase in longevity, which is reflected in a slow decrease in death rates. It should be remembered that, at best, these data are not the whole health history; intangibles such as the quality of life are very important in the people's view of what it means to be healthy.

The Australian Health Care System

A consideration of the annual expenditure on the various components of the health care system will indicate areas on which this paper should concentrate. Table 3.2 presents a categorization of annual health expenditures for a number of relevant years. Institutional care accounts for approximately one-half of the total health expenditures and by far the majority of these relate to short-term hospitals. Medications represent the next largest cost to the community, followed by medical services and nursing homes.

The basic organization of Institutional Care in Australia is different from the United States' experience. The seven state governments have the major responsibility for the provision of public health services, which include the public hospital system as well as a comprehensive mental health service. Public hospitals account for approximately 75 percent of the short-term hospital beds; the majority of the remaining are in nonprofit private hospitals, usually having a religious affiliation. In marked contrast, more than one-half of the 4.1 nursing home beds per 1000 population are based in profit-oriented institutions.

TABLE 3.2

Current expenditures on health services in Australia: 1966–67 to 1976–77 (in millions of dollars)

	1966–67	1969–70	1972–73	1974–75	1975–76	1976–77
Institutional care						
General hospitals						
Public	334 ⎫	534	771	1421	1866	2529[a]
Private	30 ⎭		95	188	248	294
Mental hospitals	60	80	120	192	233	NA
Nursing homes	62	103	180	311	378	455
Other institutions	21	30	40	78	105	128
Total institutional care	507	748	1206	2190	2830	3407
Other medical care						
Medical services	176	250	400	570	849	1035
Dental and other professional services	85	104	157	205	253	291
Medicaments	241	290	398	562	616	615
Other	48	62	83	192	269	198
Total other medical care	550	706	1038	1529	1987	2139
Public health	46	68	89	130	142	368
Teaching and research	21	NA	40	79	101	13[b]
Total	1124	1522	2373	3928	5060	5927
Percent of gross domestic product	5.0	5.1	5.6	6.5	7.2	7.2

a. Includes mental hospitals

b. Excludes teaching

Sources: 1966–67 to 1975–76: Deeble 1978, tables 1 and 2. Deeble, 1979, table 1.

N.A.: not available

The other major issue that is especially relevant to any longitudinal comparison of mechanisms of finance is the rate of increase of these expenditures. From table 3.2 it can be seen that expenditures have been generally rising out of proportion to the gross domestic product; however, there would appear to have been a quantum leap in the two-year period of 1974 through 1975. Some of this increase, which is not really peculiar to Australia, has been attributed to attainment of wage parity by the predominately female workforce, especially in the short-term hospitals. An even greater proportion can be attributed to the large increase in the number of health professionals which has been promoted since the 1960s, when the increase was seen as a major solution to the problem of maldistribution. In this paper, this increase will only be considered in so far as it could have been an outcome of the method of payment.

Australian Politics and Health

In Australia, the attitude of the early settlers, emancipationists, and colony officials has been described as a determination not to duplicate the "old poor law system" of Britain. Social goals were achieved in the early days by charitable organizations wherein help was given by the more affluent members of society, and directed through formal committees of influential citizens. Mutual aid or "friendly societies," financed by regular contributions from members, began in 1871. Governments quickly became involved in subsidizing benevolent committees, and the degree of subsidization of health and welfare has progressively increased over the years.

Over the last 35 years, social policy with respect to the amount and type of public financing of health care has been politically divisive. The major Australian political parties have markedly different approaches to running the economy. The Liberal-Country party coalition has always favored a laissez-faire system with the government intruding as little as possible. The Labor party has traditionally seen the purpose of a government as involving the setting and achieving of social goals promoted via public expenditure.

Both the federal and state Parliaments are modeled on the "Westminister" system with two houses of Parliament, both of which are elected on a regular basis (three and six years). The party or coalition of parties that has a majority in the lower house becomes the government and provides the ministry (including the prime minister or premier). In addition to the possibility of leading a minority government in the House (a situation which can occur when there are more than two parties, as seen in recent Canadian experience) it is also possible for the government not to control the Senate. If the Senate continually rejects bills from the House, a double dissolution of Parliament results.

Although the Federal Constitution of 1901 limits the power of the federal government in health as well as in other areas, from the time of the constitution the Commonwealth has grown progressively more dominant vis-à-vis the states. In 1927 the Commonwealth took over existing state debts in a power play which put all future borrowing under the jurisdiction of the federal extraparliamentary Loan Council. After the commencement of the Second World War, the Commonwealth legislated (and survived a constitutional challenge) to give Commonwealth income tax priority and to provide each state that ceased to levy income tax a reimbursement grant. The Labor government raised the issue of National Health Insurance in the 1940s and introduced legislation to subsidize health care. When this did not survive a constitutional challenge, the Labor government held a referendum (one of only four which has been successful) which extended the power of the Commonwealth under section 51 of the constitution to make laws

> for . . . the provision of maternity allowances, widows' pension, child endowment, unemployment, pharmaceutical, sickness and hospital benefits, medical and dental services (but not so as to authorize any form of civil conscription) benefits to students and family allowances.

The first National Health Bill was passed in 1948 but was not implemented by the change of government in 1949. The Liberal-Country party coalition repealed this bill and substituted a government-subsidized private indemnity insurance package. By careful exploitation of the political windfall of a split in the Labor party on religion versus communism they were able to remain in government until 1972. Although there were regular minor changes within this package during that time period, the one major change was brought about because the

Liberal coalition did not control the senate in 1967, which set up an enquiry into health insurance. The government, acting quickly to save face, instituted its own investigation, which culminated in the 1969 Nimmo Report. In 1972 the Labor party under Whitlam's leadership attained power for the first time in 23 years. The pent-up force of Labor's social policy program, so long frustrated, burst forth in what has mildly been described as a turbulent governmental period. During this period, Labor did not control the Senate and faced serious and unremitting opposition to many of its social programs, with the health insurance plan as the major focus. During the first twelve months of Labor government the Senate rejected thirteen bills, deferred another ten, and amended twenty others. After continued Senate rejection, the health bills, along with four others, were cited as grounds for a double dissolution of both Houses of Parliament. Labor survived the election, but was still without control of the Senate; it needed an unprecedented joint sitting of both Houses for the legislation to be passed. During 1975 Labor continued to push for rapid changes in public expenditure to promote social policy issues, even though inflation was running at record levels (16 percent) and the unemployment rate had doubled. When a series of scandals involved senior government ministers, the governor-general used his little-known power as queen's representative to remove the government from office. The resulting election was fought on the grounds of economic management, and the Liberal coalition won in a landslide.

This large mandate allowed the Frazer government to take a position strongly opposed to that of its predecessor. Scotton has summarized this position with respect to social policy:

> The general context within which the Frazer government's social policies have been formulated is the broad objective of reducing the size of the public sector and leaving the largest possible portion of total resources in the hands of private individuals, both as producers and consumers. The classical liberal ideology which underlines this position has been reinforced by the priority accorded to the reduction of inflation, for which the orthodox remedy is minimization of budget deficits, achieved primarily through cuts in outlays (Scotton and Ferber 1980, p. 1).

With the economy still the major election issue, Frazer was re-elected in 1978, and this was perceived as a mandate to pursue his federal austerity policies. (In a statement to the nation, Frazer actually admonished the people with "Life wasn't meant to be easy.") In discussing these austerity measures, Scotton (1980) identified that during the Whitlam term the increase in the gross domestic product absorbed by the public sector came entirely from expenditures for social purposes. As the health plan had always been one of the most politically controversial social policies, it was logical that it should be one of the principle targets for cutbacks. In tune with these economic concerns, the Frazer government also promoted a policy which Frazer entitled "new federalism." The policy's overall purpose was to clarify and minimize overlap of the respective powers of the federal and state governments, and this was operationalized by partial or total Commonwealth withdrawal from many of the social welfare and planning programs to which its power had been extended during the Whitlam government.

Since 1975 there have been a number of changes in the health care financing system which are consistent with the increasing implementation of the above two policies. Scotton, who had a major role in the development and implementation of Labor's tax-based universal health scheme, noted that the stagnant state of the economy was not fully realized in 1976 and that consequently the achievement of the above goals impelled the government to even more stringent economies in subsequent budgets (Scotton 1980). Furthermore, this has resulted in two systems of government-funding of health care being implemented since 1975. The first change provided two alternatives: a government tax-based system and a subsidized private indemnity insurance with government competition. The second change introduced what is essentially a tax-based catastrophe insurance. The Frazer government has been in somewhat of an economic dilemma with respect to its health policy, as Scotton has outlined:

> A more serious complication for economic policy has been that the reduction of public outlays on health services directly increased the net prices of health services included in the consumer price index, which is the principle measure of the rate of inflation and hence of the government's success in controlling it (Scotton 1980, p. 176).

Subsidized Indemnity Insurance: 1952–1975

Following the 1949 elections, the Liberal-Country party coalition decided against implementing the National Health Insurance plans that had been legislated in 1948. The compromise plan that they proposed attempted to ensure a wide-cover national health scheme which did not alter the private nature of professional behavior. Equity, both in terms of access and payment, was envisaged as following naturally from adherence to the professional ethic (with a certain amount of the "Robin Hood Principle") as was the issue of the overall cost of medical services. The four parts of this health plan were:

1. The Pharmaceutical Benefits scheme enacted in 1950
2. The Pensioner Medical Service enacted in 1951
3. The Hospital Benefits Act of 1952
4. The Medical Benefits Act of 1953

The Pharmaceutical Benefits scheme heavily subsidized medications, provided that they were contained in a government list and were prescribed by a medical practitioner. The Pensioner Medical Service scheme provided free general medical service for pensioners (subject to a means test) and their families, with participating doctors paid at a concessional rate.[1]

The Hospital and Medical Benefits Acts, although formerly separate, were organized in the same manner. The patient was charged by the hospital[2] or the medical practitioner for the service; if insured, the patient could then submit the relevant claim to his or her voluntary (nonprofit) health insurance fund, which then distributed both the fund benefit and the Commonwealth benefit in a single payment and sought subsequent reimbursement. In 1963, nursing home benefits were separated from the voluntary hospital insurance scheme and all patients in nursing homes became eligible for a daily payment equal to the Commonwealth insured hospital benefit, whether they were insured or not.

The relative merits of this scheme were put under scrutiny by the House of Representatives' Committee on Enquiry into Health Insurance, which tabled its report (the Nimmo Report) in 1969. This report documented seven major problems with the scheme and put forward 42 recommendations to improve it. Among the problems were:

1. The operation of the health scheme was unnecessarily complex and beyond the comprehension of many
2. The benefits were frequently much less than the cost of medical and hospital treatment
3. Contributions had increased to such an extent that they were beyond the capacity of some to pay
4. The rules of many of the registered insurance organizations permitted disallowance or reduction of claims for particular conditions,[3] the application of which caused widespread hardship
5. Nonenrollment of underprivileged groups

The major change introduced in 1970 was the development of a most-common-fee schedule with a differential benefit for specialists compared to general practitioners. On the basis of the common fee, Commonwealth and fund benefits were set so that the patient would pay directly $A.80 for a normal consultation. For more costly services, a maximum patient-direct contribution was set at $A5.00. The crux of this system was the most common fee; but the medical fraternity did not see such a concept as fitting in with their philosophy, and their compliance was not high.

The government also allowed the private insurance funds to segregate contributors to whom they could have applied maximum benefit exclusions (such as pre-existing or chronic illness) into special accounts, the operating deficit of which was subsidized by the federal government. The amount of this subsidy grew rapidly, partly reflecting increases in hospital costs and rising levels of insurance coverage, and partly reflecting the rigor with which the funds applied their own rules on eligibility.

Table 3.3 addresses the question of who paid for the medical and hospital benefits throughout the duration of this type of health insurance. A clear effect of the implementation of some of the recommendations of the Nimmo Committee can be seen in the jump in the percentage of Commonwealth to total benefits after 1969. The lack of any indexing of the Commonwealth benefits resulted in the progressive reduction of the percentage in other years.

TABLE 3.3

Voluntary health insurance scheme: contributions, benefits,
and coverage of hospital and medical costs, 1953-54 to
1974-75 (in millions of Australian dollars)

| | Contributions | | Benefits | | | Percentage of |
	Total	Est. tax relief[a]	Fund[b]	Common-wealth[c]	Total	Commonwealth to total benefits
1953-54	19.5	NA	8.4	19.5	27.9	70.0
1963-64	93.3	19	75.1	47.2	122.3	38.6
1966-67	144.1	33	113.2	67.4	180.6	37.3
1969-70	205.3	54	169.2	94.9	264.1	35.9
1972-73	315.7	100	291.3	283.3	529.6	45.0
1973-74	381.1	115	310.4	249.2	559.6	44.5
1974-75	567.2	171	469.2	308.4	777.6	39.7

a. Estimated income tax saved by taxpayers claiming deductions for contributions to funds, at marginal rates of taxation.

b. Including ancillary benefits, but net of federal government reimbursement of special account deficits and subsidized health benefits.

c. Insured benefits, including special account and subsidized health benefits plan payments.

NA: not available

Source: Scotton 1978, p. 110.

The Pharmaceutical Benefits scheme demonstrated a similar progressive reduction in the proportion of costs met by the government (see table 3.4). The original purpose of this scheme had been to provide a limited range of life saving and serious-disease-preventing drugs free to those who needed them. The government negotiated the prices of drugs included in the formulary directly with manufacturers and paid 33.3 percent mark-up reimbursement as well as a dispensing fee to pharmacists. It should be pointed out that the index presented in column 5 of table 3.4 is not a price index, but a combination of changes in price as well as composition of drugs. Discounting for this change in composition, it appears obvious that the monopsonistic purchasing power of the federal government has kept prices of most drugs below that of their North American counterparts. Over the years there was general cooperation of the medical and pharmaceutical professions with this scheme so that equity considerations were not really an issue.

TABLE 3.4

Pharmaceutical benefits scheme: expenditures, prices, and
volume of prescriptions, 1963–64 to 1975–76

	Total expenditures[a]		Average price per prescription		Average number of prescriptions per head of population
	Total ($m)	Percentage met by gov.	Amount ($)	Index (1963–64 = 100)	
1963–64	82.6	81.1	1.86	100	4.02
1966–67	104.3	82.4	1.94	104	4.59
1969–70	136.2	83.9	2.08	112	5.29
1972–73	194.2	74.9	2.64	142	5.71
1973–74	233.9	74.8	2.65	142	6.60
1974–75	278.8	76.0	2.78	149	7.25
1975–76	351.6	72.9	3.23	174	7.43
1976–77	338.0	69.5	—	—	—
1977–78	361.2	70.9	—	—	—
1978–79	391.1	69.4	4.16	224	—

a. Total cost (including patient contribution) of benefit prescriptions (i.e., excludes cost of drugs supplied through public hospitals).
Sources: Scotton 1978, p. 123, and Annual Reports of Director General of Health.

The Nimmo Committee mentioned that the hospital and medical insurance plans were guilty of nonenrollment of underprivileged and high risk groups in the population. Removing this bias is a major social goal in the provision of health insurance; and the relevant question is: What is the extent of the problem? As hospital insurance is liable to have the greater financial benefit to the consumer, it can be assumed that figures for those who were hospitalized (see table 3.5) will be an underestimate of those who were insured against hospital and medical costs. The percentage of uninsured people who were admitted to hospitals over these years (1967–71) progressively decreased from 15.6 to 12.1 percent. If these individuals represented the independently wealthy, one would expect the distribution of place of hospitalization to be skewed toward the private hospitals. Since this is not the case, the conclusion that has to be drawn is that the subsidized indemnity scheme was not meeting one of its major social goals: equality of access.

TABLE 3.5

Number and percentage distribution of days of
hospitalization—type of federal benefit entitlement—public
and private hospitals—1967–68 to 1970–71

Year ended June 30	Number of days hospitalization (thousands)			Percentage distribution		
	Public	Private[a]	Total	Public	Private[a]	Total
1968[b]						
Insured	7,287	2,753	10,040	47.0	90.2	54.1
Uninsured	2,683	213	2,896	17.3	7.0	15.6
Pensioner	4,734	—	4,734	30.5	—	25.5
Nonqualified	799	86	885	5.2	2.8	4.8
Total	15,504	3,053	18,557	100.0	100.0	100.0
1969[b]						
Insured	7,618	2,805	10,423	47.9	89.6	54.8
Uninsured	2,572	237	2,809	16.2	7.6	14.8
Pensioner	4,881	—	4,881	30.7	—	25.7
Nonqualified	823	89	912	5.2	2.8	4.8
Total	15,895	3,131	19,026	100.0	100.0	100.0
1970						
Insured	8,003	2,851	10,854	49.3	89.8	55.9
Uninsured	2,441	235	2,676	15.0	7.4	13.8
Pensioner	4,804	—	4,804	29.6	—	24.7
Tuberculosis	101	—	101	0.6	—	0.5
Nonqualified	900	87	987	5.5	2.7	5.1
Total	16,249	3,173	19,422	100.0	100.0	100.0
1971						
Insured	8,700	2,971	11,671	53.0	90.6	59.2
Uninsured	2,181	199	2,380	13.3	6.1	12.1
Pensioner	4,643	—	4,643	28.3	—	23.6
Tuberculosis	73	—	73	0.4	—	0.4
Nonqualified	825	109	934	5.0	3.3	4.7
Total	16,422	3,279	19,701	100.0	100.0	100.0

a. Pensioner Medical Service entitlement is not available in private hospitals.
b. Excludes tuberculosis patients.
Source: Annual Report of Director of General Health, 1972–73.

Medibank: A Universal Income Tax Based Health Scheme

Between 1973 and 1975, the Labor government implemented four expansionist strategies aimed at overcoming the problems related to the effective provision of comprehensive health care. These were:

1. A tax-financed national health insurance program known as Medibank. This ensured access to a basic level of hospital care for everybody, without charge, together with high levels of coverage against all medical expenses, no matter whether they were incurred in or out of the hospital.
2. A hospital development program funded out of general revenue. This was aimed at correcting the maldistribution of facilities, upgrading or replacing dilapidated stock, and achieving stated guidelines for the supply and organization of hospital services.
3. A community health plan to establish out-of-hospital services and improve the coordination of health services in the community and their links with other health and welfare services.
4. A health services research and development program.

The Hospital Development and Community Health Programs were designed to overcome maldistribution of health care facilities and services. The Community Health Program had as its main objective the improvement of "community health services to those living in areas where there is a significant unmet health service need" ("Review of the Community Health Program" AGPS 1976). It aimed at quickening the evolution of comprehensive multidisciplinary teams for primary care and provided subsidies of 75 percent of capital expenses and 90 percent of operating expenses. Both of these programs were expansionist in nature and were funded out of general revenue.

The health insurance scheme was designed to fit within the fee-for-service philosophy of the medical fraternity. It created a single health insurance fund, Medibank, which was administered by a statutory Health Insurance Commission. When this occurred in July 1975, the large number of private insurance funds were reduced to providing gap insurance.[4] The scheme covered 85 percent of the standard fee for any given medical service, on the proviso that the maximum difference between benefit and scheduled fee should not exceed $A5 for any service. As in Canada, doctors could bill the government in bulk on a regular basis as long as they were prepared to accept the benefit as full payment. Doctors, however, still had the option of charging the patient, who would then be expected to pay the extra moiety.

With respect to hospitalization, Medibank benefits entitled a patient to free treatment (by staff doctors) in standard wards of public hospitals. In addition, if an individual wished to be treated as a private patient (including the choice of his or her own doctor), there was a uniform $A16 per day subsidy to the hospital to enable a reduction of the fee. Benefits in the public hospitals were provided through agreements with state governments under which the federal government met 50 percent of the net operating costs (with no upper limit).[5]

By its very nature, Medibank increased health insurance coverage from 87.9 percent of the population in 1974–75 to 100 percent in 1975–76. As it was based on a progressive income tax, the health insurance also fulfilled the social goal of the more wealthy subsidizing the less wealthy. That leaves the question of cost, which was addressed in retrospect by Scotton, one of the codesigners of Medibank, in the following way:

> The introduction of a universal insurance program inevitably has a sizeable impact on total health costs and public outlays. Any extension of insurance raises provider incomes by reducing the incidence of bad debts and concessional fees, while the removal of financial barriers to low income patients must be expected to generate additional demand. Furthermore, the politics of changing established systems always requires that new arrangements be made more acceptable by generosity to the prospective participants. Medibank involved the incorporation of the pensioner medical service into the program at considerably enhanced benefit rates, while the hospital agreements were such as to produce considerable net savings to state governments at a time when hospital costs were growing explosively.... As part of its opposition to Medibank, the AMA pressed its fee claims during 1974 and 1975 with a singular aggressiveness. Fee inquiries established by the government awarded increases in scheduled fees for 1975–76 which were 34 percent above those of 1974–75 and 64 percent above those of 1973–74. The fees actually charged almost certainly rose more steeply still, as AMA-recommended fees anticipated and outstripped rises in scheduled fees (Scotton and Feber 1978, p. 112–13).

Legislative exploitation of the weak position of the Labor government compounded the above expansionary factors. The original design of Medibank proposed funding the program through a 1.35 percent levy on taxable incomes; however, the Labor government could not get the Senate to pass the necessary legislation. The program was consequently funded out of general revenue, thus representing an effective savings to an individual of his or her previous cost of health insurance. Such politicking helped guarantee government problems in the managing of the economy.

As the Medibank program was only in operation for a maximum of ten months, it is not possible to make definitive statements about the overall effect on utilization of doctors' services. Some expansion was an explicit objective of the program, and a sample contract survey of general practitioners in Sydney indicated an increase of 11 percent in total contacts (Richardson 1977). A more drastic change was reported in benefits paid for pathology services: an increase of over 100 percent in the year 1975–76 (*AMA Gazette*, February 3, 1977).

In the political infighting that preceded the introduction of Medibank, it was predicted that the program would especially affect public hospitals and would result in a soaring demand for casualty and outpatient services, extensive waiting lists, and a general lowering of standards as a result of an inability of facilities to cope. These predictions prompted the Australian Hospital Association and its Victorian counterpart to survey the impact of Medibank on Victorian Public Hospitals. The conclusions of the survey were:

> Increases in casualty/outpatient attendances are well within established growth patterns; waiting lists have increased by less than 10 percent; until the change in eligibility for standard admission in October 1976, the proportion of standard to private patients remained substantially the same as had been the case with public patients; by and large, hospitals are happy with receipts/ payment accounting; and although the use of overdraft financing is increasing, at 30/6/77 it was only of minor proportions ("Has Medibank Affected Public Hospitals?" 1979, p. 6).

Although there would not appear to be a change in utilization, there did appear to be a change in total costs. Scotton commented on this:

> While it is probable that the infusion of federal grants led to some

slackening in financial controls, it also appears that the reported costs of public hospitals were artificially inflated by the inclusion of previously omitted terms. The open-ended cost-sharing formula in the hospital agreements certainly offered the incentive to do this (Scotton 1978, p. 113).

With respect to the other major cost areas mentioned earlier, the government continued the Pharmaceutical Benefits scheme in essentially the same form but legislated major changes relating to nursing home benefits. Controls on admission, fees, and the number of new nursing home beds were implemented in response to the way fees had been escalating in previous years[6] (see table 3.6) as well as in response to the fact that nursing homes (56 percent profit-oriented in 1972) tended to raise their fees and to absorb increases in benefits intended to reduce the patient's out-of-pocket costs. The government's response was aimed at reducing reliance on profit-oriented providers, and the basis of federal support was changed to funding the operational deficit of nonprofit nursing homes. As a result, state- and deficit-funded homes could charge standard fees whereas the private homes often charged much higher fees. Scotton sums up the coverage of these benefits:

> In late 1976 it was estimated that the percentage of patients in each state covered by the "standard fee"—that is receiving the target level of coverage—ranged from 44 percent in New South Wales and 57 percent in Victoria to 92 percent in Tasmania (Scotton 1976, p. 122).

Reintroduction of a Major Role for Private Insurers: 1976–78

The change of government in 1975 soon led to changes in the manner of government funding of health services. A two-tiered system was developed wherein private insurance became a progressively more attractive scheme as the level of income rose. In the months that preceded the introduction of this scheme, public debate was heated particularly with respect to the size of the income tax levy that was to be introduced.[7] The rate chosen (2.5 percent) maximized the inducement for the majority of people to take up alternative insurance. The government also empowered Medibank to offer private insurance coverage, and the public was faced with a confusing array of options both within

TABLE 3.6

Nursing home benefits, 1963–64 to 1975–76 (years end June 30)

	1963–64	1972–73	1973–74	1974–75	1975–76
Number of beds (June 30)	28,685	53,416	54,420	54,756	55,578
Federal government payments (in millions of $)					
Ordinary benefit	17.9	60.2	61.2	60.6	51.3
Supplementary benefits	—	24.3	24.9	25.2	21.9
Pensioner additional benefits	—	8.5[a]	26.0	64.2	68.3
Deficit funding	—	—	—	10.1[a]	51.9
Special account deficit payments	—	—	0.7	1.5	2.3
Total federal government	17.9	93.0	112.7	161.5	195.6
Private insurance benefits[b]	—	1.1[a]	4.6	9.8	12.6
Total nursing home benefits	17.9	94.0	117.3	171.4	208.2
Average daily benefit per bed[c]	$1.80	$4.92	$5.96	$8.60	$10.31

a. New benefits payable as from January 1.
b. Net of special account deficit payments.
c. Total benefits per day divided by the mean of start-of-year and end-of-year approved bed numbers.

Source: Scotton 1978, p. 120.

Medibank as well as from the private firms. As a result, in October 1970, *Choice*, the journal of the Australian Consumers' Association, reviewed the insurance options (presented in figures 3.1, 3.2, and 3.3) to help people make the decision. The scheme was such that 35 percent of the population was expected to stay with basic Medibank and to pay (or not pay, in the case of very low incomes) the 2.5 percent levy up to a ceiling. A further 20 percent of the population was expected to opt for the levy plus hospital-only, shared-room insurance from one of the private funds. The remaining 45 percent of Australians were expected to take out full private insurance.

Government regulations of private insurance funds differed markedly in this period from pre–Medibank arrangements. As earlier, non-profit organizations were allowed to participate; however, the former federal subsidies to the private insurers were not completely reintroduced on the principle that the premiums for people choosing private insurance should cover the full costs incurred. The government made two exceptions to this principle: the introduction of a subsidy considered sufficient to keep the annual cost of supplementary hospital-only insurance close to a specified government target and the creation of a reinsurance pool, which took over the function of the earlier subsidization of special accounts deficits. The ground that a fund could transfer a contributor to this reinsurance pool was hospitalization in excess of 35 days. The government commitment to this fund had an upper limit ($A50 million) and the only liabilities that could be transferred were those from the basic table. The deficit over and above the government subsidy was paid by the insurance companies in proportion to their hospital fund membership.

With respect to the government funding of hospitals: through a legal technicality the Frazer government was able to declare all the federal-state Medibank hospital agreements invalid. From this position of power, they were able to specify that only approved net operating costs would be subsidized.

Scotton has summarized the impact of this renegotiated position:

> The federal government's right to participate in prospective budgeting on a hospital-by-hospital basis contrasted radically with its previous impotence in hospital control. The extent of its power was demonstrated in the August 1977 budget when it unilaterally—and without prior notice—cut its allocation to the

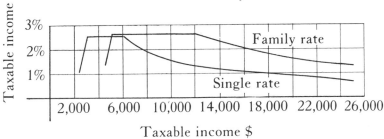

FIGURE 3.1

Medibank levy

Source: *Choice* October 1976, p. 332.

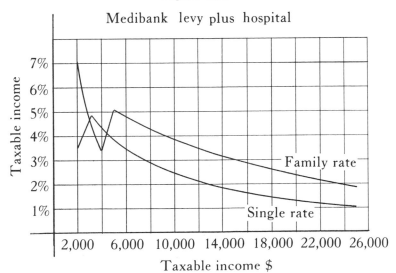

Figure 3.2

Medibank levy plus hospital

Source: *Choice* October 1976, p. 332.

Figure 3.3

Medibank private: medical and hospital package

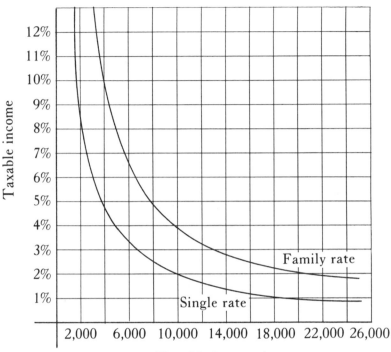

Taxable income $

Source: *Choice* October 1976, p. 332.
Editor's note: The data in Figures 3.1, 3.2, and 3.3 have been outdated by changes to the Health Insurance Act of Australia.

states by 5 percent from the amounts arrived at in federal-state officer's meetings the previous May (Scotton 1980, p. 185).

In addition to this effect, the government subsidy per occupied day was cancelled for public hospitals (but not for private hospitals), and pathology and radiology services were to be charged to patients insured for hospitalization.

In July 1976 the government appointed a committee on Care of the Aged and Infirm to report particularly on the nursing home situation. A year later the major recommendations of this committee were implemented. First of all, the amount of benefit was substantially increased by between 45 and 77 percent, depending on the state as well as the type of benefit. In addition, legislation was introduced to oblige hospital insurers to meet the full amount of benefits for all their contributors, and it was expected that these contributors would be registered with the reinsurance fund. These arrangements did not consist of an incentive for nursing home patients to become insured, for if uninsured they received the same benefits from the levy scheme. There was a built-in incentive to insurance companies, however, as the patients did not need to be transferred to the reinsurance fund; and a loophole in the legislation allowed funds the possibility of keeping the contributions and paying no benefits. This led to some active solicitation of both nursing home proprietors and patients by some of the funds. This unwelcome social practice was only short-lived because of the boomerang effect relating to the higher risk of hospitalization for the aged.

This manner of funding health care maintained the concept of universal coverage while giving a definite role to private industry. The introduction of Medibank Private, however, successfully broke up what had previously been a cartel. All the major funds used their reserves in order to undercut the government contribution rates. Once initial rates had been established, government approval was required for them to be increased. The outcome was that all the major funds incurred deficits until they were allowed to substantially increase their rates. (Permission was not given until after the government had been re-elected in 1978.) The media were highly critical of this manner of funding health care, mainly on the grounds of complexity. The *Sydney Morning Herald* summed up the general feeling on September 29, 1976: "Its complexity replaces the simplicity of Medibank Mark 1 and that alone is a step backward not forward. It has caused massive confusion." The increased complexity, as well as the development of duplicate systems, also led to substantially increased administrative costs.

The large increases in fund contribution rates decreased the incentive to withdraw from Medibank, and the government commissioned a paper on possible arrangements for health care funding in the Australian setting. As a result "A Discussion Paper on Paying for Health Care" was tabled in Parliament on March 15, 1978. In its most explicit though unsubstantiated conclusion, this paper put forward three reasons why patients should pay a larger direct share of health care costs:

- To retard rates of expansion in the use of medical and hospital services.
- To reduce the rate of growth of government expenditures on health services.
- To reduce the rate of growth in health insurance contribution rates (p. 102).

A Front-End Deductible Catastrophe Insurance

In May 1978, the government moved toward introducing a front-end deductible catastrophe insurance. This was introduced in two phases, which were widely perceived by critics to be designed to reduce organized public opposition. Although there is some reason to doubt that such a strategy was consciously planned, the fact that the second set of changes was announced only six months after the implementation of the first set is reason enough not to concentrate on the intermediate stage.

In keeping with the conclusions of the discussion paper "A Discussion Paper on Paying for Health Care," the government was determined to increase the out-of-pocket payment by the patient. The Department of Health (August 1979) had reported that approximately 85 percent of all claims were for services under $A20; and as of September 1, 1979 the government announced that it would pay all expenses above that figure for any item of service for all persons (up to the limit of the scheduled fee). The patient would pay the first $A20, unless he or she was a pensioner or disadvantaged person. Doctors were allowed to continue bulk billing for these exceptions, and their reimbursement was 85 percent of scheduled fees for those who qualified for the pensioner medical scheme (and their dependents) and 75 percent for those whom the doctor was prepared to classify as socially disadvantaged persons. At the same time, hospital fees for shared accommodation and private accommodation were substantially increased; but for insured patients, free standard ward care was still provided. The government also announced that a cost inquiry would be established to investigate hospital efficiency and administration.

The result of these changes was that the Labor party and consumer advocates began recommending that individuals should not insure. The September 1979 issue of *Choice* magazine provided a series of scenarios for people to compare the benefits of insurance or noninsurance. One of these (scenarios) is presented in table 3.7. A health insurance survey was conducted by the Australian Bureau of Statistics in March 1979, and it recorded that 30 percent of the population had taken the Labor party's advice and opted out of insurance altogether. As expected, the younger and healthier people were the ones to make the decision not to insure.

The implications of these changes for the funds are serious, particularly as their reserves had been whittled down by the previous scheme and the medical funds had reported an operating deficit of $175 million for the financial year 1977–78. The funds reacted to this problem by introducing a variety of packages aimed at attracting some of the healthier members of the population. However, the effect of these new packages has increased the complexity of the whole health insurance business and seems to have resulted in more and more people opting out. It is quite possible that the main reason that this has not resulted in a mass exodus is that the fund distributes the Commonwealth benefit with its own single payment, and as many Australians "gave up trying to understand the whole mess long ago" this payment may be seen as coming only from the fund. Of course, the funds have a vested interest in keeping this obscure.

A particularly unwelcome social effect of this latter scheme relates to the socially disadvantaged person status. As this decision is up to the individual doctor, and he, in turn, is financially penalized for making it, considerable hardship is likely to result before such a decision is made. The "Robin Hood Principle" has surfaced again, with all its disrespect for the pride of the individual.

The Future of Health Insurance in Australia

In Australia, as in America, 1980 is an election year, which means the possibility of a change in government.[8] What would happen should the Labor party be elected to office? The Labor party platform has not changed in its commitment to a universal health scheme financed by a levy on personal income tax. However, Labor is demonstrating that it has learned some lessons since its last time in office and has planned

TABLE 3.7

Scenario 3: Ten general practitioner consultations and illness requiring major surgery (e.g., breast cancer[c]), in Australian dollars

	N.S.W.[d] schedule fees ($)	Uninsured ($)	Your costs[a] if you are:	
			Insured for 75% medical and basic hospital ($)	Insured for 100% medical and basic hospital ($)
10 General practitioner consultations @ $10.19	101.90	101.90	25.48	—
1 General practitioner consultation	10.19	10.19	2.55	—
1 Specialist consultation	29.04	Free treatment and	7.26	—
1 X-ray	23.25	accommodation	5.81	—
5 Attendances for radiotherapy	83.03	in a public hospital	20.76	—
2 Full blood counts	7.23		1.81	—
1 Blood grouping	13.10		3.28	—
Biochemical analysis	19.87		4.97	—
Operation (specialist)	312.76		10.00	—
Assistance at operation	62.55		10.00	—
Anaesthetic	99.41		10.00	—
Histopathology	65.48		10.00	—
17.5 days accommodation, public hospital, shared ward, @ $50 per day	Accommodation cost 875.00		—	—

Approximate annual insurance costs (N.S.W.)[b]			
Family	—	551.20	634.40
Single	—	275.60	317.20
Total annual outlay			
Family	112.09	663.12	634.40
Single	112.09	387.52	317.20

a. Your costs will be higher if your doctor charges over-schedule fees.

b. Based on estimates that 75% medical plus basic hospital coverage will cost in the vicinity of $10.60, family rate ($5.30 single) and that 100% medical plus basic hospital coverage may cost around $12.20 weekly, family rate ($6.10).

c. Patients being treated for breast cancer should not take this list of services as an accurate guide. More or different services might be required. A modified list would not alter the fundamentals of the cost comparison.

d. N.S.W.: New South Wales—a major state in Australia.

Source: *Choice* September 1979, p. 264.

for a phased reintroduction of Medibank. The first phase of that plan has been ennunciated by the Leader of the Opposition, Mr. Bill Hayden:

> The first step in the restoration of a universal health scheme under the next Labor Government will give full medical coverage to all children under sixteen, to dependent students, and to expectant mothers . . . .
>
> People not covered directly by the scheme will continue to have their medical costs above $A20 met by the government . . . .
>
> Finally, under our plan, doctors will be reimbursed 85 percent of schedule fees for all eligible patients, eliminating the present differential rate for socially disadvantaged patients. This will create greater equity in the arrangements and encourage doctors to make more use of the provision for the socially disadvantaged (Hayden 1979, p. 2).

What would happen if the Liberals were re-elected? A trend analysis of the last four years would suggest another change in the manner of insurance within 1980. There is no conviction among the Australian public that the present system is the optimal one. Increasing disapproval is being voiced by many sections of the media, and this has reached such a level that leading writers in a number of daily papers in various cities have advocated a return to something like Medibank. A commonly held media view is that the government "has to decide whether to go on adding patches to a system which is rapidly self-destructing."

Conclusion

Having briefly reviewed the Australian experiments in government funding of health care, it is timely to ask what these have to offer to your consideration of whether to introduce national health insurance, and what aspects of any such scheme should be emphasized. Although there have been many changes in the Australian system of national health insurance, these have been made in an evolutionary manner. The question that needs addressing is, What is a politically acceptable social policy with respect to health care in Australia?

To begin with, Australian health care is firmly based on the private entrepreneurial fee-for-service system. Just as firmly, it is based on large-scale government intervention in the area of funding across all levels of health care, but with a particularly strong role with respect to institutional care. This role is feasible when the government controls these institutions or when the institutions are nonprofit organizations, but the role becomes more complicated when the government is a third-party payer to profit-oriented institutions, as was demonstrated with nursing homes.

That universality is an essential part of the Australian health care system was demonstrated in September 1979, when the Minister for Health suggested that Commonwealth subsidies might be made contingent on an individual being insured with a private fund. This created a huge public outcry, and the suggestion was quickly dropped. It would also seem that the most politically acceptable way for the government to fund such a universal health scheme is from a levy on income tax.

It is also apparent that any such government funding of health care will have to come to terms with the issue of the escalating costs of health care. Within a fee-for-service system, one major concern is who sets the fee schedule; and the government needs to be concerned with what controls can be put on this system so that fee increases are kept within the range of the consumer price increases. In Australia, this issue is extremely sensitive, as fee setting has been seen as the exclusive right of the medical profession. This profession is highly conservative and consistently opposes any innovations in social policy or in the manner that it is implemented.

But the escalating costs of health care are more the result of increasing technology and the rapidly increasing number of health professionals. The issue with respect to technology relates specifically to which technology is able to make a satisfactory diagnosis, and this has been a major focus of inquiries into pathology services in Australia for the last five years. What is not being properly recognized by the Australian government is that the number of health professionals has a major impact on the cost of health care (Pierce 1978), especially when fee setting is carried out on a target-income basis. In Australia, the number of new health professionals has been increasing substantially each year, and it would appear that the government is still working on the invalid assumption that increasing the number of professionals will solve the maldistribution problems. This issue may very well surface as a result of the Hospital Cost Inquiry that is presently underway.

When eventually confronted, this issue will be politically sensitive because of the inherent conflict between health and education goals.

The present debate about National Health Insurance in Australia revolves around whether primary care should be a completely insured service or not, and on whether there is any role for private insurance companies in future developments. This conference is addressing these very same issues, and I trust that I have demonstrated for you that Australia is a good social laboratory to which you can look for evidence to aid decision making.

Chapter 3 Notes

1. This is a very different system from the way the Commonwealth provided for those whose need for medical attention could be attributed to a war. In 1919 the Commonwealth Repatriation Department was set up to provide comprehensive care for the latter group. The Pensioner Medical Service was only to cover services of a general practitioner and did not extend to consultant specialists. The "Robin Hood Principle" can be seen in the fact that doctors were expected to be satisfied with less than the scheduled fee-for-service.

2. The costs of hospitalization to the patient were artificially low throughout this period and reflected the Commonwealth government subsidy per occupied-bed-day as well as state government social policy.

3. Disallowance categories included venereal disease, alcoholism, self-inflicted wounds, and drug addiction.

4. Gap insurance covered the difference in price between private care (more luxurious accommodation and treatment in a hospital by a doctor of choice) and standard benefits. To maintain an incentive to patients to hold private medical insurance, the funds offered a package which covered dental and other ancillary service benefits.

5. Although the Planning Committee had recommended an open-ended 50/50 sharing of net operating costs for a two year interim period, the states bargained for and got a ten-year term.

6. Control of admission was legislated as the domain of public medical officers. Conflict with the medical profession, however, led to compromises, and this aspect of the legislation was never implemented.

7. Labor had originally proposed a 1.35 percent levy in 1972. The Australian Council of Trade Unions proposed a 1.6 percent levy and Scotton proposed that the levy should be 2 percent.

8. *Editor's note:* This paper was written and delivered at the conference prior to the 1980 election.

Chapter 3 References

Commonwealth Department of Health. August 1979. "A Brief Guide to the 1979 Health Benefits Changes."

Annual Reports of the Director General of Health. Various years. AGPS.

Annual Reports of Health Insurance Commission. 1974–1978.

"Australia in Brief." Australian Government Publishing Service, 1979.

Australian Bureau of Statistics. 1979. "Health Insurance Survey, March 1979."

Australian Department of Health. 1979. "Details of Successful Prosecution of Doctors."

Australian Hospital Association, Victorian Branch. 1979. "Has Medibank Affected Public Hospitals?—A report of a survey to assess the impact of Medibank upon Victorian Public Hospitals." Mimeographed.

Australian Newspapers: 1969–79 various issues. The *Advertiser*, the *Age*, the *Australian*, the *Canberra Times*, the *Examiner*, the *National Times*, the *Sydney Morning Herald*, the *West Australian*.

Beard, T. C. Senior Medical Officer of Community Health, Commonwealth Department of Health. Personal communication. 1979–80.

Choice, Journal of Australian Consumers Association. October 1976, September 1979, and November 1979.

Constance, M. 1977. "Unravelling the Health Tangle." *National Times*, October 17–22, 1977.

Deeble, J. S. 1967. "The Costs and Sources of Finance of Australian Health Services." *Economic Record* 43: 518–543.

Deeble, J. S. 1979. Australian Health Expenditures: An Overview. Unpublished paper presented to a symposium of the South Australian Postgraduate Medical Education Society in Adelaid in July 1977.

Deeble, J. S., and Scotton, R. B. 1977. "Health Services and the Medical Profession." In K. A. Tucker, ed. *Economics of the Australian Service Sector*. London: Croom Helm.

Deeble, J. S. 1978. "Health Expenditures in Australia 1960–61 to 1975–76." Health Research Project, Report no. 1. Australian National University, Canberra.

Dewdney, J. C. 1972. *Australian Health Services*. Toronto: Wiley and Sons.

Donnison, D. 1976. "An Approach to Social Policy." Supplement to *Australian Journal of Social Issues* 11, February 1976.

Doust, K. Medical Director of Medibank. 1979. Personal interview.

Hatfield, D. 1979. "Health Insurance Policy Changes 1974–1980." Honors thesis. Macquarie University.

Hayden, Bill. 1979. "Labour's Family Health Care Plan." Press statement by the leader of the opposition, November 27, 1979.

Hospital and Health Services Commission. 1978. A discussion paper on paying for health care, AGPS, Canberra.

Kilmester, G. 1979. "The Rise and Fall of Medibank—A short history of health care funding in Australia." pp. 27–28. Panacea.

National Health & Medical Research Council. 1978. "Getting a Doctor: Access to Primary Health Care in Australia." Discussion paper. October 1978.

Pierce, J. P. 1974. "An Introduction to the Australian Health Care Delivery System for Health Care Researchers." Mimeographed. Department of Clinical Epidemiology & Biostatistics, McMaster University.

Pierce, J. P. 1978. "A Rationale and Methodologies for Health Manpower Studies." Commissioned for Hospitals and Health Services Commission. Canberra: AGSP.

Richardson, J., and Philips, T. 1977. "Report of a Survey of Sydney Medical Practitioners Before and After Medibank." Research Paper 139. Sydney: Macquarie University, March 1977.

Sax, S. 1972. *Medical Care in the Melting Pot.* Sydney: Angus & Robertson.

Sax, S., "Impact of Federal Health Insurance and Health Resource Allocation Policies in Australia 1975–1979." Presented at American Public Health Association Annual Meeting, November 4–8, 1979.

Scotton, R. B. 1974. *Medical Care in Australia—An Economic Diagnosis.* Melbourne: Sun Books.

Scotton, R. B. 1977. "Medibank 1976." *Australian Economic Review* 1st Quarter.

Scotton, R. B. 1978. "Health Services and the Public Sector." In Scotton, R. B., & Ferber, H. *Public Expenditures and Social Policy in Australia* 1. Melbourne: Longman Cheshire.

Scotton, R. B. 1978a. "Costs and Use of Medical Services." *Australian Economics Review* 2nd Quarter.

Scotton, R. B. 1980. "Health Insurance: Medibank and After." In Scotton, R. B., & Ferber, H. *Public Expenditure and Social Policy in Australia* 2. Melbourne: Longman Cheshire.

Southby, R., and Chesterman, E. 1979. *Australia: Health Facts, 1979.* School of Public Health and Tropical Medicine, University of Sydney.

Discussants' Comments on Section I

Rita Ricardo-Campbell

Stuart O. Schweitzer

Michael Zubkoff

Rita Ricardo-Campbell

I am going to devote most of my remarks to Matt Lindsay's paper because I did not fully agree with it. Matt Lindsay's paper presents a "model of bureaucratic government supply in which the implied behavior of these institutions (that is, government hospitals) differs from that predicted for similar private institutions." That governments and private institutions act differently has been documented elsewhere. The paper is drawn in some measure from chapter 4 of *National Health Issues: The British Experience*, authored by Cotton M. Lindsay with Bernard Feigenbaum, Steven Honda, Kenneth Tamor and Robert Williams (LaRoche Laboratories, 1980).

Lindsay documents that a lower quality of care is provided under the British National Health Service (NHS) than under the United States' multiple (government and private) systems. The British National Health Service's low payments to British physicians have resulted in subsequent physician emigration. Lindsay's proof that in recent years British physicians are underpaid relative to earnings by manual workers assumes that physicians have inherent capabilities

that are 20 percent higher, on the average, than manual workers' capabilities. Returns on educational investment, which is substantial in
terms of foregone earnings, are calculated here by estimating the present value of foregone earnings, using a lower discount rate the
greater the number of years spent in gaining an education. Ignored is
the substantial economic literature in the United States about returns
on professional education, to which Lindsay has contributed.

The emigration data on British physicians support the facts that
British-educated and British-born physicians have been moving out of
the United Kingdom, leaving foreign-trained and foreign-born physicians to take over an increasing share of general practice, especially in
the rural areas. Emigration and the much lower medical examination
scores by foreign physicians imply a declining quality of care. A large
part of medical care is information, and language barriers do not promote ease of communication. That care under the British NHS is of
lower quality than in the United States is also supported by Lindsay by
noting that the average total personnel per hospital bed is greater in
the United States than in the United Kingdom. The ratio in the
United States is also greater than in West Germany. I am not sure that
this latter fact, however, proves a differential in quality of care between the United States and West Germany.

A third Lindsay indicator of lower quality care in the United Kingdom is a comparison of per capita capital expenditures on hospitals
under the NHS in the United Kingdom (1951 through 1971) with
U.S. per capita expenditures for all hospitals (1951 through 1975).
The data are corrected for inflation. Lindsay's table 1.8 and figure 1.4
give data for the United Kingdom through December 1971 and for the
United States for 1975. Obviously the gap in the dollar amounts between the NHS and the United States is far less in 1971, the last comparative year, than in the first comparative year (1951). However, the
rate of growth over the twenty-year period of per capita investment in
the United Kingdom averaged 27 cents per year compared to only 4
cents per year in the United States. Lindsay's data for the United
Kingdom ended in 1971. The comparative plot for both countries
should end in 1971, and then the rates of increase would be more
easily ascertainable, even to a casual viewer, than when later data for
only the United States are included. Compare my chart (figure 4.1) to
Lindsay's figure 1.4. However, even if we include 1973-1975 U.S.

FIGURE 4.1
U.S. and NHS capital expenditures per capita

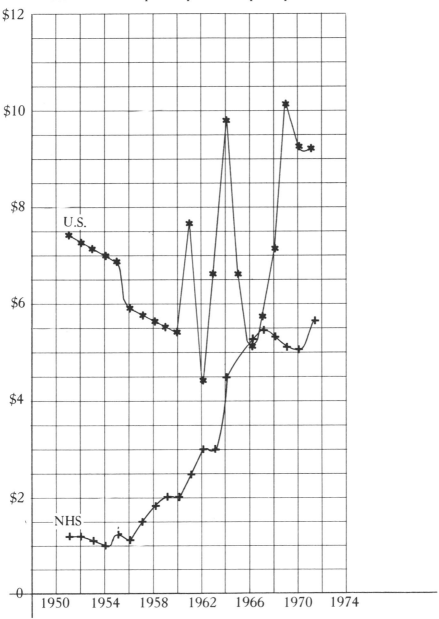

data, the average annual rate of increase in the United States (20 cents) is still less than the average (1951–1971) in the United Kingdom. The recent high rate of hospital growth in the United States (table 1.8 of Lindsay's paper) cannot be assumed for the future because of the volatile nature of the U.S. expenditures and the probable effect of the 1974 federal certificate-of-need law. This requires area or state approval prior to building new hospitals or expanding old ones as a precondition for obtaining Medicare and Medicaid reimbursement for patients using the new facilities.

The United Kingdom's hospital expenditures per capita are obviously lower under their governmental system than hospital expenditures are in the mixed government and private system of the United States. However, the United Kingdom's gross national product (GNP) per capita was, and is, also lower than in the United States. What I do not know from the data is whether British investments in hospitals would have been any higher if the hospitals had not been nationalized. One suspects that they might have been, but one doesn't know that from the data.

Opportunities for capital investment for private hospitals exist in the United Kingdom. I am surprised that there are no data included on these, especially in view of the recent publicity given to the Manor House Hospital supported by the Electricians' Union and wealthy foreigners.

To analyze only supply factors as indicators of quality, without any consideration of the demand side and especially of the well-known long waits for appointments in physician offices for surgeries or hospital beds in the United Kingdom, is disturbing. The book from which this paper draws discusses this waiting in detail under three broad groups:

1. Type 1 diseases are those with fast decay rates, for which there are substitute, out-of-hospital modes of treatment.
2. Type 2 category of diseases are those for which there are few or no substitute out-of-hospital modes of treatment, and thus individuals are willing to wait longer for treatment. These individuals have chronic diseases that are usually not curable, but the resulting pain and disability might prevent them from working, and their symptoms usually would be relieved by in-hospital care.

3. Type 3 ailments are "emergency" conditions, and it is assumed that individuals in these circumstances will have a very short waiting time.

Although these three classifications are interesting, some of the inclusions are puzzling; for example, multiple sclerosis and hypertensive diseases are placed in the emergency classification.

In 1974 persons with appendicitis, which I assume is an emergency condition, had a median waiting time for a hospital bed in the United Kingdom of 7.5 weeks; cataract cases, which both Lindsay and I would agree are not emergencies, had a waiting time of 15 weeks. Cataracts, however, do interfere with one's working ability and enjoyment of life, and a relatively long waiting period (the median wait for all cases in the United Kingdom in 1974 was 7.2 weeks) does indicate that in the United Kingdom, less attention is paid to persons suffering from nonfatal diseases. This type of poor-quality care does not show up in the mortality rates, whereas waits for hospital care of a disease that definitely affects the mortality rate, for example, cancer (median wait of 2.2 weeks for a hospital bed), do. However, a frequency distribution by selected diseases indicates that some persons with terminal disease had relatively long waits. In 1974 7.5 percent of persons with cancer waited three months or more for a bed. Queuing for hospital beds is probably inflated, however, because many individuals will queue far ahead of their need.

Recently, Ake Blomqvist published in his book, *The Health Care Business* (Vancouver, B.C.: Fraser Institute, 1979), a table indicating that "low mortality diseases . . . account for 35.5 percent of all (hospital) episodes in Canada but only for 25.6 percent of those in the United Kingdom" (p. 122). Blomqvist concludes that the data are consistent with the U.K. system being less effective in treatment of disease associated with temporary disability and pain. The Blomqvist method of computing ratios of hospital episodes per death by selected disease categories in both the United Kingdom and Canada appears to be a measurement of quality overlooked in Mr. Lindsay's paper.

The U.K. system, being a centralized system of health care, is more affected by strikes than the multiple systems in the United States. The 1975 and 1979 strikes in the health care sector in the United Kingdom were disastrous for the quality of health care in that country.

The United Kingdom and Australia illustrate how politics, rather than medical need, dominate allocation decisions. New hospitals in the United Kingdom tend to be located where there are more votes. In Australia, the size of co-payments depends on which political party is in power.

In West Germany, the early development of national health insurance under Bismarck has evolved in negotiations among government, unions, employers, providers, and private insurers of third-party payments into coverage for almost all costs of medical care under a fee-for-service system. West Germany has no co-payments and Reinhardt apparently supports this policy. Reinhardt quotes M. L. Barer, et al.: "cost sharing, coupled with third-party coverage, is believed by physicians to draw more fiscal nourishment to the physician sector than could otherwise be had from third-party payers under universal first-dollar coverage." In contrast, the ten-month-old (as of March 1980) 20 Australian dollars (26 American dollars), co-payment was imposed by politicians who believe in a co-payment's effectiveness to restrain demand. Both West Germany and Australia have a fee-for-service system of payment which, when coupled with nearly 100 percent third-party payments, means rising prices. It appears plausible that two pocketbooks, the government's and the consumer's, can be called upon to pay a larger total amount than either would separately. This does not negate the restraining effect of a co-payment on utilization. In the United States, health maintenance organizations (HMOs) are increasingly imposing such restraints. In Palo Alto, California, Take-Care has a $4 charge for each physician visit; Kaiser-Permanente has a $1 charge for its lower benefit package and a $2 charge for its higher benefit package, while Bay Pacific has a $3 co-payment fee, and a Palo Alto Medical Clinic plan had, until late 1980, a 25 percent cost-corridor. This plan has been replaced by TakeCare. Do co-payments restrain demand or only yield some direct revenues to the provider of the services? Where systems such as West Germany's do not have co-payments, these revenues are foregone.

Although Reinhardt refers to the *Wall Street Journal* (December 19, 1979) column by Jonathan Spivak, he does not quote from it. It is clear that the 1977 West German controls worked for about two years—about the same length of time that the U.S. Phase II price controls (November 1971–April 1974) worked. In both instances, when voluntary acceptance by physicians decreased, their break-out of procedures and charges for new individual items more than made up for revenue losses due to the lid on prices. The standing joke of the Health Services Industry Committee of Phase II was that the next time you go into a physician's office, he will charge you for a handshake because it is a diagnostic tool. Today in the United States some physicians are beginning to charge substantial amounts for telephone calls. The prices for individual items can remain constant, but costs will rise. In West Germany, hospitals are exempt from the controls, and their costs are rising rapidly.

Reinhardt states that resource allocation is primarily either through the market system or by government rules. To this, I would add two other forms of allocation: time-price (or waiting) and occupational status, as in the United Kingdom and the Soviet Union, respectively. In addition, bribery in various forms exists in countries where there are only government-paid physicians.

Among the interesting points made in the paper on West Germany is that civil servants are not under the otherwise all-pervasive government health insurance, but have private insurance and private physicians. To me, this is reminiscent of social security in the United States. It also raises the question of whether there are two levels of care easily identifiable, at least by the civil servants, in West Germany. Note Reinhardt's statement that it is "not uncommon for physicians to divide their day into practice hours for statutorily insured and privately insured patients and to attempt different practice styles for the two types of patients." One wonders if in the United States, physicians discriminate similarly between Medicaid, Medicare, and other patients and, further, if fee-for-service physicians discriminate between their patients who belong to different fee-for-service HMOs and their other private patients. In many areas of this country—Boston, Massachusetts and Palo Alto, California, for example—physicians have patients whose financial arrangements differ. If physicians know which HMO or insurer pays a patient's bills—and because referral practices often differ in accordance with third-party arrangements, this is probably true—then they may practice price discrimination and/or waiting-time discrimination. In addition, their modes of practice, especially with respect to tests, X rays, and referrals, may differ in accordance with reimbursement rules. This is, however, another area of research.

May I end on a note of some optimism? I believe, along with the authors of both the Australian and West German papers, that consumers could participate more sensibly in allocative decisions. The Australian articles in *Choice* did, according to John Pierce, affect the choice of insurer. It is partly through this channel that a closer approach to competitive markets might be reached in the United States.

Stuart O. Schweitzer

One of the more depressing aspects of studying the foreign experience with respect to health care, especially with regard to questions of cost, is the similarity in experiences of countries with vastly different types of structures and processes for delivering care. Conferences that bring representatives of foreign countries together invariably bring together similar experiences. No country has been visibly successful in restraining the costs of health care while at the same time satisfying its population that access to care and quality of care are adequate. This paper will not present a cure-all for this common malady, but will rather attempt a diagnosis of the problem with reference to the Australian, West German, and British experiences. If this diagnosis is successful, lessons for the United States will be indicated.

A major policy issue in comparative analyses of health systems is assumption of responsibility over the health sector—that is, determining what level of government is responsible for the health system, or whether that responsibility should rest with government at all. What makes the matter more complex is that "health services" is not a single function but has three identifiable components: financing, regulation, and delivery.

The three national systems described by Lindsay, Reinhardt, and Pierce assign responsibilities for these functions differently among national and subnational governmental units and between the public and private sectors. This marks a rather substantial departure from traditional economic thought. Only in the past few years have economists been concerned with the question of responsibility for a particular role in an economic system. There has always been an underlying assumption that relevant economic relationships, such as economies of scale and economic efficiency, are independent of the organizational structure. Whether a program is administered by the federal or the local government, or by the private sector, would not matter if one assumed the same objective function and relevant market information.

The Australian scene is an ideal example of a social experiment gone awry, with the Australians having made a number of dramatic changes in policy, but in so doing losing any means of evaluating their actions. One only wishes for an instant replay capacity to review what has gone on in Australia. What has occurred is a shifting of roles between the private and the public sectors, especially with regard to financing and, to a lesser extent, regulation. Of particular interest is the most recent shift, starting in 1976, when the government's Medibank was substantially denationalized, with increased reliance placed on payroll tax increases to fund optional insurance. Though options were introduced, perhaps the array of choices was so confusing that the role of competition among them really was not effectively increased by denationalization. It would be useful to analyze some of the Australian data to see which people shifted from one plan to another, what kind of users they were during the Medibank period, and what kind of users they were subsequent to denationalization.

Another Australian experience which could be of potential interest for policy analysts in the United States is the attempt to create catastrophic insurance. Again, the experience is not as relevant as it might have been, for the amount of cost-sharing is only $A20 per service. Thus the Australian system represents a co-payment plan more than a catastrophic deductible plan, according to the American idiom.

The West German experience illustrates an interesting model for the United States because of German reliance on the private sector for financing and regulation as well as for production of care. The federal role in Germany is relatively small, limited to arbitration in negotiations over fees between the insurers and the providers. In addition, a program is being developed to involve the federal government in financing hospital construction, which is also a current proposal in the United States.

The Health Resources Administration of the Department of Health and Human Services (DHHS) is now looking very closely at ways of regulating health facility construction, and given the confusing types of incentives, it is not unreasonable to propose that the government simply take over the funding of health facility capital, either directly at the federal level or at the local level, such as through the Health Systems Agencies (HSAs).

The West German experience permits us to consider again the role of competition among insurers, but the information presented to us is not clear. West Germany has 1,500 sick funds, which have an enormous diversity in premiums because they set rates according to the experience rating of their particular employee group. There is no effective competition because there is no effective mobility of the subscribers between one plan and another. The subscribers are assigned plans on the basis of their location, employment, or profession. The variation in premiums described by Reinhardt has little to do with competition among plans because of the inability of most German workers to actually opt for one plan or another: diversity is certainly not synonymous with competition. It would be useful to explore the degree of competition which does exist among white-collar workers who are free to choose between the statutory fund and the optional private insurance plan. The Reinhardt paper suggests that an approximately equal number of enrollees have opted for each of those plans. As with the Australian experience, one would like to examine the characteristics of those who chose each of the insurance alternatives.

A strong element of the West German program of cost containment is negotiation over physician fees. Though this process appears to be successful, these fees do not in themselves determine expenditures. Quantity of services as well must be controlled in some way. Rather than deal directly with the problem of utilization as a determinant of expenditures, the new expenditure ceiling program is an attempt to reverse the causal ordering. The ceilings were instituted only in 1977, so the results are not yet clear. This approach to expenditure control has also been adopted in Great Britain with striking results. One can avoid the more difficult questions of utilization review in only one sense: if this type of control is not explicitly incorporated into policy it enters, nonetheless, implicitly, as those organizations that are responsible for implementing the expenditure ceilings search for mechanisms for doing so. The actual regulations and programs are therefore more likely to be decentralized and less visible; but of course that does not mean that the actions do not take place.

Projections of physician supply in West Germany illustrate the need to address the quantity and utilization issues frontally, as supply is expected to increase at a staggering 100 percent in each decade up to the year 2000. There is little doubt that demand generation on the part of physicians will increase pressures on utilization of services enormously.

The Lindsay thesis concerning the British health system rests largely upon his theory of public enterprise, in which public agencies are hypothesized to engage in those types of production that are most consistent with the more visible indicators of success. According to this hypothesis, British general practitioners would be less inclined to produce the kind of caring services which are thought to be an essential component of primary care because there is no statistical procedure for ensuring that such output will be rewarded in any way. The evidence presented, however, does not seem to substantiate this assertion, and several authors have, in fact, pointed out that the evidence is just the reverse—that it is the United States system, with its fragmented form of primary-care organization between general practitioners, specialists, and hospital ambulatory clinics, that is particularly incapable of delivering continuous emotionally-supportive care. The short physician visits which are observed in Great Britain do not necessarily imply that care is in any way inadequate but might rather indicate that high-quality care can be more productively generated in a setting that is characterized by a high degree of continuity. Patients in both the United States and Great Britain have ample freedom of choice, in that patients are free to leave one physician and receive care from another in both countries.

Lindsay asserts that wage differentials are important determinants of physician mobility, especially emigration. Another cause of this, however, is the restricted opportunity for professional advancement in Great Britain, caused by the relatively small and static health sector. The length of stay in British hospitals as compared to that in the United States is another example Lindsay uses to attempt to verify his theory of public enterprise. But again, other hypotheses are equally plausible. It is obvious that there are differences in the relative factor costs across hospitals and differences between hospitals and substituting institutions and programs. This being the case, it is entirely possible that the British choose a different technique of production, relying upon a different factor-mix relative to that prevailing in the United States. Hospital stays in Great Britain may reflect management philosophy less than they reflect cost-minimizing production. The far higher cost of American hospitals, for example, might be expected to lead to shorter hospital stays in the United States than is evident in Great Britain.

There are several lessons which one can learn from the three experiences noted. The first is that if the government seeks to play a monopsonistic role in the market for health services (as in Australia), it will not function in a cost-effective manner if the administration is weak. In addition, if the program is open-ended, eligibility alone determining the patterns and cost of utilization, the government or the insurer must play an active role as regulator, or else expenditures will be essentially open-ended and uncontrollable.

If the government does not wish to play an active market role, an alternative is reliance upon competition by consumers to "regulate" the market. As numerous critics have pointed out, consumers are not likely to be well enough equipped to permit meaningful competition among individual providers. A version of competition that is feasible, however, is competition between insurers. It is more reasonable for the insurers themselves to compete for the subscriber and to deal with providers in terms of negotiating fees and charges, utilization review, and so forth. The examples we have seen of competition among insurers in Australia and West Germany are, unfortunately, not instructive for us in this regard, either because mobility among plans is lacking or information concerning subscriber characteristics is not available.

The second important lesson to be learned from the experience we have seen is that control over utilization is at least as important as control over fees, and is likely to be far more difficult if the supply of practitioners is growing rapidly. Expenditure ceilings may be effective in restricting total expenditures, but they do not solve the more important question of how health services are to be allocated among patients: the macro approach only drives the allocation process into a more decentralized form. Regulation is an alternative policy to competition, but it is terribly difficult to implement in a manner that will address both the questions of equity and efficiency.

Michael Zubkoff[1]

I would like to expand briefly upon a few things that have been said and some things that were unsaid, yet implied. Specifically, I would like to further explore with you the physician's role as related to the puzzling problem of large differences in per capita use of common surgical procedures in various settings throughout the world, particularly among populations that appear quite similar in need for and access to medical services. I would like to present briefly some evidence that suggests that variations in the amount, type, and cost of medical care relate primarily to the characteristics of the suppliers of medical care, and that the pattern of use of specific surgical procedures, when coupled with the knowledge that many medical innovations have not generally been subject to rigorous evaluation, strongly suggests to me that a major reason for differences in rates of use of medical services across communities is disagreement among physicians concerning the value of many common practices in the field of medicine. The implications of this professional uncertainty of resource use and future public policy are immense.

In considering this topic, it is not possible to avoid the controversy concerning the nature and extent of supplier influence on the demand (utilization) for medical services (Fuchs 1978). In applying the principles of supply, demand, and consumer sovereignty to health care markets, some economists feel that one foundation of consumer sovereignty, the assumption of rational consumer choice, is in jeopardy. In the case of spending decisions, it is customary to assume that: (1) consumers know what they want; (2) consumers know the effectiveness of various goods and services in attaining what they want; (3) consumers know the price at which goods or services can be obtained; and (4) each consumer uses this information to maximize his or her total satisfaction. However, it is argued that these assumptions cannot be met because, in the information-poor market for health services, consumers face considerable uncertainty in defining wants (and needs). Further, they cannot discern the value of various procedures and services in meeting needs nor can they weigh issues of utility in the usual fashion; thus they cannot buy at the lowest price. In this peculiar market, the seller (the physician) is also the agent for the buyer: he or she defines needs, evaluates therapy and prices, and, as is generally the situation in providing any professional advice, makes vicarious utility judgments for the patient. In medicine these utilities are very largely determined by the physician, in contrast to the active role the client plays in most other areas, from architecture to law. Arrow (1963) emphasizes in particular the rational nature of the delegation of the decision making to the physician who recognizes health needs and understands the value of alternative therapies. However, under these circumstances, by controlling information, the physician in his agency role is in a position to manipulate demand. To control self-serving behavior, non-market factors such as professional ethics, peer attitudes, and government regulations play a role throughout the world in trying to optimize welfare. It is thus argued that it is reasonable for government to require the medical profession to establish standards which reflect the consensus of the profession on the best way of treating patients. These guidelines, the assumption goes, will serve to weed out deviant, inefficient professional behavior (Evans 1974; Evans and Wolfson 1968; Fuchs 1978; Reinhardt 1978).

The viewpoint that suppliers can influence demand is not universal. Sloan, for example, counters this argument by asserting that standard theory does not require that everyone have perfect information, only that a "sufficient number of marginal consumers [be] able to assess output and willing to seek it out at its lowest price" (Sloan and Feldman 1978). To make the point, they quote Pauly: "I know even less about the works of a movie camera than I know about my own organs; yet I feel fairly confident in purchasing a camera for a given price as long as I know that there are at least a few experts in the market who are keeping the sellers reasonably honest" (Pauly 1974). The rationality of the delegated decision as formulated by Arrow, or the opportunity to find experts who confide rational advice under Pauly's strategy, depends on the possibilities for substantial rationality among physicians in their decision making as clinicians. In a market characterized by delegated decision making, whether through seller-agents or the independent expert-agents, the assumptions for rational agent behavior are analogous to the requisites for rational consumer choice in the classical market situation. For physicians, the ideal principles for rational agency choice may be summarized as follows:

1. Physicians know as part of generally developed and shared professional knowledge the effectiveness of various goods and services with regard to their impact on health status for various human conditions.
2. Physicians know (diagnose) what particular consumers (as their patients) want (need) and in the individual situations allocate technology and care based on knowledge about outcome probabilities.
3. Physicians use the information to maximize a patient's utility.
4. Physicians can identify the least costly methods for providing care and purchase care for their patients at the most efficient price.

It is my assertion today that the assumptions of rational agency behavior (as well as those of consumer sovereignty) are not sufficiently correct to serve as a useful basis for public regulation, at least in the current environment. Both sides of the controversy have misunderstood important aspects of the nature of physician behavior in the clinical setting by underestimating the market implications of physician (as opposed to consumer) uncertainty in diagnosing disease and prescribing appropriate treatment. The uncertainty stems in part from problems in classifying a particular patient so that the probabilities of the existence of disease, extent of disease, and value of treatment are reasonably ascertained. Uncertainty also stems from the more fundamental fact that adequate information on the probabilities for treatment outcomes under controlled circumstances commonly does not exist. Finally, uncertainty exists even when patients are appropriately classified and outcome probabilities are known; the utility of the physician who makes the vicarious decisions may not correspond to the patient's utility (McNeil, Weichselbaum, and Pauker 1978). Thus the problem of "demand shift" (at least the demand for specific procedures such as prostatectomies and tonsillectomies, when viewed as per capita rate variations among communities) is more accurately understood when it is characterized as a problem illustrating the impact on consumption rates of different belief sets as held by individual physicians than when it is put forth as an example of self-serving professional response to economic incentives. To put the problem back in Pauly's terms of reference, the complexity of human biology and human decision making in the clinical setting is such that, on net, information on the workings and repair needs of cameras is more thorough and reliable than is information on the workings of human organs and their appropriate repair.

The General Problem of Variation in Demand

As evidenced in the papers presented by Lindsay, Pierce, and Reinhardt, people throughout the world are interested in the fact that the use of medical services and expenditures varies significantly among apparently comparable populations living in neighboring communities. The phenomenon predates the widespread availability of health insurance in the United States or of national health insurance in the United Kingdom. The classic description of small-area variations is Glover's pre–World War II study of tonsillectomy among British school children, who displayed tenfold differences in per capita rates between different school districts (Glover 1938). These variations in demand persisted long after national health insurance removed any possible economic motives for tonsillectomy (Glover 1959). In more recent years, extensive variations for total surgery and for specific procedures have been documented between nations (Bunker 1970), for neighboring communities within the United States (Wennberg and Gittelsohn 1973; Wennberg and Gittelsohn 1975; Detmer and Tyson 1978; and Griffith 1978), for Canadian provinces (Vayda and Anderson 1968; Roos, Roos, and Henteleff 1977; Stockwell and Vayda 1979), for geographically separated but apparently homogeneous members of insurance plans (Lewis 1969), and for enrollees in prepaid group practices (Luft 1978). While the rates are generally lower in the United Kingdom and Norway than in North America, the range of variation within the United Kingdom and Norway appears to be of the same order of magnitude as seen among areas in the United States (McPherson, Wennberg, and Hovind 1980). See figure 4.2.

Variations in demand for surgery may occur because of four sets of factors that are intrinsic to the populations or to the suppliers of health care (Gittelsohn and Wennberg 1977). For a population, the probability of surgery of a particular type (S_K) for a particular disease (h) can be expressed as a function of the conditional probabilities of four not necessarily independent factors:

P_{hi} Probability of disease h in individual i

q_{ij} Probability individual i seeks care from physician j

$r_{jk(h)}$ Probability physician j uses condition label k for disease h

$s_{jk(h)}$ Probability physician j recommends surgery for condition k(h)

The probability S_K for a particular procedure in the population may be represented as the sum over all disease states h, of individuals i (who are members of the population) and physicians j (who are contacted by one or more members of the population):

$$S_K = \Sigma_h \, \Sigma_i \, \Sigma_j \, p_{hi} \, q_{ij} \, r_{jk(h)} \, s_{jk(h)}$$

Further, the overall rate of surgery in an area (S_t) is a function of the

FIGURE 4.2

Rates for prostatectomy (P) and inguinal hernia (H) among
subareas in Norway, the United Kingdom, and New England

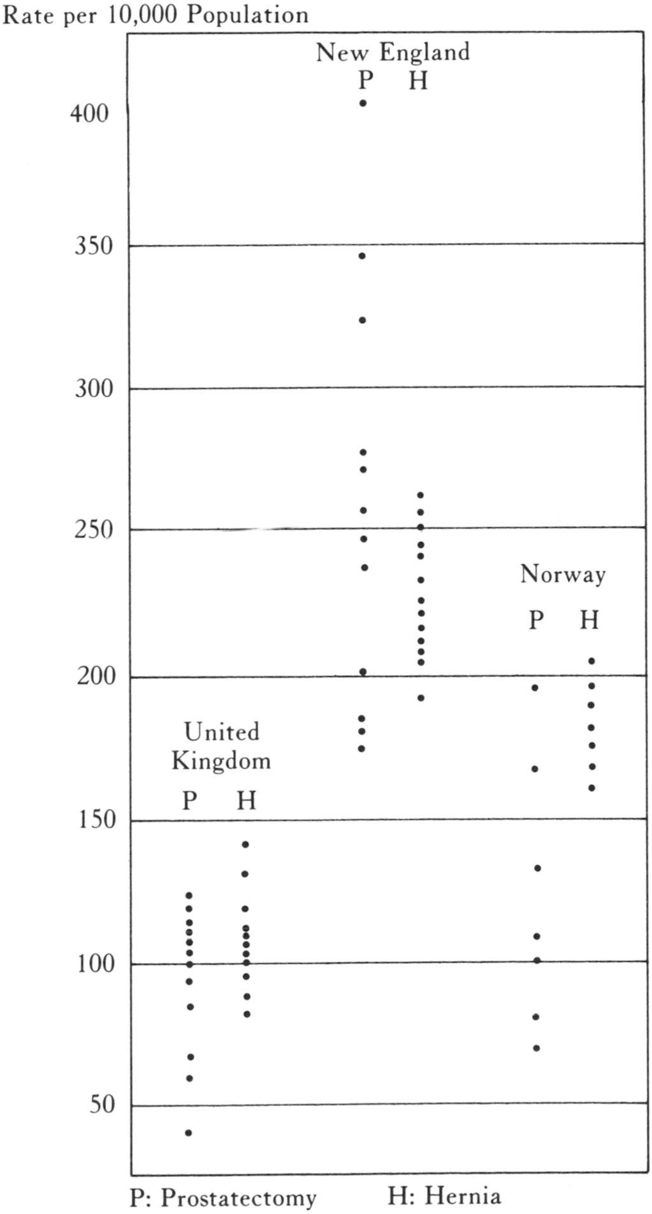

Rate per 10,000 Population

P: Prostatectomy   H: Hernia

individual probabilities associated with each of the constituent procedures that are part of current surgical practices:

$$S_t = \sum_1^n S_{K_1} + S_{K_2} + S_{K_3} + \ldots + S_{K_n}$$

This model summarizes both biological and social factors which determine total surgical utilization S_t and individual procedure use rates for
defined populations S_K. When the incidence of illness among populations is similar, when the members of the population contact (and
comply with) their physicians in similar proportions, and when the
physicians make similar diagnostic and therapeutic decisions, then the
utilization rates among the populations will be similar. When they are
not similar, the differences can be explained by differences among patients, physicians, or both. Given specific examples of variation in utilization, the problem is to evaluate the strength of the contribution of
each party.

Small-area analysis, a technique which isolates neighboring populations on the basis of patterns of use of services, provides an exceptional
opportunity for evaluating variations in utilization. In a typical small-
area analysis (Wennberg and Gittelsohn 1973), the smallest demographic units (such as zip codes or minor civil divisions) are assigned
to hospital areas, based on the place of hospitalization for the plurality
of hospital admissions from the demographic unit. The resultant populations, which usually range in size from 10,000 to 100,000 persons,
are sufficiently large to obtain statistically stable procedure rates, particularly for common procedures. However, the numbers of physicians
whose work loads contribute substantially to each area's rate are usually small. Consequently, the physician contribution to the area rate
for a particular procedure is determined by the decision of a small sample of physicians regarding the indications for the procedure.[2] When
communities with similar populations (in the sense of the probability
of illness and behavior in seeking care) are compared, the patterns of
variation of specific procedures will reflect the range of physician
choices concerning the labeling of illness and beliefs concerning the
effectiveness of specific treatments for improving health status.[3]

A further advantage of the small-area technique is that the means
for defining populations, which is based on patient flow patterns from
minor civil division to place of hospital, does not strongly bias the population selection process on the basis of illness. The process of popula-

tion definition can be viewed as a pseudorandomization based on geographic proximity to place of service. (The predominant reason for selecting a place of service, at least in the suburban, small town and rural settings, is proximity.) At least for common medical conditions as they occur in most demographic units, no overriding illness-related bias should affect people's decisions on place of residence. Perhaps the most important point is that the factors which are surrogates for illness rates (such as age, race, or ethnic composition) can be controlled for. Further, consumer contributions to demand can be directly tested by household interview techniques. Both techniques have been used to assess consumer contributions to utilization in Northern New England.

Consumer contributions to variations in demand are dependent on the disease incidence in populations and on the behavior of individuals in making choices to seek and consume care (given that a particular disease has occurred or is thought to have occurred). Direct evidence that consumer factors can be essentially constant across small population areas with striking difference in utilization rates has been obtained for selected communities in Vermont (Wennberg and Fowler 1977). Approximately 300 households were surveyed in each of six hospital service areas selected for study because of differences in size and in rate of consumption of health services. The range in utilization was nearly twofold for surgery rates and for expenditures for hospital care. The household survey could detect few differences among the populations in the distribution of consumer attributes that are usually thought to predict the use of health services (see tables 4.1 and 4.2). The differences detected could not rationally explain the differences in utilization. No differences were seen in the distribution among areas of such important predictors as the proportion of consumers with health insurance (cross-classified by type of insurance coverage), reported episodes of acute and chronic illness, poverty level, or availability of physician care. Furthermore, residents of the surveyed areas contacted their physicians in approximately equal proportions (75 percent) each year. The results indicate that these populations, while differing with regard to exposure to medical services and rates of utilization, were essentially similar in age-specific illness rates and behavior of consumers in seeking care.

In most small-area analyses, where such detailed population infor-

TABLE 4.1

Characteristics of populations living in six sampled hospital service areas

	Area I	Area II	Area III	Area IV	Area V	Area VI	Statistical comparison among areas
Socio-demographic characteristics of adults:							
Percent with one or more years of college	35	35	31	21	26	33	.05
Percent white	98	99	99	99	97	98	NS
Percent raised on farm	31	33	35	34	50	42	.001[b]
Percent Vermont- or New Hampshire-born	66	60	68	64	61	59	.05[b]
Percent living in area more than 20 years	47	49	47	57	47	47	NS
Household economic characteristics:							
Percent below poverty level	21	19	20	21	23	20	NS
Percent with health insurance[a]	83	84	83	82	84	84	NS
Percent of insurance policies Blue Cross	51	54	47	47	54	50	NS
Households with regular place of physician care	98	99	98	98	99	97	NS
Illness level:							
Percent with any restricted days in last 2 weeks for chronic condition	5	5	6	7	4	5	NS
Percent with chronic condition	26	28	29	28	23	23	.05[b]
Percent with more than 2 weeks of bed days in last year	6	6	5	7	5	4	NS

a. Excluding Medicare and Medicaid.
b. Linear trend component of chi-square statistic related to rank on expenditures and utilization of hospitals not significant.
NS: Not significant.

TABLE 4.2

Resident access to physicians and health screening services in six sampled hospital service areas

Health Service	Area I	Area II	Area III	Area IV	Area V	Area VI	Statistical comparison among areas
Percent of population with physician contact within year preceding interview	77.3	76.1	74.2	70.9	73.4	72.6	.001[b]
Percent of population with episode of illness contacting physician within 2 weeks of interview	29.3	29.3	34.1	34.4	26.1	30.2	NS
Percent of females 18 years or older receiving one or more Papanicolou tests[a] within year preceding interview	59.5	52.2	56.5	49.8	54.8	63.2	NS

a. Within one year of interview.
b. Linear trend component of chi-square significant P < .001 for hospital utilization: nonsignificant for Medicare Part B expenditures.
NS: Not significant.

mation is not available, the impact of illness rates on variations in utilization rates can be evaluated by correlating the population age-structure with utilization rates. Since age is by far the most important predictor of incidence of illness, age-structure differences among populations would be expected to bear a strong positive relation to health care utilization if variations in illness rates were a substantial reason for variations in utilization rates. Among small-area studies in Northern New England, age structure has not been generally useful in explaining variations in utilization. Indeed, the effect of age is sometimes inversely related to expenditures. For example, among thirteen Vermont areas the percent of population 65 years of age and older is negatively correlated with reimbursements under the Medicare program (Wennberg and Gittelsohn 1973).

Physician contribution to variation in demand is suggested by several studies which show that the varying composition and overall cost of health services depend upon the number, specialty, type, and other characteristics of physicians providing care. Feldstein (1977) has shown an inverse correlation between numbers of general practitioners and use of hospitals; Bunker's studies (1970) show that the difference in rate of surgery between the United Kingdom and the United States is associated positively with a difference in per capita numbers of surgeons. A similar relationship has been shown by Vayda for Canadian provinces (Vayda and Anderson 1968), by Lewis (1969) for counties in Kansas, and by Fuchs for U.S. census area (Fuchs and Newhouse 1978). The SOSSUS studies show a similar relationship (American College of Surgeons and American Surgical Association 1976).

Wennberg and Gittelsohn (1973) show that demographically similar populations living in Vermont hospital service areas that are served more by general practitioners who do not do surgery (who perform solely as family physicians) have lower per capita costs for hospitalizations and fewer surgical admissions than populations in areas served by general practitioners who perform surgery. Furthermore, areas served by general practitioners who do not do surgery have lower expenditures for diagnostic services. Areas with more internists incur greater costs for hospitalizations and receive more diagnostic tests; areas with more surgeons receive more surgery.

The correlations between physicians' supply and expenditure and service rates derive, of course, from differences in work loads under-taken by the individual physicians who make up the different spe-cialties. When these workloads are considered in terms of their specific components (the actual procedures performed) the heterogeneity of population use rates for most, but not all, services suggest that the strategy for allocation depends more on professional preferences than on patient needs or utilities. This phenomenon can be illustrated by examining the patterns of use of common surgical procedures.

Supplier-Induced Utilization
Exemplified by Surgical Practices

Case studies comparing rates in specific hospital service area popula-tions suggest that decision rules differ substantially among surgeons with regard to indications for most operations. Figure 4.3 illustrates one such study. The figure gives data for the five most populous hospi-tal service areas in Maine. The expected number is the age-adjusted number of cases that would occur in each area if the state's average rate applied. The rate at which specific procedures are performed within an area varies markedly and, to a large degree, independently of the rates of all procedures. For example, while area II and area III have the same total operation rate, area II exceeds in hysterectomies (56 percent more than the state average), and area III exceeds in vari-cose veins (89 percent more than the state average). By contrast, in area III the hysterectomy rate is well below the state average and approximately one-third the rate in area II. In each of the five areas a different procedure is performed most often; in four of the five areas, the least performed procedure is different. The number of surgeons and their specialty distribution do not vary to the same degree as the population-based rates for these operations. Also, hospital beds per cap-ita do not vary in a pattern to account for the variation in rates. Con-sequently, physician and resource supply are a less likely explanation than differences in opinions of physicians about the proper indications for surgery.

The phenomena illustrated in figure 4.3 tend to persist from year to year, and it is possible to identify epidemiological "signatures" for the medical care consumed by a community. Figure 4.4 illustrates such a signature for procedures in area I. The relationships remain nearly constant from year to year. For example, in 1973 prostatectomies in

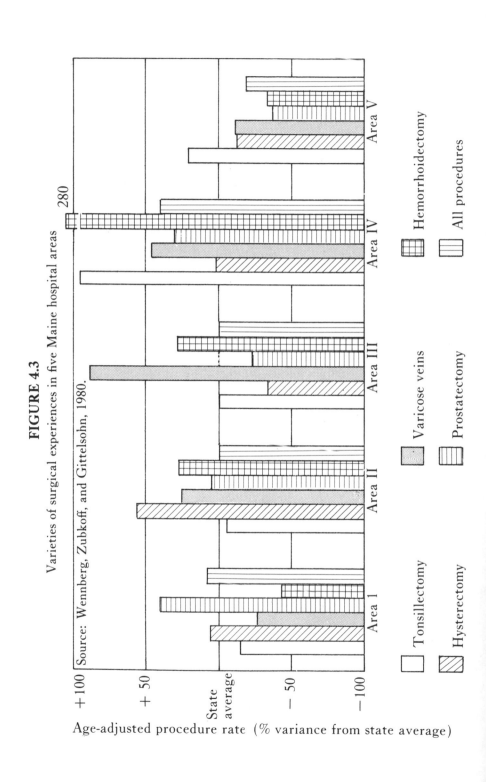

FIGURE 4.3

Varieties of surgical experiences in five Maine hospital areas

area I exceeded the state average by 40 percent. Over the next three years, the same pattern of excess for this procedure is observed; on the other hand, hemorrhoidectomy, a procedure that was done at a rate of only about 50 percent of the state average in 1973, continues through 1977 at about the same relatively low rate. The other procedures maintain their characteristic places.

For the procedures illustrated in figure 4.3 the numbers of cases in excess or deficit of that predicted by the state average can be large. Table 4.3 gives the accumulated observed and expected number of cases for each of the five areas over the five year period. Area I records 736 fewer tonsillectomies and 349 more prostatectomies than predicted; area II has 815 more hysterectomies.[4] As I have said, the small-area technique displays the impact of the clinical decision made by a small number of physicians. For example, the hysterectomy profile in area II is generated largely by six physicians who, from year to year, do

FIGURE 4.4

A characteristic surgical signature over time in one Maine
hospital area (1973-1977)

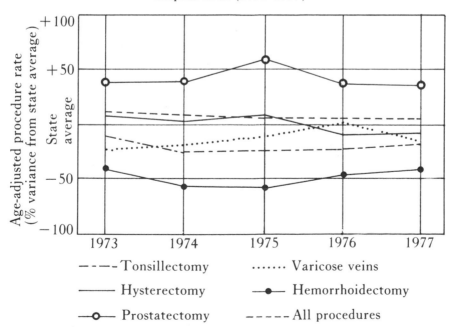

Source: Wennberg, Zubkoff, and Gittelsohn 1980.

TABLE 4.3

Number of procedures above (+) or below (−) expected[a] in
five Maine hospital service areas for selected surgical
procedures (1973–1976)

Procedure	Area I	Area II	Area III	Area IV	Area V
Tonsillectomy	−736	+ 97	+ 49	+806	+659
Hysterectomy	+ 15	+815	−140	− 62	−228
Prostatectomy	+349	− 14	− 54	+ 2	− 83
Hemorrhoidectomy	−223	+ 79	+ 79	+152	− 58

a. Expected based on accumulated numbers of cases for each year (1973–1976). State
average rate is used to estimate the expected number of cases.

about the same number of hysterectomies. Similar patterns of behavior
exist for other physician-procedure combinations. Although not without clear exceptions, a constancy rule appears to apply to work load
decisions by physicians, resulting in the community profiles seen in figure 4.4.

Other case studies show that when procedure rates change substantially in a specific area population, the changes often relate to migration of specific physicians in or out of the area (Wennberg and
Gittelsohn 1980). They can also be related to feedback of information
to physicians. Perhaps the most convincing evidence of physician influence on utilization rates comes from examples in which physicians
have been provided with information on geographic variations. In the
1950s Paul Lembke used insurance data to develop profiles of per capita rates of surgery in different communities in the Rochester, New
York area. When he showed the results of his study to the responsible
physicians, the rates in high rate areas dropped. (Lembke 1959) Similar experiences have been reported for hysterectomy rates in
Saskatchewan (Dyck et al. 1977). Providing information on tonsillectomy rates to the Vermont State Medical Society led to a decline in the
risk for children of tonsillectomy in the highest rate Vermont area
from 65 percent to less than 8 percent (Wennberg, Blower, et al.
1977). This drop occurred when local physicians responded to the information by reviewing the indications for the procedure and initiat-
ing a second-opinion procedure between a pediatrician and a general
surgeon. In the Vermont study it was widely suggested that the local

population, when expected to undergo a tonsillectomy, would go to a neighboring hospital area to demand that the surgery be done after it became relatively unavailable locally. This did not occur.

The distributional patterns of specific procedures involve greater variations for some procedures than for others, which I believe reflects the relative degree of uncertainty that physicians (as well as patients) face in making decisions to use them. This hypothesis is a reasonable explanation for the results of a study we undertook to test the utilization model summarized by the equations presented earlier. The null hypothesis states that if in a given cross-sectional comparison each of the conditional probabilities in the equation is the same between areas then the distribution of observed rates will be normal. This follows from the normal law of errors, which states that multiple independent sources of variation based on random error combine to generate normal distributions.

The normal distribution of common surgical procedures expressed in terms of Z scores performed in children are in figure 4.5. Hernia procedures in children come very close to fitting the null hypotheses: across 62 individual hospital service areas in Vermont, Maine, and Rhode Island the distribution of rates very nearly fits the distribution predicted by the null hypothesis. From an ethnic, economic, and social class point of view, these 62 areas demonstrate considerable heterogeneity with regard to their population-at-risk. This heterogeneity is also seen in the distribution of facilities, physician manpower, and expenditures for medical services. In terms of the statistical parameters of the model for hernia procedures, these differences are insufficient to generate variations beyond what chance alone may explain. In contrast to hernias in the elderly where a truss is sometimes recommended, for inguinal hernias among children there is no professionally recognized alternative to operative treatment if the child is otherwise normal. The condition is noted for its transparency; the observation of the abnormality is usually made by a family member, and the subsequent professional diagnosis generally presents no great difficulty.

Appendectomies demonstrate greater variation in rates, indicating that the conditions for the null hypothesis are not met. For appendicitis, there is nearly unanimous agreement that proper treatment is surgical excision; however, the problem, duly recorded in surgical literature (de Dombal 1972), is to know when the condition that brings the patient to the physician is truly appendicitis and not a mimic for

FIGURE 4.5

Distribution of common surgical procedures performed on children

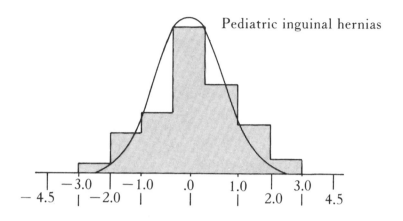

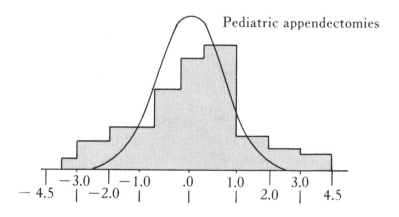

which appendectomy is of no value. The data suggest that physicians' judgments to distinguish false positive and false negative situations may vary from area to area.

In contrast to both pediatric herniorrhapies and appendectomies, tonsillectomies demonstrate a gross departure from the requirements of the null hypothesis. Rates among areas vary by amounts which are both large and highly statistically significant. The medical literature is replete with evidence of professional controversy concerning the indi-

(Figure 4.5 continued)

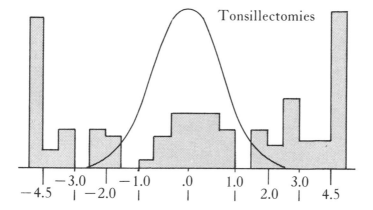

Note: These figures are histograms of the distribution of Z scores based on one degree of freedom chi-square tests in which each rate in each of 62 areas was tested against the rate for all areas. Under circumstances where the variation in rates among areas is explained by stochastic (or random) variation, the Z scores would approximate the normal distribution (mean = zero, standard deviation = ± 1). Such a distribution is expected if the null hypothesis holds: the incidence of illness, access to physicians, physician labeling, and physician choice of therapy are similar among areas.

cators for this procedure. Convincing evidence of the importance of variation in physicians' perceptions of the need for tonsillectomies is found in the 1934 study of the American Child Health Association. In a sample of 1,000 New York school children, 60 percent had already been tonsillectomized. The remaining 40 percent were re-examined by school physicians who selected 45 percent for tonsillectomy; the children without recommendation were then re-examined by a second group of physicians who recommended that 46 percent undergo the procedure. The third re-examination of twice-rejected children led to tonsillectomy recommendations in 44 percent. After three successive second opinions, only 67 out of the original cohort of 1,000 were spared a recommendation for tonsillectomy. The authors concluded that the process of recommendation depended principally on the physician rather than on the child's health status.

In studying distributional patterns, we have found that specific surgical procedures have characteristic variations. Procedure-specific patterns of variation tend to be similar throughout the world even though health services are organized and financed differently. Figure 4.6 demonstrates the pattern of variation among subpopulations of three New England states. Hernia procedures (inguinal herniorrhaphy) have a similar low-level pattern of variation in all three states; appendectomy and cholecystectomy are intermediate; prostatectomy, hysterectomy, and tonsillectomy are examples of high-order variation procedures that appear to have similar patterns of distribution in each state. The figure also illustrates that the pattern of variation within each of the states tends to be consistent from state to state. For example, for inguinal hernia procedures, the coefficient of variation is low in each state and there are no areas in any state which were significant (at p = .01). By contrast, for tonsillectomy the distribution of rates in each of the three states yields a relatively high coefficient of variation, a comparatively wide range between low and high rates, and shows 21 of the 33 areas having rates that are significantly different by the chi-square test.

In the United States, patterns of variation in procedure rates among health maintenance organizations (HMOs) appear to be similar to those seen under fee-for-service systems in Maine, Rhode Island, and Vermont. Hal Luft, who is sitting in the audience, has studied surgical services among HMOs and found overall surgical rates to be consistently lower than under fee-for-service (Luft 1978). However, the specific procedures demonstrated considerable variation between HMOs. Among the studied HMOs, tonsillectomies and prostatectomies demonstrated a much greater range of variation than did cholecystectomies or hernia:

Procedure	Ratio of High to Low Rate
Prostatectomy	3.6
Tonsillectomy	2.8
Cholecystectomy	2.0
Hernia	1.9

The results of a recent comparison of surgery rates among health regions in the United Kingdom and health districts in Norway, as seen earlier in figure 4.2, show that the pattern of procedure variation seen in Northern New England also exists under the national health ser-

FIGURE 4.6

1975 rates for six common procedures in the eleven largest
hospital areas of Rhode Island, Maine, Vermont

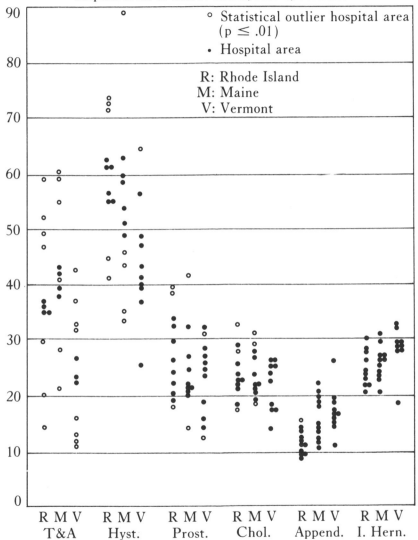

○ Statistical outlier hospital area
  (p ≤ .01)

• Hospital area

R: Rhode Island
M: Maine
V: Vermont

T&A: Tonsillectomy and Adenoidectomy
Hyst.: Hysterectomy
Prost.: Prostatectomy
Chol.: Cholecystectomy

Append.: Appendectomy
I. Hern.: Inguinal Hernia

vices of these two European countries, although the distributions are such that the United Kingdom and Norway have lower mean rates than New England (McPherson, Wennberg, and Hovind 1980, unpublished).

The evidence for the lack of professional consistency in diagnosing many illnesses and treatments is extensive and independent of the epidemiologic evidence on variations. The medical literature is clear concerning the ambiguous nature of the evidence purported to connect many commonly used medical and surgical practices with improved health status (Cochrane 1973; Bunker, Barnes, and Mosteller 1977; Wennberg, Bunker, and Barnes 1980). It is also clear concerning the variability of physicians as observers and interpreters of medical evidence (Koran 1975). Variations or disagreements among board-certified surgeons in recommending specific procedures have also been documented (Rutkow, Gittelsohn, Zuidema 1979). The distributional characteristics of specific procedures among small-area populations reflect this professional uncertainty.

Implications of Professional Uncertainty for Resource Use and Future Public Policies

With the qualified exception of certain drug outcome studies, the issue of the effectiveness of allocated services with regard to their "curing" or their "caring" expectations has not been of direct concern to public policy; nor has the issue of how resources are allocated among competing priorities (for example, between curing and caring efforts or between alternative approaches to either) been of direct concern. The issue of how and when resources designated for use in the health sector are allocated to optimize individual welfare is a responsibility tacitly delegated to the medical profession and to be resolved through the profession's traditions, which emphasize science and ethics as a sufficient means for resolving questions of fact and value. This process assumes health resource allocation based on professional consensus concerning the value of technology and the nature of patient need or utility. However, if the existing evidence is insufficient to settle controversies on the value of many common medical practices, consensus standards must represent weighted averages of the opinions of those selected to establish them and cannot serve as a basis for the rational allocation of medical care resources or technology. Indeed, without more direct information on the outcomes of alternative approaches to care, rational allocation is not possible if the criterion for rationality is the maximization of health through the efficient use of medical services.

In a similar vein, unless the choices made in resource allocation represent the informed wishes of the patient rather than of the physician, the same criterion for rationality cannot be met. An important implication is that the limits on informed decision making are more severe than generally realized, affecting physicians as well as their patients. This is a problem even when outcomes are reasonably well known: McNeil shows that the values reflected by the physician's choice of treatment do not always reflect the values of the patient; had the patient known more, he or she would have chosen otherwise (McNeil, Weichselbaum, and Pauker 1978). And when the outcomes of alternative treatments are not well understood, as is often the case, informed decision making or giving informed consent is difficult indeed.

The implication seems inescapable: it is not certain at all that the central tendency of health care markets is to provide what patients want and need, although most regulatory strategies assume so and direct their attention to possible cases of professional deviance. The epidemiological findings from throughout the world concerning variations in rates of use of surgical procedures (and medical admissions) demonstrate, at the level at which health care is used, that current case selection at the margin is discretionary: incremental spending in hospital areas is to purchase services which may appear in one area as a relative excess of tonsillectomies, in another area as a relative excess of hysterectomies, in a third as a relative excess in prostatectomies, and so on. The lack of information on long-range income also indicates discretion in the fundamental sense that it cannot be objectively shown that more care is necessarily better. Nor is it certain that more intensive care would necessarily be selected by patients were they fully informed about the possible consequences. Under current standards of practice, there is a good deal of latitude in how decisions are made and no compelling policy reason, based on evidence of consequences to the public welfare, to spend at high rates unless evidence is generated which would lead to an informed choice with regard to the cost and benefit implications.

This conclusion bears important implications for many current public policy initiatives in health care, which are based on the belief that an underlying professional consensus exists on the optimum methods for allocating medical technology. Examples include such programs as the Professional Standards Review Organizations in the United States, which assume that consensus exists on meaningful standards of care that will promote the public health by ensuring that only necessary hospitalizations and procedures are undertaken. Similarly, the development of national standards for health resources (such as numbers of physicians or beds per capita) rests on the assumption that there is an established relationship between resource input and health care outcomes. Without better information on these relationships, those efforts cannot substantially improve the rationality of medical markets.

In closing, I urge that the highest priority should be given to making a substantial investment in the assessment of the outcome of common medical and surgical practices and the development of mechanisms to assure the feedback of results to the profession and the public. While much debate has focused on the assessment of new technology prior to its implementation, the dollar mortality and morbidity implications (Wennberg, Bunker, and Barnes 1980) of uncertainties concerning the value of existing services warrant a substantial investment in studies to learn more about their outcomes so that the trade-offs under their various patterns of use may be understood by physicians, patients, third-party payers, and those responsible for public policy.

Chapter 4 Notes

1. Michael Zubkoff is Professor and Chairman of the Department of Community and Family Medicine and Professor of Health Economics, at Dartmouth College. Adapted in part from John Wennberg, Benjamin Barnes, and Michael Zubkoff, "Professional Uncertainty and the Problems of Supplier-Induced Demand," *Social Science and Medicine*, in press.

Editor's note: Zubkoff's comment is an expanded version of his original presentation in the conference, titled "Professional Uncertainty in Clinical Decision Making: Implications for National Health Policy." The corresponding general discussion, and Tom Moore's comments in particular, relate to the original presentation.

2. It is important to note that the rates of procedures are corrected for "border crossing," i.e., they are population-based, reflecting the entire experience of the population, whether the procedure was done by a local or an out-of-area physician. However, the sample of physicians who do the large major-

ity of the procedures for a particular area is usually quite small. This is because border crossing for common procedures is rare. Thus one, two, or three physicians will often be responsible for 90 percent or more of the procedures done for a population.

3. Because the community rates are based on the weighted averages of several physicians, the pattern observed among community-based populations is inevitably an understatement of the true range of professional differences. Studies based on the enrolled populations among Oxford region general practices (in which one and sometimes two primary physicians are responsible for the decisions) provide a more accurate estimate of the range (McPherson, Wennberg, Hovind, unpublished 1980).

4. In area I the population-at-risk for prostatectomy (males 65 years or greater) is about 6,000. In area II the population-at-risk for hysterectomy (women 25 years or older) is about 30,000.

Chapter 4 References

American Child Health Association. 1934. *The Pathway to Correction in Physical Defects.* New York.

American College of Surgeons and the American Surgical Association. 1976. *Surgery in the United States: A Summary Report of the Study on Surgical Services in the United States.*

Anderholm, L., and Zubkoff, M. 1980. "Small Area Variations in Use Rates: A Literature Review." In preparation.

Arrow, K. 1963. "Uncertainty and the Welfare Economics of Medical Care." *The American Economics Review* 53:941–73.

Banta, H. D., and Thacker, S. B. 1979. "Costs and Benefits of Electronic Fetal Monitoring: A Review of the Literature." National Health Care Expenditures Study Publication no. (PHS) 79-3245. Hyattsville, MD: United States Department of Health, Education, and Welfare.

Bunker, J. P. 1970. "Surgical Manpower: A Comparison of Operations and Surgeons in the United States and in England and Wales." *New England Journal of Medicine* 282:135–44.

Cochrane, A. L. 1973. *Effectiveness and Efficiency: Random Reflections on Health Services.* Condon, Nuffield Professional Hospital Trust.

de Dombal, F. T. 1972. "Computer-Aided Diagnosis of Acute Abdominal Pain." *British Medical Journal* 2:9–13.

Detmer, D. E., and Tyson, T. J. 1978. "Regional Differences in Surgical Care Based Upon Uniform Physician and Hospital Discharge Abstract Data." *Annals of Surgery* 187:166–69.

Dyck, F. J.; Murphy, F. A.; Murphy, J. K.; Raod, D. A.; Boyd, M. S.; Osborne, E.; de Vlieger, D.; Korchinski, B.; Ripley, C.; Bromley, A. T.; and Innes, P. B. 1977. "Effect of Surveillance on the Number of Hysterectomies in the Province of Saskatchewan." *New England Journal of Medicine* 296:1326–28.

Evans, R. G. 1974. "Supplier-Induced Demand: Some Empirical Evidence and Implications." In *The Economics of Health and Medical Care*, edited by M. Perlman, pp. 162–73. New York: Wiley & Sons.

Evans, R., and Wolfson, A. O. 1978. "Moving the Target to Hit the Bullet: Generation of Utilization by Physicians in Canada." Paper prepared for National Bureau of Economics Research Conference on the Economics of Physician and Patient Behavior, June 27 and 28 at Stanford, California.

Feldstein, M. S. 1971. "Hospital Cost Inflation: A Study of Nonprofit Price Dynamics." *American Economic Review* 61:853–72.

Fuchs, V., and Newhouse, J., eds. 1978. "The Economics of Physician and Patient Behavior: National Bureau of Economic Research Conference." *Journal of Human Resources*, vol. 13, supplement. Madison: University of Wisconsin Press.

Gittelsohn, A., and Wennberg, J. E. 1977. "On the Incidence of Tonsillectomy and Other Common Surgical Procedures." In *Costs, Risks, and Benefits of Surgery*, edited by J. Bunker, B. Barnes, and F. Mosteller, pp. 91–106. New York: Oxford University Press.

Glover, J. A. 1938. "The Incidence of Tonsillectomy in School Children." *Proceedings of the Royal Society of Medicine* 31:1219–36.

―――― 1959. *Monthly Bulletin of the Ministry of Health* 9:62. Cited in J. Morris. 1964. *Uses of Epidemiology*. Baltimore: Williams and Wilkins.

Griffith, J. P. 1978. *Measuring Hospital Performance*. Chicago, Blue Cross Association. An Inquiry Book.

Hirshleifer, J., and Riley, J. 1979. "The Analytics of Uncertainty and Information: An Expository Survey." *Journal of Economic Literature* 17:1375–1421.

Koran, L. M. 1975. "The Reliability of Clinical Methods, Data, and Judgments." Parts 1 and 2. *New England Journal of Medicine* 293:642–46.

Lembke, P. A. 1959. "A Scientific Method for Medical Auditing." *Hospitals* 33:65–71.

Lewis, C. E. 1969. "Variations in the Incidence of Surgery." *New England Journal of Medicine* 281:880–84.

Luft, H. S. 1978. "How do Health-Maintenance Organizations Achieve Their Saving?" *New England Journal of Medicine* 298:1336–43.

McCarthy, E. G., and Finkel, M. L. 1978. "Second Opinion Elective Surgery Programs: Outcome Status Over Time." *Medical Care* 16:984-94.

McCarthy, E. G., and Widmir, G. W. 1974. "Effects of Screening by Consultants on Recommended Elective Surgical Procedures." *New England Journal of Medicine* 291:1331-35.

McNeil, B. J., Weichselbaum, R., and Pauker, S. G. 1978. "Fallacy of the Five-Year Survival in Lung Cancer." *New England Journal of Medicine* 299:1397-1401.

McPherson, K., Wennberg, J., and Hovind, O. 1980. "Small Area Variations in Use of Surgery: An International Comparison." Unpublished.

Pauly, M. 1974. "The Behavior of Non-Profit Hospital Monopolies: Alternative Models of the Hospital." In *Regulating Health Facilities Construction*, edited by C. C. Havighurst, pp. 143-62. Washington: American Enterprise Institute.

Reinhardt, U. E. 1978. "Comment." In *Competition in the Health Care Sector*, edited by W. Greenberg, pp. 121-48. Germantown, Maryland: Aspen Systems Corporation.

Roos, N. P.; Roos, L. L.; and Henteleff, P. D. 1977. "Elective Surgical Rates: Do High Rates Mean Lower Standards?" *New England Journal of Medicine* 297:360-65.

Rutkow, I.; Gittelsohn, A.; and Zuidema, G. D. 1979. "Surgical Decision Making: The Reliability of Clinical Judgment." *Annals of Surgery* 190:409-19.

Sloan, F. A., and Feldman, R. 1978. "Competition Among Physicians." In *Competition in the Health Care Sector: Past, Present, and Future*, edited by W. Greenberg, pp. 45-102. Germantown, Maryland: Aspen Systems Corporation.

Stockwell, H., and Vayda, E. 1979. "Variations in Surgery in Ontario." *Medical Care* April:390-96.

Vayda, E., and Anderson, G. D. 1968. "Comparison of Provincial Surgical Rates in 1968." *The Canadian Journal of Surgery* 18:18-26.

Wennberg, J. E. 1979. "Factors Governing Utilization of Hospital Services." *Hospital Practice* 14:115-27.

Wennberg, J. E.; Blowers, L.; Parker, R.; and Gittelsohn, A. M. 1977. "Changes in Tonsillectomy Rates Associated with Feedback and Review." *Pediatrics* 59:821-26.

Wennberg, J. E.; Bunker, J.; and Barnes, B. 1980. "The Need for Assessing the Outcomes of Common Medical Practices." *Annual Review of Public Health 1980* 1:277-95.

Wennberg, J. E., and Fowler, F. A. 1977. "A Test of Consumer Contributions to Small Area Variations in Health Care Delivery." *Journal of the Maine Medical Association* 68:275–79.

Wennberg, J. E., and Gittelsohn, A. 1973. "Small Area Variations in Health Care Delivery." *Science* 183:1102–08.

———— 1975. "Health Care Delivery in Maine I: Patterns of Use of Common Surgical Procedures." *Journal of the Maine Medical Association* 66:123–30 and 149.

———— 1980. "A Small Area Approach to the Analysis of Health System Performance: A Practical Guide to Uses of Epidemiology for the Evaluation of Medical Markets." Final report under contract #291-76-0003.

Wennberg, J. E.; Lapenas, C.; Greene, R.; and Zubkoff, M. 1980. "Variations in Population Based Use Rates and Expenditures: Implications for Manpower Policy." A report prepared for the Geographic Distribution Panel of the Graduate Medical Education National Advisory Committee.

Wennberg, J. E.; Zubkoff, M.; and Gittelsohn, A. 1978. "A Systematic Study of the Nature, Extent, Causes, and Cost Implications of Small Area Variations in Hospital and Ambulatory Care." Grant No. 18-P-97192 from the Health Care Financing Administration. U.S. Department of Health, Education, and Welfare.

———— 1980. "A Systematic Study of the Nature, Extent, Causes, and Cost Implications of Small Area Variations in Hospital and Ambulatory Care." Progress Report, March 1980. Health Care Financing Administration. Grant No. 18P–97192. U.S. Department of Health, Education, and Welfare.

Zubkoff, M.; Carbeck, R.; Morgan, B.; Westcott, M.; and Anderholm, L. 1980. "Final Report of the Geographic Distribution Technical Panel of the Graduate Medical Educational National Advisory Committee.

Zubkoff, M.; Raskin, I.; and Hanft, R. 1978. "Hospital Cost Containment: Selected Notes for Future Policy." Milbank Memorial Fund. New York: Prodist.

General Discussion of Section I

Reinhardt[1]

One thing that occasionally puzzles me about the writing of economists, myself included, is that we're never quite clear about the most fundamental premises that people put forth when they develop a health insurance system. If you read a great deal of our writings, you will find that there is a tacit premise that health care is really like other commodities, for example hula hoops, in two important respects. The first one is that the transactions in the market for health care are very much akin to the transactions in the market for hula hoops. That may very well be true; this hypothesis is testable, and testing done now shows that in many instances it is. Physicians are like tomatoes in some respects. But we sometimes believe that health care doesn't only behave in the market like hula hoops, but that society's ethical precepts on health care are identical to society's ethical precepts for hula hoops. We call a distribution of hula hoops an efficient one when the hula hoops go to those people who value them most. Of course, we all know that the people who value things most are those who can pay the most for them. Therefore, it is very simple to tell whether the hula hoops have been efficiently distributed. And we think that hula hoops should be tailored to individual taste. If somebody wants his red, it should be red, and if somebody wants his oval, it should be oval. Perhaps we should have a whole range of hula hoops, some even square.

Surely, you wouldn't want a public enterprise to produce hula hoops. It is quite clear that if we produced them with government enterprise and distributed them free of charge, all of the precepts that we teach freshmen would be violated. In fact, how would you decide how many hula hoops to make? Some politician would decide that. What color and what shape? Again, it would be up to some politician, and I think that you could very quickly prove, without resorting to data at all, that it is conceivable that upper- and middle-class children wouldn't get quite the hula hoops they otherwise would have had and wanted, and they may have some square ones.

It seems to me that for some commodities, this analysis can be very constructive. But it misses the central point about health care. I feel that many American health economists seem to have lost sight of the central dilemma of the health care problem; namely, we don't believe that ethical precepts of hula hoops apply to health care. Economists often forget that.

There are at least two different premises that I see societies bring to health care. One is what I call the European premise, and is the principle of solidarity. It is a concept that I challenge you to find in an American economics textbook. This principle is simply not our mental compass; but in Europe, it is all they talk about. They say that everyone should be in the same boat as far as health care is concerned, but not as far as shoes and hula hoops. You ask, "Why don't you have private schools in your country?" They say, "It violates solidarity. We know it makes for a Harvard, but we don't care. We don't have a Harvard, but we have solidarity." It is an extreme premise to bring to a system, so very extreme that in reality it simply cannot be implemented. The commissar and the top bureaucrats will generally evade solidarity and say it is good for others, but not for them.

The second premise that you could apply to health care, which is different from hula hoops and, say, shoes, is that you have a maximum of tolerable suffering that you allow in society. We really don't care that much about bare feet, but we do care that there be a minimum adequate practice of health care guaranteed to every American regardless of ability to pay.

The dilemma of the health care system is, therefore, how to couple a particular ethical system with a system of production and distribution that is run on quite a different principle: the ability to pay, which in turn is determined by effort, luck, and lineage.

You could say, well, there are some Americans who don't have access to health care, who don't have health insurance. We'll cover them with the government, or we'll cover them somehow, and the rest will do as they wish. But it is hard to write it into law. Those worried about health insurance find that it is very difficult to fuse the two systems. At the point where you fuse, all kinds of absurdities may take place; for example, somebody who is working and is reasonably poor may be much worse off than somebody who isn't working at all. The agony over health care is really this coupling of two ethical systems.

Cotton M. Lindsay's Paper

Goodman

The other side of the fact that the British National Health Service has reduced the invisible services offered to the public, is that it offers a great many more visible services. This is an interesting aspect that is not touched upon in Lindsay's paper. The ambulance service in Britain operates almost like a free taxi service (there is about one ambulance ride per year for every two or three people in the country); general practitioners still make house calls, and they have home visitors; health nurses make about one visit per year for every two households. These are visible things the public wants.

Matt has not mentioned it, but I think what is visible to the public matters a great deal, and in a system like the British National Health Service, the patients have very little incentive to become well informed about health matters. What can they do with more knowledge? They can become more intelligent voters, but that doesn't help them when they are standing in line. The suppliers have very little incentive to communicate knowledge to the patients because they are not selling services: their incentive is to reduce the size of the queue, not increase it. In a system like that, you have consumers who are very ignorant about health matters, and what they want are these visible things like free ambulance rides and the general practitioner's house calls, and for a long time they wanted chest X rays. The government went all over the country giving everybody chest X rays. By contrast, most British women don't know about Pap smears (only about 8 percent of the eligible women in the country get them); they don't know anything about CAT scans, which the government doesn't provide; and they don't know what a dialysis machine is (the government buys very few of those). It is the public perception and what is visible to the voters that motivates a great deal of what goes on in the British National Health Service.

Ingbar

I was very intrigued about Matt Lindsay's point regarding what is a visible and what is an invisible sign of success in a much more bureaucratic system (than the American system). In California hospitals, according to the last statistics I saw, more spending originates in the administration and fiscal service departments than in the patient service areas. Of course, these are figures which, as you know, are normally hidden by our customary accounting system. You normally do not see direct costs, and therefore do not know what proportion of this spending in fact originated in fiscal service areas. If one moves away from looking at aggregated costs in the various countries that have been discussed this morning, and begins to look at costs for the administrative component in these institutions as distinct from inpatient costs or ancillary service area costs, I wonder what kinds of pictures we would get. In addition, when we begin to pursue this question of the visible versus the invisible kinds of output and outcome measures, what lessons do we draw from the experience of these three countries?

Ricardo-Campbell

I would like to make two brief comments. One relates to Mary Lee's comment on hospitals: 35 percent of all community hospitals in the United States are now in multihospital systems, whether nonprofit or for-profit. This indicates to me that the management of hospitals is improving in the United States. I will not address the accounting issues. The other point I would like to make is that unwritten rules apparently exist in the United Kingdom. There are unwritten rules about the use of kidney dialysis machines. The *London Times*, in May 1979, indicated that there is an informal allocation by age of kidney transplants: life expectancy is shorter for older than younger persons, and therefore the ratio of benefits to costs is less for the aged. In 1976 the number of patients per one million population treated by dialysis or a functioning transplant was 71.2 in the United Kingdom and about 140 in the United States.[2]

Fleming

I would like to ask Matt Lindsay whether his studies on Britain included any comparison of the British National Health Service with some of the older systems, like the British United Parliament Association and the United Health Services, which appeared to have some success.

Lindsay

Private health insurance is a growing industry in Britain, and it is a matter of the public being willing to pay for services that are supposed to be available free of charge. This started off, of course, with people whose time costs were high, who couldn't afford to be out of work for long periods of time waiting for surgery or other treatments. Very early on, executives began buying private insurance and became private patients in British hospitals. Since the expected wait for any hospital treatment has grown over time, the number of people who buy private insurance and seek treatment in a private hospital, or become private patients in a government hospital, has grown dramatically. A major union, the ELETPU (electricians), bargained successfully last year to provide private health insurance for their 40,000 members. Working class people are also opting out of the government-provided, so-called free service, and they are going back to the private sector.

John P. Pierce's Paper

Goldbeck

From the Australian example, I think I saw on one of Pierce's tables that 43 percent of the private hospitals were for-profit hospitals. And if it is true, that is a much larger percentage than what we have in this country. Is there any message from a cost-containment, managerial standpoint, or from a delivery-of-services standpoint?

Pierce

You should remember that private hospitals are a very small percentage of total hospitals, which are mainly state and public hospitals. And when you consider that 43 percent of private hospitals are for-profit, that seriously deflates the figure. There are 340 private hospitals in Australia. The average number of beds for private hospitals is below 100, so I think you've forgotten the first proportion from which the second proportion is taken.

Zubkoff's Comment

Moore

I would like to point out that Mike Zubkoff gives the assumptions of a competitive model. Having taught economics for a number of years, I would quarrel with those assumptions, especially assumptions two and three. Consumers don't know the effectiveness of various goods and services in any market; they don't need to, as a matter of fact. There is a variety of market devices that provide a great deal of information about goods. Nor do consumers have to know all prices; only a marginal group of consumers has to be sensitive to prices to get competitive results.

In addition, I would comment on your tables, particularly on the variety of rates of various medical practices in different areas and the data on Maine. Your data suggest to me that hospitals specialize, and from a casual look, that sounds good to me. In fact, I understand that the hospital specialization system provides better service. You get better treatment in hospitals used to doing a particular procedure than in one that is not. So, I fail to see the importance of these data.

Zubkoff

Just two informational points. On the principles of rational agency choice, all I'm trying to say with those is that if I'm turning to someone to serve as an agent for me, these are the kinds of things that I would like him to know. I would like him to know about the effectiveness of the types of services that he is going to prescribe and treatments that he is going to give me.

With respect to the main data: first, the main New England data, as I understand it, is hospital-service-area-specific with population-based data, so that if you lived in San Francisco and received care here at a hospital, you would show up in the utilization rates of this institution in Palo Alto, for example.

Second, the idea that the institutions specialize is one way of looking at it. The other way is to look at the physician's epidemiological signature, and there are case studies, at least in New England, where we followed physicians who have moved from one community to another, and what they do in community B is exactly what they did in community A.

Pierce

As an epidemiologist, I must comment that your first three tables are not epidemiological data. To say that someone who comes from San Francisco to Stanford belongs to the hospital population of Stanford is fine, but you're not counting the denominator; you're only counting the numerator. You must count both sources; it is the people who don't come as well that you need to include in calculating your rates.

Chapter 5 Notes

1. *Editor's note:* These comments by Reinhardt were made not in rebuttal to discussants' comments, but as an introduction to the oral presentation of his conference paper. Since they have evoked some reactions by participants in later sessions, I have incorporated them here in a somewhat abbreviated form.

2. John C. Goodman, *National Health Care in Great Britain* (Dallas: The Fisher Institute [n.p.] 1980), p. 101.

Section II

General Issues and Health Care Policies
in the United States

Access to Medical Care in the United States: Equitable for Whom?

*Lu Ann Aday**

Introduction

"Equity of access" to medical care has been an expressed goal of much of the effort in health policy formulation and implementation during the past 25 years. Just what is meant by this objective and how well it has been achieved have been sources of continuing debate over this period. The discussion that follows will attempt to suggest some answers to these questions, based on the most recent conceptual and empirical work in this area. Particular attention will be devoted to the extent to which the equity goal has been realized for the traditionally disadvantaged groups in our society and to identifying those groups for whom the greatest inequities persist and why. Fully understanding the current national profile of access to medical care—particularly with respect to detecting the greatest pockets of remaining inequity—

*Senior Research Associate, Center for Health Administration Studies, University of Chicago. The original research on which this paper was based was supported by a grant from the Robert Wood Johnson Foundation (Princeton, New Jersey) and Contract No. HRA 230-76-0096 from the National Center for Health Services Research (Hyattsville, Maryland).

should permit health policy makers, planners, administrators, and providers to make more informed judgments concerning the allocation of
scarce health system resources to the areas of greatest need.

The Concept of Equity of Access

Two main themes regarding the concept of access to medical care
have recurred in the professional literature of the past 25 years. Some
researchers tend to measure access by characteristics of the population
(such as family income, insurance coverage, or attitudes toward medical care) or characteristics of the delivery system (such as the distribution and organization of manpower and facilities). Others argue that
access can best be evaluated through outcome indicators of individuals' passage through the system, such as their utilization rates or
satisfaction levels. The work in this area carried out by the Center for
Health Administration Studies at The University of Chicago has attempted to synthesize and integrate these various points of view (Aday
and Andersen 1974; Aday and Andersen 1975; Aday et al. 1980).

As figure 6.1 demonstrates, our access framework implies that characteristics of the delivery system (the availability and distribution of
health care providers and facilities, for example) and characteristics of
the population at risk in an area (their age, health status, insurance
coverage, and income levels) reflect the probable, or potential, levels
of access to medical care, while utilization and satisfaction measures
may be considered indicators of actual, or realized, access to services.
Health policy efforts—such as physician manpower redistribution programs, hospital-based group practice arrangements (like those funded
by The Robert Wood Johnson Foundation [Block et al. 1978]), or
large-scale federal financing initiatives—represent efforts to influence
the characteristics of the delivery system itself (by providing more convenient facilities) or of potential users of the system (by eliminating
the financial barriers to care) and thereby ultimately influence the
probability of individuals' entering the system and their subjective
evaluations of how satisfactory they found the experience of care-seek-
ing to be. These indicators of potential and realized access to medical
care parallel the structure, process, and outcome measures of quality
described in the quality-of-care literature (Donabedian 1973). For example, structure and process measures may be viewed as indicators of

FIGURE 6.1

Framework for the study of access

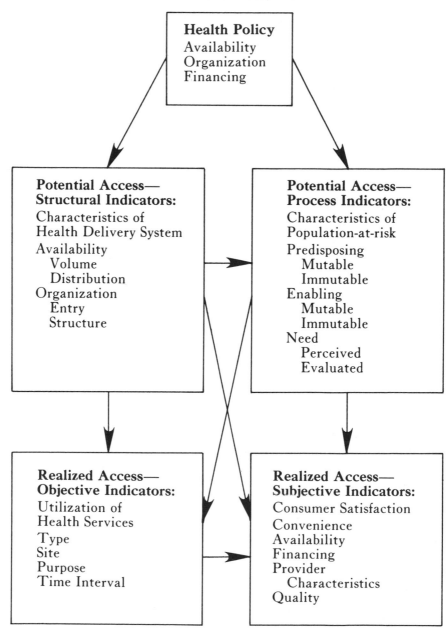

potential access in that they specify particular structures or resources (the number and distribution of physicians in an area, for example) or behaviors or procedures (average travel or office waiting time) that may ultimately influence whether or not some other outcomes of interest are realized (increased utilization rates and consumer satisfaction levels, for instance). Realized access may be measured in terms of more objective units-of-service indicators or subjective levels of expressed satisfaction with relevant dimensions of care. Basically our approach implies that, as with judgments of overall quality of care, variant conclusions regarding access levels may result, depending upon which dimension—structure, process, or outcome—one chooses to emphasize. The selection of one dimension rather than another for consideration at a particular time depends on the particular health policy outcome relevant to the access impact evaluator.

Basically then, according to our framework, *access may be defined as those dimensions which describe the potential and actual entry of a given population group to the health care delivery system.*

Utilization rates and satisfaction scores reflect the actual impact of a variety of potential system and individual determinants. These more immediate outcomes, rather than changes in health status, are taken as the end points of the access model, because a variety of factors other than contact with the health care system per se are apt to bear upon health status (heredity, nutrition and environment, for example) and because access is generally assumed to imply right of entry to the system, independent of ultimate changes in the health status of the population.

Two main categories of social indicators of the access concept may be specified on the basis of the framework: potential and realized access indicators. Figure 6.2 points up how the variables available from the 1975–76 national survey conducted by the Center for Health Administration Studies (CHAS) operationalize the different aspects of the access framework.

Of particular interest to us are the problems people experience in obtaining care once a need is perceived. The greatest equity of access is said to exist when need, rather than structural or other individual characteristics, determines who gains entry to the health care system (Andersen et al. 1975). To the extent that having a family doctor, insurance coverage, or actual utilization is a function of the person's

FIGURE 6.2
Operational indicators of the access framework [a]

I. Potential Access–Structural Indicators: characteristics of health delivery system
   A. Availability
      1. Volume
         a. Personnel
            (1) Number of physicians
            (2) Number of dentists
            (3) Number of optometrists
         b. Facilities
            (1) Number of hospitals
            (2) Number of hospital beds
      2. Distribution[b]
         a. Number of personnel per 1,000 population in county of residence
         b. Number of facilities per 1,000 population in county of residence
   B. Organization[c]
      1. Entry
         a. Convenience of regular source of medical care
            (1) Availability of services at night, on weekends, and in emergencies
            (2) Mode of transportation
            (3) Travel time
            (4) Cost of travel to facility
            (5) Special arrangements required to obtain care
            (6) Appointment system and waiting time
            (7) Office waiting time
            (8) Time doctor spends with the patient (on the average)
         b. Selecting a regular source of medical care
            (1) Reasons for choosing a regular source of care
            (2) Reasons for considering changing a regular source of care
      2. Evaluated
         a. Physician severity ratings of conditions reported for episode (two week disability)
         b. Physician severity ratings for symptoms experienced in the year

III. Realized Access–Objective Indicators: utilization of health services
   A. Type
      1. Physician
      2. Hospital
      3. Dentist
      4. Optical services

B. Site
   1. Location of nonhospitalized visits with physician in the year—home, office, telephone
   2. Location of most recent visit with a physician in the year
   3. Location of visits to a physician in connection with illness episode

C. Purpose
   1. Preventive
      a. General physical exam and related tests
      b. Pregnancy-related use
   2. Illness-related
      a. Response to symptoms experienced in the year
      b. Use in response to disability experienced in previous two weeks and in the year
      c. Whether person needed to use certain services, but did not, and why
         (1) Physician
         (2) Dentist
         (3) Optical services
   3. Custodial
      a. Nursing home stays reported in connection with illness episode
      b. Arrangements for posthospitalization care in connection with illness episode

D. Time inverval
   1. Contact
      a. Percent seeing a physician in the year
      b. Percent hospitalized in the year
      c. Percent seeing a dentist in the year
      d. Percent seeing an eye doctor in the year
   2. Volume
      a. Mean physician visits in the year
      b. Mean hospital days in the year
      c. Mean dentist visits in the year
      d. Mean eye doctor visits in the year
   3. Continuity
      a. Pattern of care in response to illness episodes
      b. Summary indexes of continuity of care

IV. Realized Access–Subjective Indicators: consumer satisfaction
   A. General attitudes (based on personal and family experiences in general)
   B. Specific attitudes (based on most recent visit to a physician)
   C. Compliance (following doctor's advice regarding use of prescribed medicines, return visits, hospitalizations in connection with illness episode)

(continued)

(Figure 6.2 continued)

a. The operational indicators listed here correspond to those collected in the 1975–76 national survey to represent the respective aspects of the framework. Findings are not presented here on all of these indicators.

b. These resource variables were obtained from the American Medical Association (AMA) and the National Center for Health Statistics (NCHS) (American Medical Association, 1975; National Center For Health Statistics 1976) for the counties represented in our sample. The county information on the actual number of resources and persons was then attached to the record of each individual selected from that county.

c. This information is not, as emphasized in the discussion in the text of the framework, actually obtained from sources using the delivery system or a particular service organization as the unit of analysis. The indicators listed were actually collected in the 1975–76 survey of consumers. They are included here under the "delivery system" subheading simply to point up the types of entry and structure data on access that might be collected, using a particular delivery organization as the observational unit. Information on sources of medical care used by those with no regular source is only obtainable from a survey of individuals in population-at-risk, however.

general physical health or of particular presenting complaints, an equitable system of health resource allocation is said to exist. Inequity is suggested, however, if services are distributed on the basis of demographic variables such as race, family income, or place of residence rather than need.

Verbrugge (1980) suggests that increasing attention should be given to measuring inequity, drawing on models of race and sex discrimination applied in other disciplines, for example. Blumstein and Zubkoff (1979) express the concern that value judgments are implicit in any efforts to define equity and that benefits must be weighed in relationship to the costs to society of pursuing this value as a major national health policy goal.

In the analyses that follow, inequity will generally be interpreted to mean that the access levels for a particular group compare unfavorably to the national average or to other groups in the population. In most cases, the results of direct adjustments for variant levels of need among the different population subgroups of interest will be discussed, so that inequity (due to factors other than illness) can be evaluated. Methodological and policy-relevant caveats concerning this approach to measuring equity will be discussed in more detail later.

The Data

The primary set of data on which the findings to be presented are based is a household survey of the United States population conducted in late 1975 and early 1976 by the Center for Health Administration Studies and the National Opinion Research Center (CHAS-NORC) at the University of Chicago.

The 1975–76 study is the fifth in a series of national household surveys of health care utilization and expenditures conducted by the Center for Health Administration Studies. The previous four surveys— conducted in 1953, 1958, 1964, and 1971—emphasized estimates of families' total health care experiences and costs (Anderson and Feldman 1956; Anderson et al. 1963; Andersen and Anderson 1967; Andersen et al. 1976), while the most recent study concerned individuals' access to the health care system and problems they encountered in obtaining care when they needed it (Aday et al. 1980).

In the 1975–76 study, interviews were conducted in 5,432 households representing the noninstitutionalized population of the United States. An adult and child under 17 years of age (if one lived in the household) were selected at random from each household, yielding a sample of 7,787 individuals. The overall response rate for the survey was 85 percent. In addition to a probability sample of the noninstitutionalized population, there was also supplementary sampling of persons (non–SMSA Southern blacks and Spanish-heritage persons living in the southwestern states) experiencing episodes of illness. These groups were thought to have special problems of access, and hence oversampling was done to ensure that a sufficient number of cases would be available for analysis. All data in the tables presented in this paper are based on weighted distributions to correct for the oversampling of these groups and to allow estimates to be made for the total noninstitutionalized population of the United States. The sampling errors associated with estimates for the minority samples are, in some cases, still quite high, however. Sampling (standard) errors are, therefore, reported in the tables so that the data can be more appropriately interpreted. See the Methodological Appendix at the end of this paper for a fuller description of the variables used in the analysis and the approach used to estimate standard errors. Generally, in discussing the findings, differences that are equal to or greater than at least two standard errors of the difference between the groups being compared (i.e., $p \leq .05$ that difference occurred by chance) are emphasized.

The Findings

Some groups that have traditionally been considered disadvantaged in our society with respect to both potential and realized indicators of access to medical care include the elderly and children (particularly poverty-income members of these age groups), farm dwellers and inner city residents, low income people in general, and racial and ethnic minorities. Data from previous national studies do show that these persons have, at least in the past, fared the worst in terms of overall access rates, relative to the national average. Evidence from the most recent national survey shows that these historical inequities may be disappearing, however.

In the analyses that follow, particular attention will be devoted to summarizing the current access profiles for these traditionally disadvantaged subgroups. Afterwards, explanations for remaining differentials for selected groups that appear to fare the worst in comparison to the nation as a whole will be pursued. Of special interest will be hypotheses relating to mutable factors which, in fact, health policy might manipulate to reduce persisting inequities.[1] In selecting the variables to examine, particular attention will be given to those factors that are representative of the broad health policy approaches currently being applied or proposed to remedy these problems. The general health policy categories to be considered parallel the availability, organization, and financing characteristics outlined in our theoretical framework.

The figures reported in the tables are not adjusted for age, sex, and need differences unless indicated. Analyses incorporating such an adjustment showed that the differences accounted for very little of the variance between the subgroups reported here.[2] The standard errors associated with any given estimate were generally higher than the variance associated with these equitable population characteristic adjustments per se. Any statistically significant variation between subgroups reported in the tables can then be interpreted as due primarily to factors other than illness, such as inequitable system or individual characteristics.

According to table 6.1, young children and the elderly in general are

TABLE 6.1

Potential access barriers for selected population subgroups (United States, 1976)[a]

Population subgroups	Percent with no regular source of medical care	Percent who wait more than 30 minutes in office to see regular source of care	Percent under 65 years of age without insurance coverage
Age and poverty level			
Young children (1–5 years)	[b]	[b]	
Poor	5 (1.1) [b	30 (2.3)	14 (1.5)
Nonpoor	6 (2.4)	38 (5.4)]b	26 (4.8)]b
	5 (1.5)	26 (2.9)	9 (2.0)
Elderly (65 years and over)		[b	
Poor	9 (1.3)	40 (2.5)	—
Nonpoor	12 (2.6)]	48 (4.1)]b	—
	8 (2.0)	36 (3.2)]	—
Place of residence			
Rural farm	7 (1.5)[b]	47 (3.4)[b]	17 (2.7)[b]
Urban inner city	15 (1.0)	33 (1.7)	14 (1.0)
Suburban	13 (0.8)	31 (1.2)	10 (0.8)
Family income			
Low	14 (0.8)[b]	43 (1.3)[b]	28 (1.2)[b]
High	11 (0.8)	32 (1.2)	5 (0.6)
Race			
Urban black	16 (2.0)	38 (3.3)[b]	16 (2.0)[b]
Rural Southern black	10 (2.3)	56 (3.8)	21 (3.0)
Spanish-heritage, southwest	17 (4.6)	35 (5.4)	35 (5.4)
Majority white	12 (0.6)	35 (1.0)	10 (0.6)
National average	12 (0.5)	36 (0.8)	12 (0.5)

a. Numbers in parentheses are the standard errors of these estimates.
b. Highest and lowest categories of this variable differ significantly (p ≤ .05).

not disadvantaged with respect to the national average in terms of having a regular point of entry to the health care system or the convenience of the wait they usually experience before actually seeing the provider when they go for care. Among the elderly who do have a regular source of health care, a larger proportion of the poor than the nonpoor have to wait more than half an hour to see the doctor, however. Poor children also average longer waits than children from higher income families. Children in poor families are also more likely to have no form of third-party health insurance in contrast to those from more well-to-do homes.

There is a somewhat greater tendency for urban inner-city dwellers to lack a regular source of care, particularly compared to people who live on farms in rural areas. Rural farm dwellers tend to experience much longer waits at their regular source of care before seeing the physician, however. Larger proportions of the rural farm and urban inner-city populations are uninsured in comparison to suburbanites. Farmers are probably less likely as a group to have health insurance because most are self-employed, and therefore are not as apt to be covered through their jobs as people in other professions. Some "working poor" inner-city minorities may not be able to afford private insurance but are not poor enough to be eligible for Medicaid benefits.

Differences in the proportion of low and high income persons who reported not having a regular source of medical care still exist; 14 percent of low income persons and 11 percent of high income persons cannot identify a routine point of entry to the health care system. This gap between the high and low income groups has narrowed since 1970, when the proportions were 16 percent for the low income group and 8 percent for the high income group (Aday et al. 1980).

A larger proportion of the low income group experiences long waits to see a doctor compared to their high income counterparts, however. This, to some degree, is a function of where they go more often for care (hospital outpatient departments and emergency rooms, for example) and the fact that they are less apt to make an appointment to see the doctor for that visit. Despite the advent of Medicaid, larger proportions of the poor, compared to the nonpoor, have no form of health insurance coverage. Having coverage (particularly private coverage) is highly associated with whether and in what type of job the person is employed. Many marginally poor also do not qualify for Medicaid.

Among people with a regular source of care, rural Southern blacks experience the longest waits compared to any of the other groups. All of the ethnic minorities are less likely to have any form of third-party coverage against the potentially high cost of serious illness than majority whites. This is particularly true for the rural Southern black and Spanish-heritage groups.

Table 6.2 provides an overview of how different groups fare in respect to objective and subjective indicators of realized access. As with the process indicators just examined, young children and the elderly, in general, are not significantly below the national average. The score on a physician-norm based indicator of the proportion of necessary services received for symptoms experienced does, in fact, show that young children tend to be substantial overutilizers of services compared to what a panel of physicians deemed appropriate.[3] This is undoubtedly to some degree a function of the large number of routine visits usually required for this age group, in which existing symptoms might also be treated, and to the higher rates of phone calls to physicians from parents worried about their child's illness. The higher rates of nonuse of dental services for the very young and the very old, relative to the national average, is a function of the lower need for dental care on the part of these age groups, compared to older children and young and middle-aged adults. As was the case with the potential access barriers, it is the low income people in each age group who deserve attention the most with respect to identifying unfavorable realized access rates. Compared to their higher income counterparts they have poor scores on all of the indicators of realized access. More dissatisfaction seems to be registered by parents about the amount of time they have to wait to obtain care for their children than by the elderly who voiced lower levels of dissatisfaction with the amount of time they had to wait. Poor parents tend to register more dissatisfaction than do well-to-do parents—especially concerning their out-of-pocket cost of their child's most recent visit to a physician.

Rural farm dwellers do not do as well as urban residents with respect to physician contact rates in general and in terms of actually seeking care when they experience symptoms of illness.

There is still a differential in overall physician contact rates by income. This gap has narrowed substantially over the past fifteen to twenty years, however. For example, during the year 1963, 44 percent of low income persons had not seen a doctor compared to 29 percent of the high income individuals. By 1970 the proportion of low income

TABLE 6.2

Realized access indicators for selected population subgroups (United States, 1976)

Population subgroups	Objective (Utilization) Indicators[a]			Subjective (Satisfaction) Indicators[a]	
	Percent with no doctor visit in year	Percent seeing doctor for symptoms more or less often than "necessary"	Percent with no dentist visit in year	Percent dissatisfied with cost of most recent medical visit	Percent dissatisfied with office waiting time on most recent medical visit
Age and poverty level					
Young children (1–5 years)	[b]13 (1.5)	[b]+20[c]	[b]76 (2.2)	43 (3.3)	[b]30 (2.3)
Poor	25 (3.7)[b]	+5	84 (3.4)[b]	59 (7.9)[b]	39 (5.4)
Nonpoor	8 (2.0)	+25[c]	72 (3.1)	39 (3.3)	28 (3.1)
Elderly (65 years and over)	21 (1.7)	−1	67 (2.0)	37 (3.2)	24 (2.2)
Poor	28 (3.9)[b]	−8	78 (2.7)[b]	40 (5.4)	29 (3.9)
Nonpoor	18 (2.0)	+3	62 (2.5)	36 (4.1)	22 (2.7)
Place of residence					
Rural farm	32 (3.1)[b]	−12[c]	55 (3.4)	36 (4.1)	27 (3.7)
Urban inner city	23 (1.2)	−4[c]	49 (1.4)	40 (2.1)	29 (1.6)
Suburban	22 (1.1)	−5[c]	48 (1.4)	36 (1.7)	27 (1.5)

Family income					
Low	27 (1.2)[b]	−5[c]	67 (1.3)[b]	42 (1.7)[b]	33 (1.6)[b]
High	21 (1.1)	−6[c]	39 (1.3)	35 (2.0)	25 (1.5)
Race					
Urban black	23 (2.0)[b]	−2	61 (2.5)[b]	43 (5.4)	37 (3.2)[b]
Rural Southern black	35 (3.6)	−1	82 (3.0)	45 (6.3)	39 (5.0)
Spanish-heritage, southwest	35 (5.4)	−10[c]	69 (5.4)	39 (8.9)	32 (6.2)
Majority white	23 (0.9)	−6[c]	48 (1.1)	37 (1.3)	27 (0.9)
National Average	24 (0.7)	−5[c]	51 (0.8)	37 (1.0)	28 (1.0)

a. Numbers in parentheses are standard errors of these estimates.

b. Highest and lowest categories of this variable differ significantly (p ≤ .05).

c. This indicates that people's actual behavior in response to symptoms and what physicians thought appropriate differed significantly (p ≤ .05) based on a modified chi-square statistic. Standard error estimates per se are not available for this ratio. See the Methodological Appendix for a discussion of the index and test of significance.

persons in this category was reduced to 35 percent, while the high income group rate remained relatively constant. In 1976 the rates were 27 percent for low income persons and 21 percent for high income persons (table 6.2). Similarly, while in years prior to 1976 the indicator of necessary services received showed substantial gaps between high and low income persons (with the low income group having much lower scores [Aday et al. 1980]), the 1976 data show that there is essentially no difference with respect to this particular indicator of realized access. Substantial income differentials persist for dental services utilization. This particular service is still not covered by most of the major health care financing and program initiatives introduced during the past ten to fifteen years. Many other educational and attitudinal factors are also associated with the utilization of this particular type of service, which may help to account for this continuing income differential. Low income people also continue to be more dissatisfied than higher income individuals with the cost and convenience of obtaining care.

The rural Southern blacks and Spanish-heritage groups in the Southwest tend to have the highest proportions of people who did not see a doctor or dentist during the year. Significantly more urban blacks than majority whites also had no contact with a dentist in the year. Because of the sampling error associated with the "necessary" care index for the racial minority groups in particular, caution should be exercised in generalizing from the findings for these groups. It does appear, however, that the Spanish-heritage group may tend to have lower scores (they see a doctor less often than they should), especially compared to nonwhites. As with the variation noted earlier for different income groups, the realized access differentials for whites and nonwhites on these particular indicators compare much more favorably in 1976 than in previous years. For example, in 1963 the proportion of nonwhites not seeing a doctor was around one-half (51 percent) compared to about one-third (32 percent) of the whites. By 1970 the rates had narrowed to 42 percent and 30 percent, respectively; and by 1976 the white–nonwhite differential had effectively disappeared: 26 percent of the nonwhites had not seen a doctor compared to 24 percent of the whites (Aday et al. 1980). As with physician contact rate differences, the white–nonwhite gap in dental services utilization has been reduced over time, though differences still remain. Nonwhites, especially rural Southern blacks, tend to see a dentist substantially less often than do majority whites. The Spanish-heritage group in the Southwest also contained a large number of people who had not seen a dentist during the year. There is a tendency for nonwhites to be more dissatisfied than whites with the cost and convenience of the care they receive. The proportion of urban and rural Southern blacks dissatisfied with their waiting time to obtain care, in particular, differs in a statistically significant way from the level of dissatisfaction expressed by majority whites with this aspect of care.

The preceding summary has suggested that there are groups in our population for whom pockets of inequity of access remain. In tables 6.3 through 6.10 the impact of the characteristics of the population-at-risk and the delivery system, which may help account for these differences (for the racial groups in particular), is explored. Inequity of access to medical care (and other services) for different racial subgroups in our society has been a prominent source of concern since the birth of the civil rights movement some twenty years ago. There is evidence, as we have seen, that many of the overall white–nonwhite medical access differentials that existed when this movement began have narrowed or even disappeared. For certain subgroups (rural Southern blacks and Spanish-heritage persons in the Southwest, for example) some apparent inequities remain, however. Special oversampling of these groups in our study permits their access situation to be brought into clearer focus, so that reasons for the remaining inequities can be identified and, eventually, more informed solutions to their problems be undertaken.

Decisions concerning which variables to consider in examining particular access indicators were guided by (1) our analytic framework outlined earlier in figures 6.1 and 6.2, (2) previous empirical research on the correlates of these indicators, (3) those target groups which have been the special focus of health care program design in recent years, and (4) the extent to which the variable represents a current health policy or program emphasis. For example, low income groups traditionally have been the focus of health policy efforts, and there has been evidence in the past that poor people encounter more access barriers than the well-to-do. Therefore, in each of the tables, the effect of family income levels on the different racial groups' access experience will be presented. In addition, other variables which identify target groups that may have special access problems along the dimensions being considered are examined. Most major health policy emphases at the present time involve some effort to influence either the availability, the organization, or the financing of medical care by increasing the supply of providers, enrolling individuals in formal primary care arrangements such as health maintenance organizations (HMOs), or extending coverage against the financial hardships of catastrophic illness. As appropriate, factors representative of these broad health policy emphases are examined in relationship to the access dimensions being considered here. In general, variables for which the categories of the variable having the highest and lowest scores on the access indicator differ by at least two standard errors of their difference ($p \leq .05$) for the population as a whole or one of the racial subgroups are reported in tables 6.3 through 6.10.

According to table 6.3, poor people are less likely to have a regular family doctor than the more well-to-do. The findings for the availability factor—the distribution of physicians in the area in which the person resides—are in a direction opposite from that which might be predicted. The proportion of people without a regular source of care tends to be higher in areas with the highest concentration of physicians. This finding undoubtedly reflects the association of the physician distribution variable with the rural–urban character of the place in which individuals live and the forms of care generally available in those areas. Places with low physician-to-population ratios tend to be rural, whereas the concentration of physicians is higher—and also the distribution of specialties much different—in densely settled urban areas. People in rural communities that have few physicians are more likely to identify some provider they would go to for care regularly than are people in large cities, because of the different models of care generally available in those areas. In rural communities there tend to be few physicians (most are in solo practice) who can be readily named by area residents; in contrast are the plethora of large-scale institutional providers (such as hospital outpatient departments and emergency rooms or public health clinics) to which people may go in urban areas.

Whether a person has health insurance is also associated with whether he or she can identify a particular person or place to go to if care is required. The correlation of insurance coverage and having a regular source of health care is registered most clearly for the majority whites and Spanish-heritage persons living in the Southwest, though the relationship for this latter group is not statistically significant be-

TABLE 6.3

Potential access barriers: Percent with no regular source of medical care by race by selected subgroup characteristics (United States, 1976)[a]

Subgroup characteristics	Majority white	Urban black	Rural Southern black	Spanish-heritage, Southwest	National average
Poverty Level					
Poor	13 (1.3)[b]	20 (3.4)	12 (3.0)	20 (7.3)	15 (1.0)[b]
Nonpoor	11 (0.6)	14 (2.0)	7 (2.9)	14 (2.3)	11 (0.6)
Physician-to-Population Ratio					
0–66 physicians/100,000	10 (1.3)[b]	NA	7 (2.9)	13 (7.0)	10 (1.0)[b]
67–110 physicians/100,000	10 (1.0)	8 (4.1)[b]	12 (3.0)	6 (6.5)	10 (0.8)
111+ physicians/100,000	13 (0.8)	18 (2.7)	NA	21 (5.4)	15 (0.8)
Insurance Coverage					
Uninsured	22 (2.7)[b]	27 (7.0)	17 (8.1)	31 (10.5)	23 (1.9)[b]
Insured	11 (0.6)	14 (2.0)	9 (3.0)	11 (4.1)	11 (0.5)
National Average					
Unadjusted	12 (0.6)	16 (2.0)	10 (2.3)	17 (4.6)	12 (0.5)
[Adjusted for equitable population characteristics]	[11 (0.6)]	[16 (2.0)]	[11 (2.3)]	[16 (4.6)]	NA

a. Numbers in parentheses are standard errors of these estimates.

b. Highest and lowest categories of this variable differ significantly (p ≤ .05).

NA indicates that estimate was based on fewer than 25 observations when it appears in the "Subgroup Characteristics" breakdowns and for the "National Average" it means the adjustment for equitable population characteristics was not applicable to the national average.

TABLE 6.4

Potential access barriers: Percent who wait more than 30 minutes in office to see regular source of care by race by selected subgroup characteristics (United States, 1976)[a]

Subgroup characteristics	Majority white	Urban black	Rural Southern black	Spanish-heritage, Southwest	National average
Poverty Level					
Poor	43 (2.5)[b]	48 (5.5)[b]	60 (5.0)	38 (8.9)	45 (2.1)[b]
Nonpoor	34 (1.0)	32 (3.1)	50 (6.5)	32 (4.7)	34 (1.0)
Physician-to-Population Ratio					
0–66 physicians/100,000	41 (2.1)[b]	NA	62 (6.3)	41 (14.6)	42 (2.1)[b]
67–110 physicians/100,000	20 (1.4)	28 (7.4)	53 (5.1)	38 (14.6)	40 (1.3)
111+ physicians/100,000	29 (1.2)	40 (3.3)	NA	33 (6.2)	31 (1.2)
Location of Regular Source of Care					
Hospital OPD or ER	46 (4.3)[b]	53 (5.5)[b]	68 (14.7)	44 (21.3)	49 (3.4)[b]
Doctor's office or private clinic	35 (1.0)	31 (3.1)	55 (5.1)	33 (6.2)	35 (0.8)
Type of Regular Source of Care					
Does not see particular doctor	44 (3.3)[b]	48 (5.5)[b]	54 (16.1)	52 (18.4)	46 (2.6)[b]
Does see particular doctor	34 (1.0)	33 (3.2)	57 (5.0)	33 (6.5)	35 (0.8)
Specialty of Regular Source of Care					
General practitioner	37 (1.3)[b]	36 (5.3)	61 (6.3)[b]	35 (8.6)	38 (1.3)[b]
Specialist	32 (1.2)	29 (3.9)	49 (6.5)	29 (10.5)	32 (1.2)

Appointment Arrangements at

Regular Source of Care				
Just walks in	56 (2.5)[b]	46 (5.5)	65 (6.2)	44 (8.9)	55 (1.7)[b]
Arranges appointment in advance	31 (1.0)	35 (3.2)	49 (6.5)	30 (8.4)	31 (1.0)
Insurance Coverage				
Uninsured	41 (2.5)[b]	38 (6.6)	65 (8.0)	39 (8.9)	41 (1.7)[b]
Insured	35 (1.0)	38 (3.3)	55 (5.1)	34 (6.5)	36 (0.8)
National Average				
Unadjusted	35 (1.0)	38 (3.3)	56 (5.0)	35 (5.4)	36 (0.8)
[Adjusted for equitable population characteristics]	[35 (1.0)]	[37 (3.3)]	[54 (5.0)]	[35 (5.4)]	NA

a. Numbers in parentheses are standard errors of these estimates.

b. Highest and lowest categories of this variable differ significantly ($p \leq .05$).

NA indicates that the estimate was based on fewer than 25 observations when it appears in the "Subgroup Characteristics" breakdowns and for the "National Average" it means the adjustment for equitable population characteristics was not applicable to the national average.

cause of the large standard errors associated with the estimate for the group.

Table 6.4 shows that there is a tendency for poor people to average longer waits in providers' waiting rooms compared to people with higher incomes. Health care system resource availability and organizational factors are particularly important in understanding which groups may experience the most inconvenience along this dimension and why. The supply of physicians in the community, the type of facility to which the person usually goes for medical care, whether he or she generally sees a particular doctor there, the specialty of the attending physician, and whether visits to the facility are usually scheduled in advance—all these factors influence to some degree how long the patient has to wait before receiving treatment from the provider.

In general, when the supply of physicians in an area is relatively high, fewer people have long waits (except for the urban black group). Though this relationship is not a statistically significant one, it suggests, as did the data on this indicator in table 6.3, that the impact of the supply of providers in an area on the convenience of medical care must be considered in the context of the actual institutional arrangements in place for delivering these services. Urban blacks, it seems, would have shorter waiting times if they made less use of hospital emergency rooms and outpatient departments, or if they more often had available to them forms of care in which they could see one particular doctor when they went. Having an appointment arranged in advance of a visit to the physician generally means that the patient will not have to wait as long to be seen. Though the statistical significance of this difference is less for blacks than for majority whites, both urban and rural Southern blacks would appear to benefit from institutional arrangements in which their visits were scheduled in advanced rather than physicians' seeing them on a first come–first served basis. That general practitioners in rural areas of the South have particularly high patient loads and/or poor appointment scheduling systems is suggested by the high proportion of rural Southern blacks who have to wait more than half an hour to be seen when they go to such providers. There is also a tendency for people without insurance coverage to average longer waits.

According to table 6.5, some target groups which should receive particular attention in any efforts to expand insurance coverage benefits are the poor and those who are in families in which the main breadwinner has less than a high school education, is not employed, or, if working, is self-employed or in a nonprofessional-type job. Larger proportions of the poor of all racial groups are apt to have no insurance against the potentially high costs of serious illness. This is particularly the case for poor Spanish-heritage people. In all racial groups, the proportion of people without insurance also tends to be higher in families whose head has a grammar school education or less compared to those in families whose head is college educated. The statistical significance of the impact of whether the head of the family is employed, and the professional or nonprofessional nature of his or her job, on whether family members are insured is the clearest for the majority white and urban black groups. Because of the small number of people who are self-employed in most of the minority groups, the impact of this factor on whether people are insured is the clearest for the majority white category. The fact of being poor, poorly educated, working in a nonprofessional job or in one's own business has an especially dramatic effect on whether Spanish-heritage people have insurance coverage—compared to their majority white counterparts—even taking into account the large standard errors associated with these estimates for the Spanish sample.

In table 6.6 we see that the poor are, in general, less likely to have seen a physician in the past year than those who have higher incomes. It seems that living in areas that have a shortage of physicians, not having a regular source of medical care or any general health insurance coverage are important policy-relevant correlates of physician noncontact rates.

On this indicator of realized access, too, urban blacks in areas of high overall physician concentration appear still to be at a disadvantage compared to those who do not reside in such areas. The sample sizes and associated standard errors are an issue in interpreting the findings for this and the rural Southern black group—for whom the same direction may be observed in this relationship. Once again, these findings suggest that in interpreting the impact of availability on access it may be important also to consider the types of institutional arrangements in which physicians' services are delivered in these areas.

Whether people can identify a particular place they go to when the need arises is a particularly important correlate of whether care is sought.[4] This effect is especially dramatic for the Spanish-heritage group. Furthermore, among urban blacks who can name some place

TABLE 6.5

Potential access barriers: Percent under 65 years of age with no insurance coverage by race by selected subgroup characteristics (United States, 1976)[a]

Subgroup characteristics	Majority white	Urban black	Rural Southern black	Spanish heritage, Southwest	National average
Poverty Level					
Poor	24 (2.2)[b]	28 (5.1)[b]	27 (5.6)[b]	47 (9.2)[b]	28 (1.6)[b]
Nonpoor	8 (0.6)	10 (2.0)	10 (3.9)	21 (3.0)	8 (0.6)
Education of Family Head					
8 years or less	21 (2.0)[b]	29 (7.4)[b]	27 (5.6)[b]	45 (9.2)	25 (1.5)[b]
9–11 years	15 (1.5)	19 (4.4)	15 (6.2)	23 (11.9)	16 (1.7)
12 years	8 (1.0)	16 (4.4)	6 (4.5)	30 (10.5)	10 (0.8)
13+ years	6 (0.8)	8 (3.3)	NA	17 (11.9)	7 (0.6)
Employment Status of Family Head					
Not working	21 (2.0)[b]	32 (5.1)[b]	24 (7.2)	34 (11.1)	23 (1.5)[b]
Working full or part time	8 (0.6)	11 (2.0)	20 (4.1)	35 (6.5)	10 (0.5)
Occupation of Family Head					
Not professional or managerial	12 (0.8)[b]	15 (2.0)[b]	23 (4.4)	39 (6.8)	14 (0.5)[b]
Professional or managerial	5 (0.8)	6 (3.5)	NA	16 (14.6)	6 (0.8)

Self-employment Status of Family Head

Self-employed	17 (2.0)[b]	34 (12.9)	46 (16.1)	69 (20.0)	20 (2.0)[b]
Not self-employed	9 (0.6)	12 (2.0)	20 (4.1)	30 (6.2)	10 (0.5)
National Average					
Unadjusted	10 (0.6)	16 (2.0)	21 (4.1)	35 (5.4)	12 (0.5)
[Adjusted for equitable population characteristics]	[10 (0.6)]	[16 (2.0)]	[21 (4.1)]	[34 (5.4)]	NA

a. Numbers in parentheses are standard errors of these estimates.

b. Highest and lowest categories of this variable differ significantly ($p \leq .05$). NA indicates that the estimate was based on fewer than 25 observations when it appears in the "Subgroup Characteristics" breakdowns and for the "National Average" it means the adjustment for equitable population characteristics was not applicable to the national average.

TABLE 6.6

Realized access (objective indicators): percent with no doctor visit in year by race by selected subgroup characteristics (United States, 1976)[a]

Subgroup characteristics	Majority white	Urban black	Rural Southern black	Spanish-heritage, Southwest	National average
Poverty Level					
Poor	27 (1.9)[b]	25 (3.7)	36 (4.8)	44 (8.9)	29 (1.2)[b]
Nonpoor	23 (0.9)	22 (2.7)	33 (6.2)	26 (3.3)	23 (0.9)
Physician-to-Population Ratio					
0–66 physicians/100,000	28 (1.6)[b]	NA	25 (5.6)	42 (11.3)	28 (1.6)[b]
67–110 physicians/100,000	24 (1.5)	13 (4.1)[b]	41 (5.0)	35 (14.3)	25 (1.2)
111+ physicians/100,000	21 (1.1)	25 (2.9)	NA	34 (6.5)	23 (0.9)
Type of Regular Source of Care					
No regular source	46 (2.6)[b]	52 (6.8)[b]	63 (11.9)[b]	67 (14.3)[b]	49 (2.1)[b]
Regular source, but does not see particular doctor	23 (2.9)	23 (4.8)	32 (14.7)	28 (13.8)	23 (2.2)
Regular source, does see particular doctor	20 (0.9)	15 (2.0)	32 (4.7)	29 (6.2)	20 (0.6)
Insurance Coverage					
Uninsured	32 (3.1)[b]	41 (7.9)[b]	45 (9.9)	54 (11.6)[b]	36 (2.0)[b]
Insured	23 (0.9)	20 (2.7)	33 (4.8)	26 (5.9)	23 (0.7)

National Average

Unadjusted	23 (0.9)	23 (2.2)	35 (3.6)	35 (5.4)	24 (0.7)
Adjusted for equitable population characteristics	[23 (0.9)]	[23 (2.2)]	[36 (3.6)]	[34 (5.4)]	[NA]

a. Numbers in parentheses are standard errors of these estimates.

b. Highest and lowest categories of this variable differ significantly (p ≤ .05).

NA indicates that the estimate was based on fewer than 25 observations when it appears in the "Subgroup Characteristics" breakdowns; for the "National Average" it means the adjustment for equitable population characteristics was not applicable to the national average.

they generally go to for medical care, those who see a particular physician average higher contact rates than those who do not.

Having general health insurance coverage seems to be associated with whether majority whites, urban blacks, and the Spanish-heritage population see a doctor during the year. The impact of this financial barrier and, to some degree, low income status in general, is particularly apparent for the Spanish-heritage group when comparing the proportion of low income or uninsured people in this racial group who did not see a doctor during the year to majority whites.

According to the physician-based norm indicator of necessary use (table 6.7) there is no systematic difference by income level with respect to whether people have contacted a doctor appropriately in response to symptoms. Though there is some indication that poor Spanish-heritage people tend to utilize services at lower rates than their higher income counterparts, the sampling errors associated with this estimate for this and the other ethnic minority groups is apt to be quite high. The impact of not having a regular source of care is quite substantial for most of the racial groups, however. Much larger proportions of people who do not have a regular point of entry to the system use fewer services in response to symptoms than the panel of physicians thought was appropriate. It appears that people residing in areas of physician manpower shortage see a physician less often than they should and that people who have no form of third-party coverage also seek fewer services for symptoms than those who do have such coverage. The sampling errors associated with the minority sample estimates in particular are apt to be quite large and should, therefore, be cautiously interpreted.

From table 6.8 we see that income continues to be a strong correlate of whether dental care is sought, as does the educational level of the head of the family and whether the family has dental visit insurance coverage. Further, people in areas of dental manpower shortage tend to average lower rates of dentist contact. The dramatic impact of low income and low educational levels on the propensity not to contact a dentist is borne out for most racial groups. The noncontact rate for poor and poorly educated rural Southern blacks is particularly striking in comparison to their majority white counterparts. The dental access rates of the Spanish-heritage group would appear to increase substantially if more of them were insured for the high cost of these services. The fact that there are fewer dentists available in an area also affects

TABLE 6.7

Realized access (objective indicators): Percent seeing a doctor for symptoms more or less often than "necessary" by race by selected subgroup characteristics (United States, 1976) [a]

Subgroup characteristics	Majority white	Urban black	Rural Southern black	Spanish-heritage, Southwest	National average
Poverty Level					
Poor	−8[b]	−2	+2	−13[b]	−7[b]
Nonpoor	−6[b]	−3	−8	−6	−6[b]
Physician-to-Population Ratio					
0–66 physicians/100,000	−12[b]	NA	+2	−5	−11[b]
67–110 physicians/100,000	−5[b]	+2	−3	−22[b]	−5[b]
111+ physicians/100,000	−3	−3	NA	−9[b]	−3[b]
Type of Regular Source of Care					
No regular source	−45[b]	−19	−29[b]	−49[b]	−42[b]
Regular source, but does not see particular doctor	−20[b]	−11	−5	−9	−18[b]
Regular source, but does see particular doctor	+1	+4	+3	−2	+1
Insurance Coverage					
Uninsured	−17[b]	−21[b]	−3	−29[b]	−19[b]
Insured	−4[b]	0	−1	−1	−3[b]
National Average	−6[b]	−2	−1	−10[b]	−5[b]

a. Numbers in parentheses are standard errors of these estimates.

b. This indicates that people's actual behavior in response to symptoms and what physicians thought appropriate differed significantly by chance (p ≤ .05) based on a modified chi-square statistic. Standard error estimates per se are not available for this ratio. See the Methodological Appendix for a discussion of the index and test of significance.

NA indicates that the estimate was based on fewer than 25 observations when it appears in the "Subgroup Characteristics" breakdowns and for the "National Average" it means the adjustment for equitable population characteristics was not applicable to the national average.

TABLE 6.8

Realized access (objective indicators): Percent with no dentist visit in year by race by selected subgroup characteristics (United States, 1976)[a]

Subgroup characteristics	Majority white	Urban black	Rural Southern black	Spanish-heritage, Southwest	National average
Poverty Level					
Poor	63 (2.0)[b]	70 (3.9)[b]	86 (3.0)[b]	77 (7.8)[b]	67 (1.3)[b]
Nonpoor	46 (1.1)	55 (3.3)	74 (5.6)	59 (3.8)	47 (0.8)
Education of Family Head					
8 years or less	70 (2.0)[b]	72 (6.2)[b]	85 (5.1)	75 (7.8)	72 (1.6)[b]
9–11 years	60 (2.5)	58 (5.4)	81 (8.1)	65 (14.3)	60 (2.1)
12 years	48 (1.7)	65 (5.3)	84 (8.1)	65 (14.3)	51 (1.4)
13+ years	35 (1.5)	54 (5.5)	61 (11.8)	56 (14.5)	36 (1.3)
Dentist-to-Population Ratio					
0–33 dentists/100,000	60 (2.5)[b]	70 (4.9)[b]	85 (3.0)	85 (9.1)	64 (1.7)[b]
34–55 dentists/100,000	50 (1.7)	65 (6.5)	77 (5.5)	73 (9.9)	52 (1.4)
56+ dentists/100,000	44 (1.3)	60 (2.5)	NA	64 (6.4)	48 (1.1)
Dental Visit Insurance Coverage					
Not covered	50 (1.1)[b]	64 (3.2)[b]	83 (3.0)	73 (5.1)	53 (0.8)[b]
Covered	43 (2.1)	52 (5.5)	NA	44 (14.6)	44 (1.7)
National Average					
Unadjusted	48 (1.1)	61 (2.5)	82 (3.0)	69 (5.4)	51 (0.8)
[Adjusted for equitable population characteristics]	[48 (1.1)]	[62 (2.5)]	[83 (3.0)]	[70 (5.4)]	NA

a. Numbers in parentheses indicate standard errors for these estimates.

b. Highest and lowest categories of this variable differ significantly (p ≤ .05). NA indicates that the estimate was based on fewer than 25 observations when it appears in the "Subgroup Characteristics" breakdowns and for the "National Average" it means the adjustment for equitable population characteristics was not applicable to the national average.

TABLE 6.9

Realized access (subjective indicators): Percent dissatisfied with cost of most recent medical visit by race by selected subgroup characteristics (United States, 1976)[a]

Subgroup characteristics	Majority white	Urban black	Rural Southern black	Spanish-heritage, Southwest	National average
Poverty Level					
Poor	46 (3.4)[b]	52 (10.7)	51 (8.3)	37 (14.3)	46 (2.6)[b]
Nonpoor	35 (1.3)	40 (5.4)	32 (9.3)	41 (6.3)	36 (1.3)
Insurance Coverage					
Uninsured	46 (4.3)[b]	NA	42 (15.8)	38 (17.8)	46 (3.4)[b]
Insured	36 (1.3)	41 (5.4)	45 (8.1)	40 (11.3)	36 (1.3)
Actual Out-of-pocket Cost of Most Recent Medical Visit					
$25 or more	57 (3.3)[b]	61 (10.5)[b]	81 (16.2)[b]	54 (28.9)	57 (2.5)[b]
$11–$24	41 (2.1)	54 (8.1)	59 (11.9)	53 (14.9)	43 (1.7)
$1–$10	26 (1.5)	25 (5.9)	33 (7.7)	20 (11.9)	26 (1.5)
National Average	37 (1.3)	43 (5.4)	45 (6.3)	39 (8.9)	37 (1.0)

a. Numbers in parentheses indicate standard errors for these estimates.

b. Highest and lowest categories of this variable differ significantly (p ≤ .05).

NA indicates that the estimate was based on fewer than 25 observations when it appears in the "Subgroup Characteristics" breakdowns and for the "National Average" it means the adjustment for equitable population characteristics was not applicable to the national average.

TABLE 6.10

Realized access (subjective indicators): Percent dissatisfied with office waiting time on most recent medical visit by race by selected subgroup characteristics (United States, 1976) [a]

Subgroup characteristics	Majority white	Urban black	Rural Southern black	Spanish-heritage, Southwest	National average
Poverty Level					
Poor	34 (2.4) [b]	36 (5.3)	44 (6.3) [b]	28 (8.4)	35 (1.7) [b]
Nonpoor	25 (1.2)	38 (4.2)	29 (7.7)	35 (4.8)	26 (0.9)
Location					
Hospital OPD or ER	29 (3.1)	48 (6.8) [b]	40 (15.8)	42 (2.1)	34 (2.0) [b]
Doctor's office or private clinic	26 (0.9)	33 (3.9)	40 (6.3)	31 (8.4)	27 (0.9)
Appointment Arrangements					
Just walked in	31 (2.3) [b]	41 (6.6)	38 (8.1)	34 (11.1)	33 (2.0) [b]
Arranged appointment in advance	26 (0.9)	36 (3.2)	39 (6.3)	31 (8.4)	27 (0.9)
Office Waiting Time					
More than one hour	86 (2.0) [b]	83 (6.5) [b]	78 (9.8) [b]	80 (14.6) [b]	85 (1.5) [b]
31 minutes to one hour	59 (2.5)	65 (7.7)	52 (10.2)	48 (18.4)	59 (2.1)
30 minutes or less	13 (0.8)	20 (3.4)	17 (5.1)	15 (5.4)	13 (0.6)
National Average	27 (0.9)	37 (3.2)	39 (6.3)	32 (6.2)	28 (1.0)

a. Numbers in parentheses indicate standard errors for these estimates.

b. Highest and lowest categories of this variable differ significantly ($p \le .05$).

whether care is sought by some of the racial groups, though dental noncontact rates tend to be highest for rural Southern black and Spanish-heritage residents of dental manpower shortage counties.

Table 6.9 examines the relationship between (1) the cost of the most recent medical visit and various family economic status indicators and (2) levels of satisfaction. People who are poor and have no general health insurance coverage tend to be more dissatisfied with the cost of care. The strongest predictor of satisfaction with the cost of the visit, however, is the actual out-of-pocket cost of the visit itself. The greatest dissatisfaction was registered by those who paid the most ($25 or more). The impact of income and insurance coverage status is strongest statistically for the majority whites. For this group and for urban and rural Southern blacks also, the actual cost of the visit has a substantial influence on whether people are satisfied. Though the standard errors are higher and hence the statistical significance lower, rural Southern blacks paying $25 or more for a visit seemed particularly dissatisfied compared to majority whites who had to pay this much or more, for example.

The most consistent correlates of whether people are satisfied with the time they have to wait when they go for care are their income level, where they go for care, whether they arrange an appointment in advance, and the actual time they have to wait before seeing the doctor (table 6.10). The specialty of the provider did not have a significant effect and, hence, is not reported here. As we saw earlier (in table 6.4) where people go and whether they set up appointments in advance influence the amount of time they actually spend waiting to see the doctor. For the various racial groups, it is the time people ultimately spend "cooling their heels" which is the strongest determinant of how satisfied they are with the experience. Dissatisfaction is much higher for those who must wait an hour or more compared to those who see the doctor within half an hour. Urban blacks who go to hospital emergency rooms or outpatient departments can be expected to be much more dissatisfied with this aspect of their care than those who see private physicians.

Conclusions and Implications

In the preceding analyses, those groups having the greatest differentials in potential and realized access to medical care were examined.

In the discussion that follows, these findings will be reviewed, and their implications for the design of public policy solutions to deal most effectively with these persistent inequities will be discussed.

On most indicators, the rural farm population, ethnic minorities, and economically disadvantaged groups as a whole continue to experience the lowest rates of potential and realized access to medical care. The inequity gaps have narrowed considerably over the past fifteen to twenty years, however. For example, there is some evidence now that high and low income people contact doctors at similar rates when they experience symptoms of illness and that there is very little difference in the rates at which whites and nonwhites contact a physician for medical care.

The method used to explore the inequities that continue to exist (particularly for selected racial and ethnic minority groups) may be viewed as a way of translating the various health policy options being considered into an empirical language that can then be used to understand and predict better the probable contribution of these alternative solutions to the remaining problems. The broad health policy areas that are considered in dealing with the inequities parallel the availability and organizational and financial dimensions of access outlined earlier (figure 6.2). Specific programs have been developed or are proposed, which attempt to operationalize these various approaches. Examples are the following:

Health Policy Emphasis	**Program Examples**
Availability:	Health planning
	Certificate of need
	Hospital construction or conversion
	Expansion of medical schools
	National Health Service Corps
	Allied Health Training Programs
	Design of targeted services (migrant health, maternal and infant, Indian Health Service)
Organization:	Health maintenance organizations (HMOs)
	Hospital sponsored ambulatory care program

Community health centers
Emergency medical systems
Development of family practice
specialty

Financing: National Health Insurance
Medicaid
Medicare

The descriptive analyses reported here are suggestive of the kinds of programs that may be most effective in reducing remaining differentials on the respective equity indicators. More comprehensive analyses controlling for the relative contribution of these various factors would provide clearer evidence of the probable independent impact of these and other alternatives, however. Furthermore, though these analyses point out the associations among the various potential and realized access indicators, the precise cause-and-effect relationships between them remains to be specified.

Several caveats concerning the approach to measuring equity employed here should be mentioned. For example, as noted earlier, Blumstein and Zubkoff (1979) point out that value judgments concerning a right to health are implicit in any attempts to redistribute services equitably. Different types of medical providers, and consumers themselves, may well differ with respect to norms of adequate or appropriate medical care. An alternative approach to equity may focus on the equality of inputs or resources available for the purchase of care (for instance, income), rather than on consumption relative to some standard of need or medically appropriate care. Furthermore, different types of indicators, such as doctor contact rates rather than satisfaction levels, may well yield different conclusions about whether the equity goal has been achieved. Caution should also be exercised in concentrating upon a single indicator in making judgments of equity. Though mean rates of physician visits may be very similar for the high and low income groups, the proportion of the low income group that had not seen a doctor at all during the year is still greater. Focusing on the mean estimates alone, which are much more a function of unmet need levels and physician decision making once entry is gained, would not provide the most accurate access profile for these groups. In addition, whatever criterion is adopted for judging the achievement of the equity goal must still be evaluated in the context of the monetary and nonmonetary (for example, queuing) costs to the consumers and to the health care system itself in achieving that goal.

The analyses reported here suggest that efforts to increase the supply of providers must take into account the existing forms of service delivery if the greatest improvements in potential and realized access are to be achieved. For certain access indicators (dental care use, for example), income and educational considerations as well as direct third-party coverage issues also loom as important factors to consider in designing ways to improve the existing profile of care, particularly for minority groups.

Great possibilities for improving the potential and realized access to general health care services would seem to be available through various health care reorganization strategies. People who do not have a routine place to go to for medical care are much less likely to see a doctor, generally or when they need specific care. System reorganization approaches (such as enrolling groups of individuals in health maintenance organizations or converting the fragmented services of hospital outpatient departments to comprehensive, family-centered group practice models) may help to reduce the inconvenience and dissatisfaction which the poor and ethnic (especially urban and rural Southern black) minorities now frequently experience when obtaining care through existing arrangements. Encouraging physicians and patients to set up appointment systems to reduce the queues for care in big-city outpatient departments and overcrowded solo general practitioners' offices in the rural South may bring about improvements in access, as would efforts to insure that patients are able to have one provider they can identify and relate to as their family doctor.

Major financing initiatives (Medicare and Medicaid) have been credited with reducing many of the historical inequities—by race and income in particular— over the past two decades. There is evidence that the relative status of certain groups could still be enhanced if more universal third-party financing were available. Ethnic minorities, especially the Spanish-heritage population, have lower rates of third-party coverage than does the majority white population. Educational and occupational status differences help explain these differentials. Poorly educated ethnic minorities are less likely to be in jobs that provide such coverage. Furthermore, the marginal working poor are still not "poor" enough to qualify for Medicaid. In designing new federal financing initiatives, special attention could be devoted to those groups that fall between the cracks of existing third-party schemes. There is evidence that financial barriers significantly affect individuals' potential and realized access and how satisfactory they consider their experience in obtaining care to be. Options that focus on providing coverage to those persons who currently have no protection against the potentially high cost of illness, and the integration of these financing mechanisms with models of service delivery that attempt to contain the cost and ensure the quality and convenience of care to consumers, are needed to reduce the persisting inequity.

In summary, it is clear that any discussion of "equity of access" must take into account what dimension of access is being considered, as well as which target groups are of interest. In general, the plethora of existing and proposed health care programs represent a variant range of problems and target populations. Broadly applied financial initiatives such as Medicaid and Medicare have contributed substantially to improving the access of many traditionally disadvantaged groups. Inequities remain, however. For many individuals the design and convenience of the care systems available to them inhibit their seeking care or diminish their level of satisfaction when they do seek care. The analyses reported here suggest that the most cost-efficient health policy approach to these problems would be to focus on the remaining pockets of inequity and on the systematic integration of both financial and organizational solutions to dealing with them.

Chapter Six Methodological Appendix: Variable Definitions[5]

Population Subgroups

Age Age refers to the person's age as of the actual date of the interview.

Poverty level The poverty level cutting points were based on a table of "Poverty Cutoffs" for 1975, published in *Current Population Reports,* series P-60, no. 103 (September 1976), adjusted for family size, sex of the family head, and farm–nonfarm residence. The income levels provided in table 16 of that report were multipled by 1.25 to include more of the marginal poor in the poverty level category.

Place of residence A rural farm resident is one who resides in a place described as a farm by the interviewer (based on Census Bureau definition as a guide) and which is outside SMSAs or unincorporated areas within SMSAs that are in counties in which more than 50 percent of the population is defined as rural by the Census Bureau. Urban inner-city residents are those who reside in the central city of an SMSA. Suburban residents are those who reside in the urban part of the suburbs of an SMSA.

Family income A family's total annual income from all members was classified as a low income if it were less than $8,000 and a high income if it were $15,000 or more.

Race Rural Southern blacks are blacks who reside outside SMSAs but within the Southern states; the Spanish-heritage, Southwest group was made up of persons residing in the Southwestern states (Arizona, California, Colorado, New Mexico, and Texas) who had Spanish surnames or who were from families in which the head or spouse spoke Spanish as a child. Urban blacks are actually all other nonwhites besides those in the rural Southern black group. A small proportion (around two percent) do not actually reside in urban areas. The majority whites are all those who are not in any of the other three racial groups.

Potential Access Barriers

Percent with no regular source of medical care Respondents were asked, "Is there one person or place in particular you usually go to when you are sick or want advice about your health?" People who said they went to chiropractors, nurses, or other medical care providers that are not M.D.s or D.O.s (doctors of osteopathy) were excluded from the observations on which the percentages reported here are based.

Percent who wait more than 30 minutes in an office to see a regular source of care Respondents with a regular source of care were asked how long they usually had to wait to see the doctor once they got there. This referred to the amount of time he or she waited before seeing the doctor, including any time spent waiting in an examining room before the doctor came to see him or her.

Percent under 65 years of age without insurance coverage A person under 65 years old was said to have group coverage if he or she reported that health insurance was provided through a place of work or other group membership (Grange, Farm Bureau, Medical Society, group retirement plan, etc.). Respondents were characterized as having Medicaid or reduced-price care if they were covered by Medicaid, Public Aid, or other health care center where they could get care at no cost or reduced rates and they had no group coverage. Persons who said they bought their health insurance directly and had no group policy, Medicaid, or other reduced-price care were reported to have "individual" coverage. The uninsured reflected in these percentages were those who reported none of the other three types of coverage. People 65 and over were not included in this variable as this age group effectively has "universal" coverage through the Medicare program.

Realized Access Indicators

Percent with no doctor visit in the year A physician visit includes seeing either a medical doctor or osteopath or his nurse or technician at the following sites: patient's home; doctor's office or private clinic; hospital outpatient department or emergency room; industrial, school, camp, or college health service; or any other clinic such as a board of health clinic or neighborhood health center. The variable reported here refers to the proportion of the sample who did not have at least one contact of this kind with a physician during the survey year.

Percent seeing a doctor for symptoms more or less often than "necessary" (symptoms–response ratio) The index (sometimes referred to as the symptoms–response ratio) is computed as follows:

$$\text{Symptoms–response ratio} = \frac{A - E}{E}(100),$$

where A is the actual number of persons that contact a doctor at

least once for symptoms and E is the MD estimates of the number
of persons that should contact a doctor for symptoms.

The MD estimates were obtained from a panel of practicing community physicians. They were asked to estimate how many people out
of 100 in a given age group with a particular symptom should see a
physician about it. See Appendix E in Aday, et al. (1980) for a fuller
description of how these physician norms were obtained. The ratio
basically reflects the difference between the actual number of visits
people had for symptoms of illness compared to the number the panel
of physicians recommended. A negative value means they saw a physician less often than the doctors thought necessary and a positive value
more often. The absolute scores on the index should be interpreted
with caution since the values contain a certain amount of sampling
error which cannot be readily estimated because of the integration of
data from these two data sources (doctors and patients) in the construction of the ratio. A and E were adjusted for age and sex using
Multiple Classification Analysis (MCA).

Percent with no dentist visit in the year Sample people were asked
whether they had visited a dentist within the survey year. Infants were
excluded from this variable however.

Percent dissatisfied with cost of the most recent medical visit
People who had a visit to a physician within the survey year were
asked how satisfied they were with various aspects of their most *recent*
visit (completely, mostly, moderately, slightly or not at all satisfied).
People who were "completely" or "mostly" satisfied were characterized as being "satisfied" with that aspect of the visit. All others
were classified as being "dissatisfied." Only people who paid something out-of-pocket for their most recent visit were asked how satisfied
they were with the cost of that visit. Proxy respondents who accompanied the sample person reported how satisfied they were with the
care the person received during that visit to the doctor.

**Percent dissatisfied with office waiting time on most recent medi-
cal visit** See the previous discussion on measurement of satisfaction
with the cost of the most recent medical visit.

Subgroup Characteristics

Poverty level See the description under "Population Subgroups."

Insurance coverage See the description under "Potential Access Barriers." People 65 years and over are included in this variable, however. Those with Medicare are classified as being insured.

Physician to population ratio Data on the number of patient-care physicians in the county in which a person lived were obtained from AMA's *Physician Distribution and Licensure in the U.S., 1974* (AMA 1975).

Type of regular source of care See the description under "Potential Access Barriers." Those respondents who said they had some place they usually went for medical care were asked, "Is that a medical doctor, an osteopath, a chiropractor or what?" Respondents who reported they saw a medical doctor or osteopath were queried further: "Is there one doctor in particular you usually see at (place)?" In 1976 respondents who said they used medical doctors (M.D.s) or osteopaths and said "yes" to the question concerning whether they saw "one doctor in particular" were characterized as having a "particular doctor" care source.

Specialty of regular source of care The specialty of the regular source of care was determined for persons who reported seeing a particular medical doctor or osteopath by first seeing if the physician's name was listed in the *AMA Directory of Physicians, 1973.* If so, the primary specialty recorded there was used to characterize the physician. If the physician's name could not be located in the directory, then the sample person's response to the following question was used to assign a specialty status: "Which of the specialties listed (on card handed respondent) best describes this doctor's *major* specialty?" Possible responses were general (family) practice, internal medicine, pediatrics, surgery, obstetrics-gynecology, or some other specialty.

Appointment arrangements at regular source of care To determine whether a sample person generally had an appointment at his regular source of care, he or she was asked, "Do you usually have an appointment ahead of time when you go to (place) or not?"

Location of regular source of care Persons who reported having a regular source of care were asked, "Where do you usually go—to a doctor's office, a clinic, a hospital, or some other place?" The responses for a doctor's office and hospital (OPD or ER) are reported here.

Education of family head The person identified as the head of the family was asked how many years of schooling he or she had.

Employment status of family head The head of the family was asked, "Which number (on card handed respondent) *best* describes your current employment situation?" The response categories provided were as follows: work full time, work part time, laid off or on strike, unemployed (looking for work), unemployed (not looking for work), retired, unable to work (disabled), keeping house, full-time student.

Occupation of family head Those persons who were currently working full or part time or others who had ever had a regular job or who had earned $500 or more from working in the past year were asked, "For whom (do/did) you work?"; "What kind of business or industry is this?"; "What kind of work (are you/were you) doing?"; "What (are/were) the most important activities or duties?" This information was then used to classify individuals according to the 1970 Census Occupational Categories.

Self-employment status of family head Heads of the families who were asked about the nature of their present or past occupation (see "occupation of family head") were queried, "Are you/were you . . . (1) an employee of a *private* company, business, or individual for wages, salary or commissions?; (2) a government employee (federal, state, county, or local)?; (3) self-employed in your own business?; (4) working *without pay* in family business or farm?"

Dental visit insurance coverage Persons who reported they had health insurance through work or a union, health insurance through some other group, or health insurance they bought directly as an individual or family were asked to tell us which of the following kinds of coverage their plan(s) provided: hospital expenses, surgical expenses, charges for prescribed medicine taken outside the hospital, charges for dental care, charges for visits to a doctor's office, and major medical expenses. People who had CHAMPUS (Civilian Health and Medical Program of the Uniformed Services) were assumed to have dentist visit coverage.

Dentist-to-population ratio The dentist-to-population ratio was computed by determining the number of dentists in the county in which the individual resided from the *Health Manpower: A County and Metropolitan Area Data Book, 1972–75* (National Center for Health Statistics 1976), dividing that number by the population in the county, and multiplying the result by 100,000.

Actual out-of-pocket cost of most recent medical visit Respondents who had a doctor visit in the year were asked how much they had to pay for their most recent visit after the amount covered by insurance was deducted.

Location (most recent medical visit) See discussion of "Location of regular source of care."

Appointment arrangements (most recent medical visit) Adult sample persons or proxies for children were asked whether they had an appointment for their most recent visit to a physician in the year or simply walked in.

Office waiting time (most recent medical visit) Information was elicited on how long the sample person had to wait before actually seeing the physician on his or her most recent visit to a physician.

Standard Error Computations

Approximate standard errors for the percentage estimates were computed using the unweighted numbers of observations on which the percentages were based and table 6.11 with design effect adjustment (as necessary) for the Spanish-heritage, Southwest, and rural Southern black groups. The table value "N" and "percents" below closest to the actual values were used in arriving at the standard errors reported in tables 6.1 through 6.10.

Test of Significance for Symptoms–Response Ratio

The symptoms-response ratio reflects the difference between the actual number of physician visits in response to symptoms and the expected number of physician visits in response to these symptoms (using norms from a group of physicians).

A statistically significant finding on the symptoms–response ratio means that the difference between the actual and estimated number of visits for symptoms by people in that population subgroup was greater than one would expect by chance, with a given probability of being in error ($P \leq .05$). The computational formula for the symptoms-response ratio, $(A - E)/E$, approximates that of a chi-square test statistic

$$\Sigma \frac{(O - E)^2}{E}$$

where O = observed frequencies and E = expected frequencies in the cells of a contingency table.

The following statistic, based on the formula for the symptoms–response index and the chi-square statistic, was computed for each population subgroup reported in the tables and was compared with the values in a chi-square distribution table (degrees of freedom=1) to see if the difference between the actual and expected values in the ratio differed significantly from chance for each group:

$$\frac{(A - E)^2}{E} .$$

Prior to computing the test statistic itself, the actual and estimated number of visits for each symptom for each subgroup were divided by the mean sample weight for that subgroup. This procedure serves to reduce values on the test statistic, inflated by the sample weighting factors. As such, it tends to make the significance test more conservative, i.e., it is more difficult to reject the null hypothesis that there is

TABLE 6.11

Standard errors[a] of estimated percentages: 1976[b]

Number of persons	Estimated percent								
	2 or 98	5 or 95	10 or 90	20 or 80	25 or 75	30 or 70	35 or 65	40 or 60	50
25	3.8	5.9	8.1	10.8	11.7	12.4	12.9	13.3	13.5
40	3.0	4.7	6.4	8.6	9.3	9.8	10.2	10.5	10.7
70	2.3	3.5	4.9	6.5	7.0	7.4	7.7	7.9	8.1
100	1.9	3.0	4.1	5.4	5.9	6.2	6.5	6.6	6.8
150	1.5	2.4	3.3	4.4	4.8	5.1	5.3	5.4	5.5
250	1.2	1.9	2.6	3.4	3.7	3.9	4.1	4.2	4.3
400	0.9	1.5	2.0	2.7	2.9	3.1	3.2	3.3	3.4
700	0.7	1.1	1.5	2.0	2.2	2.3	2.4	2.5	2.6
1,000	0.6	0.9	1.3	1.7	1.9	2.0	2.0	2.1	2.1
1,500	0.5	0.8	1.0	1.4	1.5	1.6	1.7	1.7	1.7
2,500	0.4	0.6	0.8	1.1	1.2	1.2	1.3	1.3	1.4
4,000	0.3	0.5	0.6	0.9	0.9	1.0	1.0	1.0	1.1
7,000	0.2	0.4	0.5	0.6	0.7	0.7	0.8	0.8	0.8

a. For the Spanish total and the Spanish below poverty: multiply by 2.7. For the Spanish above poverty, the nonwhite total, the Southern rural black total, and the Southern rural black below poverty: multiply by 1.5.

b. This table is based on an estimated design effect of 1.83 ($\sqrt{\text{DEFF}} = 1.35$).

no difference between the actual and expected values in the ratio because the magnitude of the test statistic becomes smaller.

A standard error cannot be computed on the ratio per se because information from two data sources (physicians and patients) were used in constructing the index.

Chapter 6 Notes

1. For a further explanation of the mutability concept in the context of determinants of medical care utilization see Andersen and Newman (1973).

2. This is apparent from the adjusted figures reported for the racial groups in tables 6.3 through 6.8. In all cases, age and sex and the need measures (e.g., perceived health level, amount of worry over health, number of disability days in the year, etc.) most highly correlated with the access indicator (Pearson r of at least .10 or higher) were incorporated in these MCA-based adjustments. These factors had very low correlations with patient satisfaction, and hence were not used to adjust those indicators.

3. See the Methodological Appendix for chapter 6 for a more detailed discussion of this index.

4. There is the question, of course, of whether having a regular source of care tends to lead to greater utilization, or whether people who have recently been ill and sought the services of a physician will be more likely than non-recent users to remember and claim they have a regular source of care. These relationships are very difficult to test using cross-sectional data. In a recent article applying a path analysis approach to operationalizing aspects of the framework, however, Andersen and Aday (1978) noted that the indirect effects of regular source of care through illness on utilization were relatively small compared with its large direct effect. They conclude that "even if the causal specification between regular source of care and illness in the model were totally incorrect the variable would still seem to have policy relevance because of its large direct effect."

5. Variables are generally arranged in the order in which they appear in the tables.

Chapter 6 References

Aday, L. A., and Andersen, R. 1974. "A framework for the study of access to medical care." *Health Services Research* 9 (Fall 1974): 208–20.

Aday, L. A., and Andersen, R. 1975. *Development of Indices of Access to Medical Care*. Ann Arbor: Health Administration Press.

Aday, L. A., et al. 1980. *Health Care in the United States: Equitable for Whom?* Beverly Hills: Sage Publications.

American Medical Association. 1975. *Physician Distribution and Licensure in the U.S., 1974.* Chicago: Center for Health Services Research and Development, AMA.

Andersen, R., and Aday, L. A. 1978. "Access to medical care in the U.S.: realized and potential." *Medical Care* 16 (July 1978): 533–46.

Andersen, R., and Anderson, O. W. 1967. *A Decade of Health Services.* Chicago: University of Chicago Press.

Andersen, R., and Newman, J. 1973. "Societal and individual determinants of medical care utilization." *Milbank Memorial Fund Quarterly* 51 (Winter 1973): 95–124.

Andersen, R., et al. 1975. *Equity in Health Services: Empirical Analyses in Social Policy.* Cambridge: Ballinger Publishing Co.

Andersen, R., et al. 1976. *Two Decades of Health Services: Social Survey Trends in Use and Expenditures.* Cambridge: Ballinger Publishing Co.

Anderson, O. W., and Feldman, J. J. 1956. *Family Medical Costs and Voluntary Health Insurance: A National Survey.* New York: McGraw Hill.

Anderson, O. W., et al. 1963. *Changes in Family Medical Care Expenditures and Voluntary Health Insurance.* Cambridge: Harvard University Press.

Block, J. A., et al. 1978. "Physicians and Hospitals: Providing primary care." *Medical Group Management,* 25 (March/April 1978): 35–38.

Blumstein, J. F., and Zubkoff, M. 1979. "Public choice in health: problems, politics and perspectives on formulating national health policy." *Journal of Health Politics, Policy and Law,* 4 (Fall 1979): 382–413.

Donabedian, A. 1973. *Aspects of Medical Care Administration.* Cambridge: Harvard University Press.

National Center for Health Statistics. 1976. *Health Manpower: A County and Metropolitan Area Data Book, 1972–75.* Washington, D.C.: U.S. Government Printing Office.

Verbrugge, L. 1980. "Equity of access to health care: A research review and prospectus." Paper prepared on request for the National Institute of Medicine. Ann Arbor: Institute for Social Research, University of Michigan.

Labor's New Approach
to National Health Insurance

*Stanley B. Jones**

The Health Care for All Americans Act is an attempt by the nation's labor unions, and others, to accomplish classic social welfare goals in the area of health care through private insurance by the use of regulation and market incentives.

The social welfare goals of the bill have historically been linked with social security type government programs, such as the Kennedy-Corman or Health Security proposal. This new labor–Kennedy proposal moves away from the social security approach. It sets out to: (1) minimize the amount of public tax revenues required for the program; (2) maintain a major role for the private insurance industry; and (3) strengthen competition in the health care sector.

The labor unions have taken this course in order to make the proposal more politically viable. In fact, they have responded directly to the conditions for a workable national health insurance bill laid down by President Carter in his campaign in 1976. I believe the labor unions' change represents a historic change of great political importance.

If you want to understand this legislation, you must understand this

*Consultant, Blue Cross/Blue Shield Association

change of union course, as well as its political underpinnings. Otherwise, one is apt to see or hear the classic social security approach lurking behind every provision, especially when all the rhetoric used to describe the proposal emphasizes the classic social welfare goals (and how this new approach will accomplish them) and when many of the advocates of the proposal still think and argue in social security terms and are still struggling to adjust to their own new rubrics and concepts. One doesn't change several decades of thinking overnight.

Of course, it is not necessary to look at this new proposal in the way I'm going to describe it here. The marketplace for ideas, happily, is the freest of all markets in our nation. But I would submit that it is at least more interesting to look for what is new, inventive, and even promising in this proposal than it is to resort to the standard criticisms of the social security approach that we have all heard to the point of weariness. But looking at this proposal is more than a matter of interest. I believe that this new proposal narrows the political polls in the national debate and opens some possibilities for compromise that one day will need to be explored.

Goals of the Proposal

The Health Care for All Americans Act's basic goals are the same as those advanced by the labor unions for their Health Security Act. They are:

1. To assure that all residents of this country can afford to purchase all needed health care
2. To assure that needed health care is accessible to all
3. To assure that individuals pay for their insurance on an equitable basis
4. To assure that the health care received by all is of comparable quality and desirability
5. To assure that long-term increases in national health care costs grow no faster than the rate of increase of the GNP

The Health Care for All Americans Act would work toward these goals through federally mandated, comprehensive health insurance coverage (with no coinsurance or deductible) for all residents of the country. With the exception of the elderly and disabled, who are covered by a separate and equal Medicare program, all residents, regardless of income or employment status, would be covered by private health insurance. This insurance would be sold by private insurance companies and HMOs under federal regulation. The employers, employees, and other individuals who are required to purchase insurance would pay for it on the basis of their payroll or income. Finally, through competition among insurers and among providers, through negotiations on providers' budgets and fees, and through state and national planning and budgeting, the proposal aims at making health care more evenly accessible throughout the nation and at controlling health care costs.

Major Provisions of the Proposal

Benefits Covered

The proposal would include the same comprehensive services covered by both Medicare and private insurance plans. The proposal would require plans to cover hospital, physician, and laboratory services on an unlimited basis.

On a limited basis, it would cover preventive services for pregnant women and children through age 20, home health care, nursing home care, mental health care, and prescription drugs (Medicare only).

No deductibles or coinsurance (indeed, no out-of-pocket costs) could be required by insurers or providers for covered services, except in cases such as prescription drugs and hearing aids where a maximum payment is set. This provision grows out of the long-standing convictions in the unions that deductibles and coinsurance discourage low-income individuals from seeking needed care and are therefore inherently unfair. All in all, the benefits are somewhat narrower but still comparable to those of the Health Security Program.

Eligibility for Coverage

As a matter of basic principle for the labor unions, all residents of the country would be entitled to have third-party payments made on their behalf for covered services—solely by virtue of their being residents. It wouldn't matter whether they were employed or by whom they were employed. During open season, all residents—even those who have no income with which to pay a premium—would be entitled to enroll with any insurer. Individual subscribers could choose among all insurers and HMOs operating in the area. Employees could choose among the multiple offerings required of all employers. Also, mechanisms would be established to ensure that any resident who walks into a doctor's office, or is carried into a hospital, would have covered services paid for by some insurer; similarly, the bill guarantees providers that they will be paid for covered services to residents. The intent is (1) to eliminate any need by the individual to hesitate to enroll with an insurer or hesitate to seek health care because of a lack of ability to pay and (2) to eliminate any need by the provider to check on an individual's ability to pay as a condition to providing covered services.

How are these goals to be accomplished? All aged and disabled Americans would be enrolled in Medicare programs. All other U.S. residents would be required to enroll in private insurance plans certified by the government.

1. During an annual open season employed individuals would choose among the two or more insurance and HMO plans which every employer would have to offer all of their employees (including part-time and seasonal employees).
2. The nonemployed, including welfare eligibles, would have to enroll (during open season) in a certified plan in their area.
3. The Medicaid program would be converted into a premium subsidy mechanism (described later in this paper), except for a residual program of long-term care and other benefits not included in the new plan. The residual program would be state-administered.
4. Employed and nonemployed alike would be enrolled with the same private insurance carriers for comprehensive benefits, with no way for providers to distinguish them by income or any other factor.

Of course, not everyone would enroll; some will intentionally or unintentionally fall in the cracks. For patients who appear at a provider's door with no proof of coverage, the provider will bill a government agency, which will help the individual enroll in a plan (or Medicare if he is eligible), will pay the bill, and collect premiums back to the last open-enrollment period from whoever is liable. For employers, or others, who default on premium obligations, the government would pay the premium and collect through the tax system. The insurer would not be permitted to expel enrollees for failure to pay.

These provisions are intended to guarantee all residents payment for covered services under either Medicare or a private insurance plan by providing mechanisms ensuring that everyone actually enroll with an insurer or health maintenance organization (HMO), and ensuring that whoever is liable for the premium actually pays it. Let's look more closely at these mechanisms.

Liability for Premiums

For the Medicare system, the costs would be paid through existing payroll taxes. The addition of new Medicare eligibles would in fact increase the current revenues into the program in anticipation of their eligibility at age 65. Part B enrollment under Medicare and its premiums would be made mandatory.

For private insurance coverage all employers would be required to pay a wage-related premium, based on a percentage of their total payroll, to private insurers or HMOs on behalf of all their employees. The estimated size of the wage-related premium for the first year of the program is approximately 7.5 percent.

Employers could require employees to pay 35 percent of this wage-related premium, or an estimated 2.6 percent of the employees' wages, for the first year of the program.

All individuals, whether employed or nonemployed, would also be required to pay an income-related premium on nonwage income of over $2000 per year at a rate equal to one-half the wage-related premium rate. This would be approximately 3.75 percent in the first year. However, no individual or family would be required to pay a total premium in excess of the community-rated value of his coverage in his area of the country. Credits for overpayments would be made through the federal income tax system. This limitation would not apply to the employer's premium.

State and federal governments would make lump-sum payments to insurers to cover the costs of insurance for Aid to Families with Dependent Children (AFDC) and Supplemental Security Income (SSI) eligibles who have chosen to enroll with them. These payments would be made directly to private insurers based on a sampling of the insurers' roles for welfare eligibles.

This private insurance system would be self-supporting except for the payments made for AFDC and SSI eligibles. That is to say, the wage-related premium rate would be set by the federal government in negotiation with insurers at a level sufficient to cover a community-rated premium for all residents who enroll with private insurers, except AFDC and SSI eligibles. This means the wage-related premium covers the cost of insurance, not only to full-time employees, but also to part-time employees, the seasonally employed, the unemployed, and all others who are not eligible for welfare assistance. All residents of the United States (except AFDC and SSI eligibles) would be insured through private revenues paid primarily by employers and employees. You will recall that the proposal would entitle all residents of the United States who are not eligible for Medicare to enroll with a private insurer or HMO, and the insurer or HMO must take them, even though many will pay little or no premium, or pay it only when they have income. You now know how the proposal would pay for these individuals. If the wage-related premium rate did not produce enough revenues to pay the community-rated premiums negotiated by government with insurers for all these people, the government, under the proposal, would be liable to make adjustments.

The intent of this approach to premium payment, of course, is to soften the premium burden on low-wage employees and their employers. It would eliminate experience rating as a factor in the premium payment, and it would go one step beyond even community rating. By making the premium more affordable in this way, the plan is freer to make enrollment and premium payment mandatory for employers, employees, and others. Also, this wage-related approach is simpler and fairer in the minds of the unions.

Enrollment and Underwriting Through Insurers

Under the proposal, insurers would enroll subscribers, set and collect premiums, engage in marketing, design competing health programs, and process claims.

Insurers and HMOs would be required, during an annual open season and on other specific occasions, to enroll all applicants openly who approach them in a plan certified as covering the mandated benefits. No one could be turned away, except for specific reasons such as limited capacity of an HMO. No charge in excess of the wage-related and income-related premiums prescribed in the proposal could be made for mandated benefits.

All wage-related and income-related premiums are paid by employers, employees, and other individuals to insurers, not to government. I am told by constitutional lawyers that this means it would not be a tax. In order to convert these admittedly "unusual" premiums into a form insurers and HMOs can work with, the premium would be turned over to national banks or "consortia" operated by insurers, HMOs, and self-insurers. These banks would use the incoming revenues to pay their member insurers or HMOs an experience-rated premium for each individual or family they enroll. (The flow of funds is illustrated in figure 7.1.) This process is intended to discourage risk selection and to protect insurers from the obvious possibilities of adverse selection implicit in an open-enrollment system. The criteria used by the consortia for determining these experience-rated premiums would be set by the insurers or HMOs themselves—who operate the consortia. They would have to use criteria, however, that assured that all who enrolled in member plans of the consortia were insured at a total cost equal to the number of enrollees multiplied by the community-rated premium negotiated with government. The intent here is to give insurers maximum incentive to market health insurance to everyone, not to practice risk selection, and to police their own ranks. No one will be more anxious to eliminate creaming (selecting only the good risks) and ensure fair criteria for converting wage-related to experience-rated premiums than the insurers in the pool.

Insurers and HMOs are free to market their insurance to all groups and individuals in an area with assurance that they will receive from their bank or consortia an experience-rated premium for each enrollee. Bear in mind that from the employer, employee, or other individual's perspective, the premium must be paid—the only issue is what insurer or HMO to choose. If an individual insurer or HMO can provide the required coverage to its enrollees for less than the consortium's experience-rated premium, it can offer enhanced benefits or an actual tax-exempt rebate to anyone who enrolls in the plan. In fact, it can use these funds in any way it chooses. The only restriction is that any such rebate or expansion of benefits must be offered to all subscribers; that

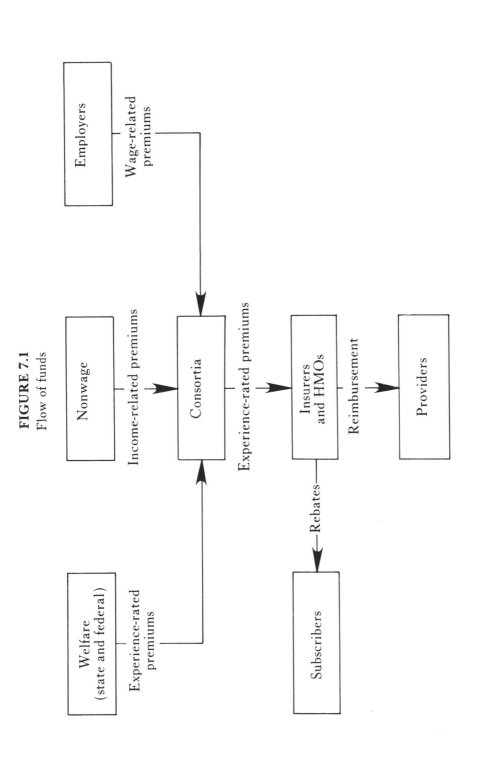

FIGURE 7.1
Flow of funds

is, it must be a community-rated rebate. The intent here is to give insurers and HMOs profit incentives to develop with providers more cost-effective health care financing arrangements by giving individual purchasers a clear cash or benefit incentive to enroll with cost-effective plans.

Finally, insurers and HMOs would pay hospitals, physicians, and other providers for all covered services for their enrollees. They would pay them at or below fee schedules and budgets negotiated for their area. These negotiations would be convened by the government, but would be carried on by the purchasers of health insurance and insurers on the one side, and the providers of health care on the other. An insurer or HMO would be free to negotiate a lower rate with these providers, however, and to pass the savings on to enrollees in the form of enhanced benefits or rebates. The intent of these provisions is to establish outside constraints on payments to providers through negotiations with the purchasers of insurance, but to allow insurers and HMOs room for competition under them.

These provisions regarding insurance and HMOs aim at (1) preserving a maximum role for private insurers and HMOs in the system, (2) encouraging insurers and HMOs to compete on the basis of cost-effective delivery of care rather than experience rating, (3) giving insurers themselves major responsibility and incentives for monitoring and enforcing the regulations to this end, and (4) using negotiations between purchasers of insurance and providers of care to set outside limits on provider fees and budgets paid by insurers.

The Government Role

I have delayed describing the government role under this program in order to keep your minds as open as possible for as long as possible under the circumstances. But I'm near the end now, and you know it's coming. There are four types of government roles.

First, government would establish and monitor procedural regulations on insurers, providers, and purchasers of health insurance. The federal government would have basic responsibility for ensuring that employers, employees, and others comply with the requirements to enroll in insurance plans and pay required premiums. The federal government also would oversee insurer and HMO compliance with open enrollment, standard benefits, and a variety of other requirements relating to fair marketing. State governments would assist individuals in enrolling with an insurer or HMO, oversee the negotiations between providers and purchasers of insurance, and monitor compliance with regulations relating to providers generally.

Second, government would assume new fiscal responsibilities. As mentioned above, the federal government would guarantee insurers that the wage-related premiums would raise enough revenues to cover the costs of the community rate it negotiates with the insurers. It also would guarantee insurers collection of bad premium debts.

Third, the federal government would offer resource development funds in the form of grants to encourage start-up of services in underserved areas, consistent with state plans and budgets.

Finally, government would assume stronger regulatory roles that set limits—or at least set targets for expenditures—on the health care and health financing system. To control costs and improve the distribution of health care resources, the proposal would establish a national planning and budgeting system. The system would involve participation by insurers, purchasers of insurance, and providers of care. It would produce projections of national health care costs based on the current state and local health planning system and other factors. Based on these plans, each state would be allocated a budget (or target) for coming years, so that the total national expenditure for covered services would rise no faster, on average, than the GNP. This budget (or target) would determine the speed with which new health services resources could be developed in a state or area; and it would be skewed to favor areas that are underserved. (Incidentally, in states or areas where tough negotiations with providers result in lower expenditure under this target, employers, employees, and individuals would pay lower wage-related premiums.) This plan and budget for projected expenditures would serve as the basis on which the federal government and insurers would negotiate the community rates for the nation and each state, which would then be guaranteed insurers through the government-set, wage-related premiums. Figure 7.2 describes the administrative structure of the proposal.

Many of the comments on this new proposal have focused on the government role in the plan, and especially on the new planning and budgeting roles of government. Clearly, these are major elements of the proposal, and no doubt deeply troublesome to those of you who favor a market incentives approach. I would like to offer the following

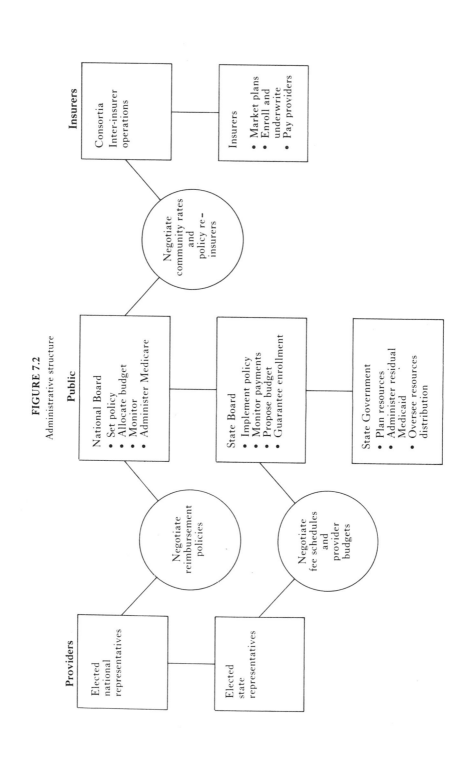

FIGURE 7.2
Administrative structure

Insurers

Consortia
Inter-insurer
operations

Insurers
- Market plans
- Enroll and underwrite
- Pay providers

Negotiate community rates and policy re-insurers

Public

National Board
- Set policy
- Allocate budget
- Monitor
- Administer Medicare

State Board
- Implement policy
- Monitor payments
- Propose budget
- Guarantee enrollment

State Government
- Plan resources
- Administer residual Medicaid
- Oversee resources distribution

Negotiate reimbursement policies

Negotiate fee schedules and provider budgets

Providers

Elected national representatives

Elected state representatives

observations, however. First, given state-of-the-art in planning and the complexity of the various political interests involved, it is really more of a public targeting process than a budgeting process. In the end, it would be through negotiations with insurers that the federal government would attempt to influence expenditures—negotiations, not budgets. Second, the potential for competition to reform health care delivery under the proposal would seem to be very strong and might prove to be the most effective part of the program. Third, the local negotiations between purchasers and providers proposed under the plan could have an impact independent of the success of the national budgeting process. Finally, as a political reality there will be a combination of regulation with any market incentives approach set in place in the years ahead. It seems to me that the idea of payment limits negotiated by purchasers of insurance and providers of care, and of planning and budgeting targets influenced by these same parties of interest, may be the basis for a compatible mixture of competition and regulation.

Costs of the Proposal

The proposal would add approximately $40 billion to the nation's total public and private expenditures on health care in 1983 (figured in 1980 dollars). The federal on-budget costs would rise roughly $30 billion, with $20 billion of this going for improvements in Medicare.

Private expenditures by employers, employees, and individuals would rise by a total of $11 billion by labor union estimates and $8 billion by Department of Health, Education and Welfare (DHEW) estimates. Within this private increase, however, because of the huge transfers of costs from out-of-pocket payments by individuals to employer premium payments, employer payments would increase some $33 billion and individual payments would drop some $25 billion according to DHEW. The exact figures calculated by the labor unions and by DHEW are presented at the end of the paper.

Concluding Observations

This is the least costly NHI bill, in federal budget terms, ever proposed by the labor movement. It is the first bill that increases the amount of funds flowing through the private insurance industry; indeed, they would easily double. It is also the first bill supported by the unions that does not make the Social Security Administration the health insurer for the nation. The proposal therefore warrants examination.

Moreover, while the labor movement would object to it on equity grounds, I believe their proposal could be made to work using community-rated, rather than wage-related premiums, with premium subsidies to lower-income individuals through the tax system. If reasonable deductibles and co-insurance were also allowed, the cost of the proposal for employers would likely be reduced by almost half. You might want to evaluate the new proposal with these possibilities in mind.

Chapter 7 Appendix: Labor Union Estimates[1]

Summary of Cost Estimates for Fiscal Year 1983[2] (in billions of 1980 dollars)

1. Total spending for services covered by the plan:

Present law	Kennedy plan	Difference
$171.4	$211.4	+$40.0

2. Total on-budget federal cost:

Present law	Kennedy plan	Difference
$51.0	$79.6	+$28.6

3. Total nonfederal cost:

Present law	Kennedy plan	Difference
$120.4	$131.8	+$11.4

Actuary estimates an employer–employee premium of 7 to 8 percent, depending upon the success of cost-containment programs.

Crossover Point[3]

The crossover point is the year in which, under this plan, the nation spends less on health care than if it enacts no legislation. Crossover:

four years after passage. In 1988, for example, the nation would spend $38 billion less than if no law is enacted.

Chapter 7 Appendix: DHEW Estimate of Costs[4]

Comparison of the Costs of President Carter's National Health Plan Legislation (Phase I) with the Health Care for All Americans Act

The Carter administration's legislative proposal and the proposal for the Health Care for All Americans Act present their costs in two different ways. In order to understand the differences between the two proposals it is helpful to compare them both ways. The following explanations assume 1980 dollars and 1980 population counts.

When the Health Care for All Americans Act was announced, it was costed in 1980 dollars using estimated 1983 population counts. By using 1980 population counts, the estimates below reduce the costs of the Health Care for All Americans Act slightly.

The Carter administration's approach looks primarily at net federal budget and employer costs because taxpayers and employers are the ones being asked to shoulder the cost of new benefits. The costs to employers are especially vital in determining the employment and inflation effects of national health plan proposals. When viewed this way, the net costs of the two proposals are as follows:

	Phase I	Health Care for All Americans Act
Federal	+$18.2	+$30.7
Employer	+$ 6.1	+$33.1
Total Cost	+$24.3 billion	+$63.8 billion

The approach taken by the advocates of the Health Care for All Americans Act is to look at these federal budget and employer costs (and other costs now borne by individuals and state and local governments as well) in order to determine the effect of National Health Plan proposals on total health system costs.

	Phase I	Health Care for All Americans Act
Federal	+$18.2	+$30.7
Employer	+$ 6.1	+$33.1
Individuals	−$ 4.0	−$25.4*
State/Local	−$ 2.0	−$ 2.7
Total Cost	+$18.3 billion	+$35.7 billion

*Includes reduced out-of-pocket and premium costs.

Chapter 7 Notes

1. From press release from Senator Edward Kennedy's office.

2. All estimates prepared by Gordon Trapnell of Actuarial Research Corp.

3. Figures prepared by Professor Isidore Falk, Professor Emeritus, Yale School of Medicine.

4. From Department of Health, Education, and Welfare press release (1979).

A Tax Credit for Catastrophic Health Insurance—An Alternative to Health Sector Regulation

*Laurence S. Seidman**

What would happen if health insurance were left to the private sector? At this stage of the national health insurance debate (when the choice may appear to be among alternative governmental interventions) the question of whether any intervention is necessary may seem academic. In my view, however, asking this basic question is a useful way to begin the analysis. In this paper, I will explain why many (although not all) health economists believe that a limited intervention—an income-related tax credit for catastrophic insurance—is the most desirable approach to the health insurance problem.

Genuine Governmental Neutrality: The Repeal of Current Tax Subsidies for Health Insurance

The case for governmental intervention usually begins by citing the exceptional cost inflation in the health sector over the past two decades. Some advocates correctly emphasize the role of insurance, private and public, in fueling the inflation. Over 90 percent of all hospital

---

*Department of Economics, Swarthmore College

revenues from patient care come from third parties. Given this extensive coverage, it is little wonder that physicians, acting on behalf of their fully insured patients, show little concern for cost when they select a hospital, order hospital services, or decide the length of stay. One response to this inflationary process is to conclude that governmental regulation is necessary to control health sector costs.

An alternative response, however, is to ask: Why is health insurance so extensive? It is no mystery that most people value major-risk (catastrophic) insurance to protect them against a financial burden that would be large relative to their income. It is far less obvious why most households have obtained private insurance policies with much higher premiums that provide nearly complete hospital coverage—"first dollar" ("shallow")—as well as major-risk coverage.

It is now widely recognized that federal tax policy has significantly encouraged first dollar coverage. If an employer compensates an employee with $100 of cash or salary, the $100 is, of course, taxable income to the employee, so that he perhaps receives $75 after taxes. If the employer instead compensates him with $100 of additional health insurance, the $100 is excluded from the employee's taxable income. This employer exclusion clearly provides a substantial inducement to additional insurance. Instead of the choice of $75 in cash versus $75 additional insurance, the choice is between $75 in cash and $100 of additional insurance.

A recent survey by the Congressional Budget Office estimates the magnitude of this tax subsidy for insurance to be $9.6 billion in fiscal year 1980.[1] Together with the medical deduction for the employee's own expense on health insurance, the total subsidy for insurance is $12.7 billion, almost one-fourth of the federal government's direct expenditure on health care.

A policy of genuine governmental neutrality towards health insurance would require the repeal of these tax subsidies: the inclusion of employer contributions to health insurance in the taxable income of each employee; and the elimination of the employee's medical deduction for health insurance.

What would happen if these tax subsidies were repealed? It seems likely that many individuals would prefer more cash, and therefore would accept less first-dollar insurance, though most would still find major-risk insurance worth its cost. In response, most employers and unions would probably seek major-risk insurance policies with lower premiums, and insurance companies would respond by offering such policies.

The reduction in shallow coverage would mean that, in sharp contrast to the current situation, many persons seeking hospital care would pay a fraction of the cost of their own service. On behalf of their cost-sharing patients, it seems likely that many physicians would begin to weigh cost against benefit and avoid cost that is unnecessary for achieving desired quality. In turn, hospitals would be compelled to respond to this new concern of physicians by attempting to achieve a given quality at minimum cost in order to attract physicians and their patients.

Would consumer cost-sharing really improve efficiency in practice? I will provide a more detailed defense later. For the moment, suppose cost sharing works as many economists expect, so that health expenditures begin to reflect a weighing by each physician, on behalf of his patient, of cost against benefit. Would the policy of government neutrality be satisfactory?

Universal Major-Risk Protection

Although a majority of households would probably obtain adequate catastrophic insurance under a policy of neutrality, a minority would not. Why would some households obtain little or no coverage, so that they are unable to afford the care they need when a serious illness strikes?

First, there will be individuals whose work place provides no insurance. Because of economies of scale in enrollment, group insurance is less expensive than individually-purchased insurance. The person not covered at his work place must therefore buy a more costly policy to obtain the same coverage. Second, private insurance companies, in a competitive market, must set premiums according to the expected medical cost, which determines the liability they will bear. They cannot vary premiums according to household income. (A company that set its premium below expected cost for low-income households, and above expected cost for high-income households, would soon lose its high-income enrollees to competitors, and therefore be unable to sustain its sliding scale.)

Consider, therefore, the individual with poor health who earns a low wage at a small firm with no health insurance policy. To obtain adequate major-risk coverage he would have to pay a premium that is large relative to his low income. An adequate policy would in itself impose a severe financial burden.

One response is that the predicament of such households is no reason to abandon strict governmental neutrality. It might be argued that the inability to afford insurance would provide the necessary incentive for the individual to increase his effort to raise his earnings; and that inadequate insurance, like inadequate income, is a stimulus to self-discipline and increased productivity.

An alternative response—which I find compelling—is that such households should be provided financial assistance to obtain adequate major-risk protection. From this perspective, the fact that a given household may find it difficult to afford adequate protection is regarded as at least partly involuntary. If the economic aptitude of the individual is modest, and his health is poor, even exceptional work efforts may leave him facing an insurance premium that is large relative to his income. Many would sympathize with such an individual if a serious illness were to strike and he was either unable to afford the care he needed or was left nearly bankrupt by the episode.

Several aspects of this philosophical position deserve emphasis. First, the primary concern of others is that this individual be able to afford the care he needs, and not be financially overwhelmed by his misfortune. This concern does not imply that medical care must be made free to the household; rather, the concern is that the individual's financial burden be tolerable, given his income.

Second, major-risk protection must be income related. An insurance policy that limits a household's liability to $3,000 may be adequate for a high-income household, and inadequate for a low-income household. Thus, a policy instrument must be used that can vary assistance inversely with household income, so that a low-income household can afford a major-risk policy with a sufficiently low out-of-pocket ceiling.

Such assistance can be achieved by a federal tax credit for each household for its expense on a major-risk private insurance policy. The credit would be largest for a low-income household, and be gradually phased out as the income rises. The size of the credit would be determined as follows. At each income level, an estimate would be made of the burden regarded as tolerable for the household and for the liability of an insurer who offered a policy with such an out-of-pocket ceiling for the household. For example, suppose a ceiling of $3,000 was deemed tolerable for a household with an income of $20,000. A private policy might require the household to pay a $1,500 deductible, and 20 percent of the next $7,500 of medical bills, until its total burden for the year reached $3,000; the insurer would then pay 100 percent of any additional medical cost.[2]

Suppose the expected liability of an insurer offering such a policy was estimated to be $300. (The insurer's liability would be much less than today's average premium for policies with little or no patient cost sharing.) One approach would be to set the federal tax credit at $300 for a $20,000 household. It could be argued, however, that a substantially smaller credit (such as $100) would be adequate, since each household might be expected to contribute towards its own major-risk protection.

The credit would be "refundable," and therefore potentially universal in its coverage. If the credit to which a household were entitled exceeded its tax liability, it would receive a check from the Internal Revenue Service (IRS) for the difference. Moreover, eligibility for credit should not depend on whether the taxpayer itemizes his tax deductions or uses the standard deduction. Thus, the tax credit is envisioned as a substitute for Medicaid, because all low-income households (whether or not they receive public assistance or earn sufficient income to pay tax) would be able to obtain credit by filing a tax return (perhaps a special simplified return designed for this purpose).

To receive a credit, the household must buy a policy that provides an out-of-pocket ceiling and covers specified services, including inpatient, outpatient, physician, and nursing care. The reason for these conditions is that the aim is not to encourage insurance per se, but only major-risk protection.

A complementary policy can substantially raise the ceiling regarded as tolerable at each income level, thereby reducing the required tax credit, and the budgetary cost of the program. The availability of medical loans, at moderate interest rates and with sufficiently long repayment periods, should be guaranteed to households. As I have explained in detail elsewhere ("Medical Loans and Major-Risk National Health Insurance"),[3] the federal government could enter into contracts with private insurers and loan institutions to administer the program.

The guaranteed availability of a loan, with sufficient time to repay, would enable each household to bear a substantially higher ceiling. For many households, a costly episode occurs infrequently. If a loan enables the household to spread the burden over several years, the household can bear a greater share without hardship. Although it is inevitable that a certain percentage of loans will not be fully repaid, the loan program will still reduce the budgetary cost of the government, because the smaller tax credit for the majority who do repay will greatly outweigh the loss on defaults.

Insurance of Last Resort

Would a tax credit for expense on a private major-risk insurance policy be sufficient? Let's examine the likely consequences.

Because of the large economies of scale of group enrollment, many people would continue to obtain insurance through their work place. The employer contribution would now be taxable income to each employee. But as long as the group policy provided an out-of-pocket ceiling, each employee would be eligible for a tax credit for his employer's contribution.

It is unlikely that most work places would retain the high premium, first-dollar coverage so prevalent today. Repeal of the employer exclusion implies that the difference between the high premium of such "complete" insurance and the low premium of a catastrophic policy would be fully borne by each employee. Each additional $100 of insurance would cost employees $100 (not $75) in take-home pay.

It seems plausible that most work places would offer a minimum policy with a moderately high ceiling and the option of supplementary coverage that would lower the ceiling. Low-income employees with a larger tax credit might elect the supplementary policy because it would be subsidized. Higher income employees would do so only if they valued the lower ceiling enough to pay the full additional premium cost without subsidy. Few work places would offer the option of a ceiling near zero.

Although the majority of households would probably obtain adequate major-risk protection, it is doubtful that such coverage would be universal. First, some work places might offer only a minimum policy with a ceiling that would be too high for some low-paid employees. It may be difficult for these employees to seek out supplementary insurance that integrates efficiently with their work place policy.

Second, some individuals will incur a costly illness of a household member while they are between jobs. In retrospect, they will regret their failure to buy temporary individual insurance. They may have simply forgotten to buy such insurance, or made a conscious decision to risk being uncovered for a short period, given their lack of income during a spell of unemployment. Whatever the reason, few people will judge them harshly; most people will sympathize with their plight.

Third, imperfect information will inevitably cause some individuals to have inadequate coverage. Some may falsely assume that their work place policy provides a sufficiently low ceiling, discovering only after a costly illness that their ceiling is very high relative to their income. Some people without work place insurance will be unaware of the existence of the tax credit and assume they cannot afford adequate coverage. Others may incorrectly assume they must owe federal tax to be entitled to a credit. Still others will simply fail to make the effort required to seek out and buy an individual policy, regretting their negligence only after it is too late.

One possible response to that is that the availability of a tax credit fulfills society's obligation. It is then up to each individual to be sufficiently informed, alert, and prudent. An alternative view, however, is that public policy ought to take one further step. Through a tax credit, the federal government can provide major-risk insurance of last resort to those who, for whatever reason, did not obtain an adequate private policy. This is the view I will adopt here.

Any household without private insurance would be eligible for a tax credit for its expenses on medical care. For example, a household with an income of $20,000 might have to bear the first $1,000 of its annual medical bill. It might then be entitled to a tax credit equal to 80 percent of its additional bill until its out-of-pocket burden reached $3,000, which would occur when its annual bill reached $9,000. It would then be entitled to a tax credit equal to 100 percent of its bill in excess of $9,000, so that its ceiling would be $3,000 or 15 percent of its income.

These specific numbers are given only for illustration. The actual tax credit schedule for each income class should be based on careful budget studies. The aim should be to set the ceiling for each income class so that, given the guaranteed availability of medical loans, the maximum burden is tolerable. The tax credit would be refundable, so that a household with a credit greater than its tax liability would receive a check from the Internal Revenue Service (IRS). Coverage would therefore be universal. The credit would be intended to replace Medicaid.

As long as the last resort credit sets the ceiling for each income class at the highest level regarded as tolerable, most households will choose to obtain private insurance that provides a lower ceiling. The tax credit for the purchase of private, major-risk insurance will encourage private coverage, even in the presence of the last resort credit. Thus, the last resort ceiling should be low enough to adequately protect the minority with too little (or no) private coverage, but high enough to encourage the purchase of private, major-risk policies.

The discouragement of reliance on the last resort credit can be justified on several grounds. First, private insurers can more effectively monitor the medical bills of their enrollees, and verify expenditures, than can the IRS with its current manpower. Given the scope of the private insurance sector, and its experience in monitoring and processing medical bills, it is sensible to try to limit the administrative burden imposed on the IRS and continue to rely on private insurers for the vast majority of households. Second, it is desirable to avoid dislocation to the private insurance sector. Unlike many other dislocations in a dynamic economy, displacement of private policies by the IRS policy would not promote welfare; it would harm that sector unnecessarily.

Another function of the last resort credit is to assist an individual whose work place policy contains a ceiling that is too large for his income. Consider an employee earning $20,000 whose work place policy has a $4,000 ceiling for all its employees. Suppose that the last resort credit (for a $20,000 household with no private insurance) would provide a ceiling of $3,000—judged to be the maximum tolerable burden. It would then clearly be inequitable to allow the partially insured $20,000 household to bear a burden of $4,000.

It is therefore natural to establish the following rule for any household with private insurance. A household with private insurance will be entitled to additional tax credit so that its burden for a given annual medical bill does not exceed the burden it would have incurred if it had no private insurance. Thus, the $20,000 employee with work place insurance with a $4,000 ceiling would receive sufficient tax credit so that its burden did not exceed $3,000, no matter how large its annual medical bill. The interaction of the tax credit for private insurance, and the last resort credit, is further delineated in the appendix to this paper.

Finally, consider an individual who buys shallow private insurance that provides only first-dollar coverage, relying on the last resort credit to provide major-risk protection. Because the private policy provides no out-of-pocket ceiling, the person would not be entitled to any tax credit for expense on the premium. This rule reflects the underlying perspective that the only justification for a tax credit is to enable major-risk protection to be obtained. Given this denial of a tax credit, as is shown in the appendix, the purchase of shallow insurance would probably be unattractive to most households.

To summarize: under the proposed policy, government would depart from complete neutrality to provide a tax credit for catastrophic insurance through either a credit towards the purchase of a private policy or a credit for out-of-pocket expenses for a household without private insurance. A complementary medical loan program would enable a smaller credit to provide adequate protection, thereby substantially reducing the budgetary cost of the program.

The Impact on Efficiency

If the proposed policy were introduced, some households would be satisfied with minimum major-risk protection, while others would want more extensive coverage. For example, a $20,000 household with a last resort ceiling of $3,000 might be willing to pay the premium of a policy that provided a $1,000 ceiling. Because additional insurance would no longer be subsidized (by the employer exclusion or medical deduction), each household considering more extensive coverage would bear the full additional cost of the higher premium. The guaranteed availability of loans would remove the cash flow motive for complete insurance. It therefore seems doubtful that many households would obtain complete insurance with no cost sharing.

Suppose, however, that despite the high premium and lack of subsidy, a household chooses to obtain complete insurance. It is sometimes thought that this is socially undesirable because complete insurance reduces the effective price of medical care to zero, causing an inflation of demand by the household. It must be recognized, however, that this inflation of demand will be reflected in the premium charged to the household. For example, suppose complete insurance causes the expected medical cost of a household to rise $300 above its expected cost under a major-risk policy. Then the insurer will have to include this

$300 in the price of the premium. If a household is so risk averse that it is willing to bear the additional cost without subsidy, on what ground should it be discouraged from doing so?

According to normative economic analysis, the only justification for discouragement would be the existence of an externality. The special role of the physician may in fact create such an externality. It is plausible that the average physician, who may be viewed as an imperfect agent for his patients, develops practices and procedures with the average insurance status of his patients in mind. It may be awkward for an MD to discriminate perfectly among patients according to each one's insurance status. Thus, when subset A of an MD's patients becomes completely insured, he may somewhat inflate the service he orders for all his patients. Thus, the inflation of demand spreads to subset B, which has only major-risk protection. Thus, when A obtains complete insurance, a cost is imposed on B—an external cost not borne by A.

The standard remedy for an externality is a tax imposed on the buyer of such insurance that will internalize the cost imposed on others, so that this cost is weighed in the decision to get completer coverage. Under our tax credit, an appropriate implicit tax can be imposed on the buyer of extensive insurance by gradually phasing out the credit as the household's insurance premium increases. For example, suppose a $20,000 household receives a $100 credit if it buys a major-risk policy with a $300 premium. If instead it buys complete insurance for $1100, an implicit tax of $100 could be imposed by eliminating the credit. (For each dollar of premium above $300, the credit could be cut 20 cents.) Thus, phasing out the credit can properly discourage extensive insurance that imposes a cost on others.

It should be noted that the externality argument seems plausible only for fee-for-service insurance. If the household obtains complete insurance through an HMO, in which providers are prepaid, and then absorb the cost of service, it is unlikely that an inflation in demand will spread to others. Under prepayment, providers have an incentive to resist an inflation in demand by the insured enrollee; similarly, they will also resist any transmission of inflationary pressure to cost-sharing members. Thus, the full credit should be retained for complete insurance through a prepaid HMO.

Given the credit phase-out for fee-for-service insurance, it seems likely that most will find complete insurance not worth its cost, and prefer a policy with significant consumer cost sharing. I now want to explain why most (though not all) health economists believe that consumer cost sharing will promote efficiency in the health sector and that it represents a genuine alternative to governmental regulation.

The opponent of cost sharing is fond of the following caricature. The patient is told by his doctor that his problem is serious and surgery is required. The patient's immediate reply is, "Doc, can you show me a price list of area hospitals?"

The image is of the "cost-fanatic" consumer, shopping around for hospitals, asking the price of each test from his hospital bed, reading his *Consumer Reports* as the anesthesia takes effect—this image is embraced only by opponents of cost sharing. If cost sharing required such behavior to promote efficiency, who wouldn't be skeptical?

For advocates as well as opponents, the key decision maker in the health sector is the physician. At the time most medical decisions are made, the patient, preoccupied with his problem, places his trust in his physician. Inpatient versus outpatient, tests, length of stay—these decisions are delegated to the physician. Today, each physician knows that his average patient, even after recovery, will never care about hospital cost, because an insurer—private or public—will pay the bill. Under the proposed tax credit policy, however, each physician will soon recognize that his average patient now bears a fraction of his own hospital cost. Upon receiving his hospital bill—with the emergency being over—the average patient will want to know whether unnecessary costs were avoided.

Today, anecdotal evidence suggests that physicians do consider the financial burden on their patient. An MD tells a patient, "I will treat you as an inpatient, which your insurance fully covers, rather than as an outpatient, which it does not." Or, "I want you to stay a day or two longer in the hospital; your insurance will cover it, but won't cover nursing care at home." Most econometric studies also detect a responsiveness of utilization to out-of-pocket price, implying physician sensitivity to the burden on the patient.

Because patients must rely on their physician, they prefer MDs who are not only highly competent, but also seem genuinely concerned about their welfare. An MD who saves them unnecessary expense, without sacrificing desired quality, is appreciated. His concern becomes one more reason for the patient to recommend the MD to others.

Thus, self-interest alone would prompt many physicians to weigh cost in response to patient cost sharing. Moreover, an important fraction of physicians do take seriously the trust relationship. These physicians would find it unethical to place a patient in hospital X rather than hospital Y, if hospital Y is more efficient, less costly, and provides identical quality of care for the patient's problem.

A combination of self-interest and ethics would cause at least a significant fraction of physicians (not patients) to shop around for a hospital. The choice of these well-informed consumers will determine whether particular hospitals in an area run surpluses or deficits. Gradually, a radical change in the pressures on hospital managers will occur. Today, physicians prefer hospitals that provide advanced technology and facilities regardless of cost. Hospitals compete to satisfy physicians, who in turn bring patients. When an important fraction of physicians begin to prefer hospitals that provide a given quality at minimum cost, that avoid the purchase of technology that will be seriously underutilized, then hospital managers will be compelled to improve efficiency.

Because the hospital sector has operated for nearly two decades in an environment in which most patients are fully insured, many have concluded that health services are immune to the market mechanism and that only regulation can contain cost and improve efficiency.

Too often there is a failure to recognize that any other sector with fully insured, or subsidized, consumers would also appear immune to the market mechanism. Let food be free to the consumer, and there would be a national food cost crisis. Let stereos be free to the consumer, and we would observe extravagant technology and cost in the stereo sector. The market mechanism cannot work for any good or service where the consumer is completely subsidized.

The current inefficiency in the hospital sector does not imply that the market mechanism cannot be made to work in that sector. Extensive insurance, induced by federal tax policy, has undermined the market mechanism by removing a crucial ingredient: consumer cost-sharing. The sensible inference is that removal of the tax subsidy is likely to restore the potency of the market mechanism.

Consumer Cost-Sharing Versus Regulation

The assumption that the market mechanism cannot work in the health sector has stimulated support for a regulatory approach. Advocates of health sector regulation sometimes cite public utility regulation as evidence that this approach can produce satisfactory performance. The comparison with public utilities, however, ignores a fundamental distinction: the presence of consumer cost-sharing in the public utilities and its absence in the hospital sector.

In the utilities, each consumer pays for his own use of electricity, water, natural gas, and phone service. Consumer cost-sharing automatically restrains demand. The purpose of regulation is to prevent monopoly pricing. In contrast, health sector regulation tries to combat the symptoms of free service. The experience of utility regulation therefore cannot be extrapolated to the health sector, where the task will be far more difficult. How satisfactory would telephone regulation be if all long-distance calls were free?

Concrete examples facilitate a comparison of cost sharing and regulation. Consider whether patient X should stay the ninth day in a hospital. Suppose patient X is covered by major-risk insurance; his income is $20,000; his deductible is $1,500; his coinsurance rate is 20 percent; and his liability ceiling is $3,000, so that he will bear at least 20 percent of additional cost until his annual medical bill reaches $9,000. If physician charges are $1,500, and the hospital's charge per day is $300, then he will not reach his ceiling until the 25th day. (The mean hospital stay is approximately eight days. See note 1.)

Patient X's physician would recognize that X will bear a fraction of the cost of each additional day (in this case, $60 per day). This cost will be weighed, by X and his MD, against the benefit as they perceive it. Suppose X lives alone, but requires someone else's presence at all times in case of a relapse. Then despite the cost, they may choose to extend the stay. On the other hand, suppose X has a spouse who can be present at all times. In this case, they may decide to end the stay and avoid the cost.

Cost sharing automatically constrains demand. Without regulation, the supply of hospital facilities would match an aggregate demand for service that reflects the weighing of cost against benefit by each physician and patient. As in other sectors of the economy, the demand that emerges from such a weighing is regarded as legitimate, and it is desirable to allow supply to respond freely to satisfy that demand. A crucial corollary is that each patient and physician, once they make their decision, will generally be able to obtain the service they desire, as promptly as they desire it, in return for bearing at least a fraction of the cost. If the physician and patient X decide the ninth day is worthwhile, their decision will not be challenged.

Now contrast the same decision under regulation. In the absence of cost sharing, neither X nor his physician has any incentive to weigh cost against benefit. Because aggregate demand for hospital services is not constrained by a financial deterrent, it would be socially wasteful to allow the supply of hospital facilities to accommodate this inflated demand. The regulatory strategy fully accepts this premise. Its aim is to restrain supply to less than the inflated demand and to allocate the limited supply according to the genuine urgency and need of patients.

How well can the regulators succeed? The crucial handicap of the regulators is that, with "free" service, there is no reliable way to ascertain the degree of genuine urgency of each physician and patient. Under cost sharing, X and his physician will choose to leave the hospital if the cost borne by X outweighs the benefit as they perceive it. Thus, if X stays, his choice reveals that he and his MD regard the benefit of the ninth day (given X's circumstances) as worth a sacrifice of $60. Cost sharing compels a revelation of the degree of urgency of each patient's preference.

With free service, X will seek the ninth day as long as it offers any positive benefit. Naturally, X and his MD will call the ninth day necessary. How can regulators ascertain the urgency of preference? Suppose they take a hard line. They devise a permissible length of stay for various medical conditions and require hospitals to enforce it. Thus, if X's condition (as defined in the regulation) prescribes a limit of eight days, then X would be pressured to leave.

It seems inevitable that an appeal would be permitted. But if X's MD appeals, how will the appeal board determine whether X is a legitimate exception? Clearly, thorough investigation of each appeal would be very costly. Manpower would be diverted to serve on hospital appeal boards. Equally important, physicians' time would be consumed in the process. (The MDs would naturally bill the third parties for their time.)

To make a sensitive decision, the board would need to become aware of whether X has a spouse, relative, or friend who could be present at all times in case of emergency, or whether a 24-hour nurse could be hired who X could trust. Moreover, X's particular attitude about hospital versus home nursing care affects his urgency of demand. How is this to be detected?

In my view, the fundamental weakness of the regulatory approach, in contrast with the cost-sharing approach, is its inability to discern sensitively the differing preferences of individual patients. It will simply be too costly to attempt to distinguish feigned urgency from genuine urgency. Thus, regulations will be written for the average patient in a category, without adequate allowance for individual differences.

Consider another example: the hospital admission decision. Person Y has been told by his MD that he may have serious disease D, though the probability is very low. The MD presents the following choice: Y can wait several weeks to see if the symptoms vanish, as is probable; or a battery of tests can immediately be done on him as a hospital inpatient.

Under cost sharing, if Y is not inclined to worry prematurely, he may well decide to wait several weeks, thus avoiding the cost. On the other hand, if Y will not be unable to enjoy life until the possibility of disease D is conclusively rejected, he may choose to have the tests done immediately, despite the cost he must bear.

Without cost sharing, even an unworried Y might elect to have the tests done immediately. In fact, Y's MD, knowing that cost is irrelevant to his patient, may simply order an immediate battery of tests, without even presenting the option.

The aim of regulation, however, is to provide only enough facilities to handle genuinely urgent demand. If facilities are adequate to handle both an unworried and a worried patient Y quickly, then supply is excessive. Unworried Y does not value the services for his case as much as it costs society to provide it; it would therefore be inefficient to allocate costly resources for this purpose.

Suppose, then, that regulators limit the supply of hospital facilities so that it is adequate only to handle worried Y's case quickly. Their intention is that unworried Y should wait, because his demand is less urgent. The problem, however, is that there is no way to assure that worried Y gets quick treatment, while unworried Y waits. With lab tests free, both will request speedy tests and express urgency if such expression is required. How can regulators detect genuine urgency? It is quite possible that unworried Y will obtain speedy tests, while worried Y will suffer a significant delay.

There is irony here. Everywhere else in the economy, Y would be free to indulge his preference for luxury, or prompt service, without any regulatory obstacle, provided he is willing to bear the cost. But in an aspect of his life that matters most, the regulatory strategy may prevent him from satisfying his preferences. He can eat at an extravagant restaurant, buy a luxurious car, but may be unable to buy a prompt battery of tests to determine whether he has a serious disease.

At first glance, cost sharing strikes some observers as insensitive to patients, while free care appears compassionate. When the consequences are examined, however, it becomes apparent that cost sharing preserves the ability of the patient, guided by his MD, to obtain the service he wants as quickly as he desires it. The price of seemingly compassionate free service is a diminution in the power of each patient over the medical service he is able to obtain.

When patients cost share, supply can be allowed to respond freely to demand, and each patient and MD can be permitted to exercise their own choice over resource use. When service is free, regulators cannot permit all demand to be satisfied, and must, by various methods, create obstacles to the attempt to obtain service. Regulators may be well-intentioned and seek to allocate resources where they believe they are most needed. But they cannot have sufficient information to tailor resources according to genuine urgency. Moreover, each patient and MD no longer have full control over access to medical resources.

If cost sharing were unrelated to ability to pay, then it too would present inequitable barriers. The income-related tax credit, however, assures that cost sharing will be geared to ability to pay. The use of a modern public policy instrument—the tax credit—enables cost sharing to be equitably implemented.

It is often argued (by opponents as well as advocates) that the regulatory approach should be judged by its ability to slow the growth rate of national medical cost. Most economists, however, would emphasize that this is the wrong criterion. The goal should be to achieve the optimal rate of growth—neither too high nor too low—both in the aggregate and for each individual consumer. It is just as inefficient to have too few resources devoted to medical care as too many.

Today, in a climate of "free" hospital service, the growth rate is surely above the social optimum. Regulation can reduce the growth rate. But the issue is how can regulators achieve the socially desirable growth rate, both in the aggregate and for each person?

The optimal growth rate cannot be decided solely on technical grounds. For all goods and services, including medical care, the optimal growth rate depends on subjective consumer preferences as well as objective production conditions. If the average individual, confronted with the cost of medical care as well as other goods and services, prefers R percent more medical care this year than last year, then a growth rate either greater or less than R percent entails a misallocation of resources.

Cost sharing automatically reveals consumer preferences and induces each person to trade off medical service against other goods and services. This process causes technical information, reflected in cost, to be combined with preference information, so that the two determine resource allocation. The aggregate growth rate reflects the sum of individual decisions in which objective cost is weighed against subjective benefit.

The fundamental shortcoming of the regulatory strategy is that it has no mechanism for revealing genuine consumer preference. It therefore cannot tell whether the regulated medical cost growth rate is socially optimal, either in the aggregate, or for each individual.

Thus, the important issue is not whether regulation can reduce the growth rate of national medical cost. It can, and it has in some countries. Rather, it is whether regulation or consumer cost-sharing is more likely to accomplish the socially optimal growth rate, both in the aggregate and for each individual. The argument for cost sharing is not that it will necessarily achieve a lower growth rate, but that it will be more likely to approach the right growth rate for each person and for the whole society.

Conclusion

The analysis began by asking what would happen if the government followed a policy of genuine nonintervention towards health insurance. Such a policy would require the repeal of current tax subsidies for health insurance. It is now increasingly recognized that these substantial subsidies have encouraged shallow, first-dollar hospital insurance, helped eliminate consumer cost-sharing from the hospital sector, and therefore fueled hospital sector inefficiency and inflation. Repeal of these subsidies would induce most households to prefer less costly, major-risk (catastrophic) insurance and would therefore restore substantial consumer cost-sharing to the hospital sector. Most health economists believe that the restoration of cost sharing would cause most physicians, on behalf of their patients, to begin weighing cost against benefit as they make decisions. The result would be a reduction in hospital cost inflation and inefficiency.

Despite the improvement in efficiency, it is doubtful that universal income-related catastrophic protection would result. For example, unhealthy low-income persons, not covered by work place insurance, would only be able to obtain adequate protection by spending a large fraction of their income on health insurance. Some might be unable to obtain insurance.

A limited governmental intervention is therefore proposed: a tax credit for the purchase of private major-risk insurance. The credit would increase, the lower the household's income was, so that each household would be able to afford a major-risk policy with a sufficiently low out-of-pocket ceiling to provide adequate protection. A complementary medical loan program, implemented by private insurers and loan institutions under government contract, would enable each household to bear a higher ceiling; it would therefore enable the government to assure adequate protection with a smaller credit and a smaller total budgetary cost.

To guarantee universal catastrophic protection, it is further proposed that the government provide "major-risk insurance of last resort" through a tax credit for medical expenses of households not covered by private insurance. For example, an uninsured household with $20,000 of income might have to bear the first $1,500 of its annual medical bill; it would then be entitled to a credit equal to 80 percent of its additional medical bill, until its out-of-pocket burden reached $3,000; it would then be entitled to a credit equal to 100 percent of its additional medical bill. The credit would be "refundable," so that a person would be entitled to the full credit even if his tax liability was less than the credit (through a refund from IRS). Thus, universal, income-related catastrophic insurance would be assured.

The consumer cost-sharing that would result from this governmental policy is preferable to regulation as a method of promoting health sector efficiency. The fundamental weakness of the regulatory approach, in the absence of cost sharing, is its inability to ascertain the degree of urgency of individual patients and guide resource allocation according to genuine urgency. There is no effective way for regulators to assure that a limited supply, confronted with inflated demand, is in fact allocated to those who value it most. In contrast, cost sharing induces physicians, on behalf of their patients, to weigh cost against benefit. The resulting demand reflects urgency and assures that supply is allocated to those who value it highly.

Finally, cost sharing promotes the ability of each patient, guided by his physician, to obtain the service he desires as promptly as he desires it. Because demand reflects urgency, supply can be allowed to meet demand, so that it is available for patients who seek it after weighing the cost. Without cost sharing, demand is inflated and regulators must limit supply below demand and place obstacles in the path of physicians and their patients as they seek service. The price of "free" hospital service is, therefore, some loss of freedom and control by the patient and his physician over access to medical care.

Income-related consumer cost-sharing, implemented by a modern public policy instrument (the tax credit) offers the prospect of improving efficiency without sacrificing equity. A tax credit for catastrophic insurance, a medical loan program, and the repeal of other tax subsidies for insurance are preferable to regulation as a strategy to treat the health insurance problem.

Chapter 8 Appendix:
The Tax Credit for Major-Risk Insurance

A household should never bear a greater burden under private policy cost-sharing than it would have borne if it had no private insurance and relied on the last resort tax credit.

Thus, the last resort credit schedule should provide a maximum burden for all households. This principle can be implemented by entitling any household with private insurance to a tax credit equal to the difference between its out-of-pocket burden under its private policy, and the burden it would have borne under the last resort credit for the same medical bill.

For example, suppose a $20,000 household without any insurance was required to pay the first $1,500 of its annual medical bill, and was then entitled to a tax credit equal to 80 percent of the additional bill until its annual burden reached $3,000 (when its annual medical bill reached $9,000); it would then be entitled to a 100 percent credit for any additional bill, so its ceiling would be $3,000 (15 percent of its income).

Consider a $20,000 household having private insurance with 20 percent patient cost-sharing and no ceiling. If the household's annual medical bill is $10,000, its burden would be $2,000. If it had no private insurance, its burden under the last resort credit would have been $3,000; it would therefore not be entitled to any tax credit. Suppose, however, that its income was $10,000: its ceiling under the last resort credit would have been $1,500. In that case, it would be entitled to a $500 credit—the difference between its $2,000 burden under its private policy and the $1,500 burden it would have borne under the last resort credit.

Thus, no household—whatever its private policy cost-sharing—can ever incur a burden greater than its burden under the last resort credit schedule.

"First-dollar-only" private insurance should be ineligible for tax credit.

The rationale for the tax credit is to ensure that every household can afford the medical care it needs and that none is severely burdened by medical bills. A first-dollar-only policy does not provide the protection sought; it should therefore be ineligible. For example, a private policy that covers 100 percent of the first $1,500 of a household's annual medical bill, but 0 percent thereafter, would be ineligible for credit.

Such "shallow-only" coverage, without tax credit, is not likely to prove attractive to most households. For example, consider a $20,000 household that would have to bear the first $1,500 of its annual medical bill under the last resort credit. Is it likely to buy a shallow-only policy that covers 100 percent of its first $1,500, and 0 percent of any medical bill above $1,500? Consider the following example:

		Size of Bill	
Health state	Percent chance	Last resort credit	"Shallow-only insurance"
1.	40%	$200	$300
2.	40%	$1,000	$1,500
3.	20%	$10,000	$10,000

To simplify, it is assumed that the household may experience one of three possible health states: it has a 40 percent chance of 1, a 40 percent chance of 2, and a 20 percent chance of 3. If it relies on the last resort credit, and state 1 is experienced, it will incur a $200 bill. With shallow-only insurance, however, if state 1 occurs, it will incur a $300 bill, because the 100 percent coverage will induce it to inflate its bill; the same would happen should state 2 occur. The bill is the same in state 3—$10,000—because the shallow coverage terminates after $1,500.

The insurer's expected liability—$E(L)$—under the shallow policy is:

$$E(L) = .4(300) + .4(1,500) + .2(1,500) = \$1,020$$

The "pure" premium (ignoring administrative cost and minimum profit margin) would therefore be $1,020. Does it seem likely that a household would be willing to pay more than $1,020 just to obtain coverage for the first $1,500, especially when it would still remain vulnerable to a maximum burden of $3,000?

In principle, if shallow insurance imposes an external cost on others (via physician behavior transmitting inflation from the insured to the uninsured) then an explicit tax should be imposed on such insurance. In practice, it may be difficult to explain the externality rationale for such an explicit tax. As the above example suggests, however, ineligibility for tax credit should discourage most households from obtaining such insurance.

One possible definition for an ineligible shallow policy is a policy in which the patient cost-sharing rate, at some point, increases as the medical bill increases. It would not be satisfactory to define it as a policy without a ceiling, because the policy described above could circumvent this by promising a ceiling of $1 million.

The ceiling need not be specified to define eligibility for tax credit.

Given the last resort ceiling, there is no reason for a household to buy a major-risk, private policy unless its ceiling is less than the last resort ceiling. Thus, as long as the private policy covers the required services, has a ceiling, and never increases the patient cost-sharing rate as the medical bill increases, it should be eligible for credit. If the ceiling is too high, households will choose not to buy it.

Nevertheless, it would be possible to specify that a household would be unable to obtain credit if the ceiling exceeds its last resort ceiling. The problem here, however, is that many will obtain a private policy through their work place; the ceiling for the single work place policy may suit the average employee, but not every employee. Thus, an employee may be compelled to pay for a policy with a ceiling above his last resort ceiling. To avoid denying credit in such cases, it might be best to refrain from specifying any constraint on the ceiling.

The credit should be phased out as the size of the (fee-for-service insurance) premium increases for a given household.

Although households will not want private policies with a ceiling higher than their last resort ceiling, many will want a lower ceiling, and some will want a ceiling of zero, that is, complete insurance. The lower the ceiling, the higher the premium. Since the tax credit does not increase with the premium, a household would bear the full cost of the higher premium. If there were no externality associated with "complete" insurance, there would be no valid reason to discourage a household from obtaining such coverage. Such insurance should cause the household to inflate its medical bills; but this inflation would be reflected in the premium.

An externality, however, may exist. When some patients become completely insured, physicians may inflate orders for all patients; thus a cost is imposed on those not fully insured. It is therefore appropriate to confront the potential purchaser of complete insurance with this external cost. This can be done by phasing out the credit as the premium increases for a given household; the reduction of credit constitutes an implicit tax on additional insurance.

For example, budget studies may imply that an adequate ceiling for a $20,000 household is $3,000, the required premium $300, and the proper credit $100 (the household would be expected to contribute $200). For a $10,000 household, the analogous figures may be $1,500, $375, and $200 (with an expected household contribution of $175). For the $20,000 household, for each $1 by which the premium exceeds $300, its credit would be reduced perhaps twenty cents, and its credit would vanish if its premium reached $800. For the $10,000 household, for each $1 by which the premium exceeded $375, its credit would be reduced twenty cents, and its credit would vanish if its premium reached $1,375.

The credit should not be phased out for a prepaid health maintenance organization (HMO).

Only the existence of an externality justifies the phasing out of credit. Under fee-for-service, inflation may be transmitted by physicians from the insured to the uninsured; under prepayment, physicians have an incentive to contain demand for all patients. Thus, an implicit tax is not warranted.

Chapter 8 Notes

1. *Editor's note:* These estimates, based on Treasury Department files, have been revised upward by their original authors. See note 11 of Ehrlich's paper (chapter 9) in this volume. For alternate estimates, see table 9.3 of Ehrlich's paper.

2. Under such a policy, the household would bear a fraction of the cost until its annual medical bill reached $9,000. It is important to recognize that only a small minority of households have annual medical bills in excess of $9,000. In 1978, the American Hospital Association reports that the average inpatient revenue per inpatient day in community hospitals was $220. Therefore, 41 days would be required for the hospital bill to reach $9,000. But approximately 99 percent of all hospital stays are less than 41 days; the mean stay in 1978 was 7.4 days (U.S. Department of Health, Education and Welfare, National Center for Health Statistics, *Utilization of Short-Stay Hospitals,* [1978], table D and table 3). Again, if the physician bill is $220, 34 days are required to reach a hospital bill of $7,500; 97 percent do not exceed 34 days. I am indebted to Dorothy Rice, director of the National Center for Health Statistics, for providing me with this data.

3. Laurence S. Seidman, "Medical Loans and Major-Risk National Health Insurance." *Health Services Research,* 12 no. 2 (Summer 1977): 123–28.

On the Rationale
for National Health Insurance:
Where Did the Private Market Fail?

*Isaac Ehrlich**

The call for national health insurance in the United States goes back as far as the 1930s but has received great momentum over the last decade. In the Ninety-fourth Congress alone, 45 separate bills were introduced under some variant of a national health insurance (NHI) title,[1] ranging from plans to provide federal tax subsidies that would encourage people to buy private health insurance, to plans to replace most private health insurance with a public plan. There are many questions that can be raised in connection with the specific detail of alternative plans. But the major one is the following: does government have a special role to play in health insurance, or the health care sec-

---

*Melvin H. Baker Professor of American Enterprise and Professor of Economics, State University of New York at Buffalo.

I would like to thank Ross Arnett III, Charles Phelps, Gordon Trapnell, and Eugene Steurele for the useful information and suggestions they have provided. I have also benefitted from the dedicated research and computational assistance of Fred Floss, Jr., and Kenji Yamamoto.

This paper grew out of my initial comments on papers delivered in this session of the conference. Its main focus, however, is the general rationale for a national health insurance system, rather than the merits of any specific plan.

tor in general; and if so, what is it and how does it differ from its role in other sectors of the economy? A systematic evaluation of this issue is a prerequisite for determining the merits of specific plans.

A frequent theme in the literature and conferences on health care is that health is a very unique commodity (unlike mechanical gadgets or hoola hoops, for example) and that ultimately this alone may justify a reorganization of the markets for health insurance and medical services under the guidance of the visible hand of government. It is, of course, easy to agree that health care is different from hoola hoops. But isn't almost any other good and service also different, at least in some respects? Clearly, essential food items, housing, fire-alarm systems, home heating and cooling in extreme weather conditions, and higher education are different. More important, they may not be less essential than medical services in determining the amount of good health individuals actually enjoy.[2] Yet we do not propose to abolish free markets in these goods (including related insurance services), or otherwise provide them under a "socialized" system because of their uniqueness. Is the case of health care services radically different?

Much has already been written about the more specific reasons for a greater role for the state in health, beyond the provision of undisputed public health services and the modification of recognizable externalities; and this paper is not intended to provide an in-depth review of all or most of the arguments.[3] My analysis here has been motivated primarily by my interest in the latest NHI bill introduced by Senator Kennedy (United States Senate Hearings, 1979, pp. 435–98), which is the subject of the paper by Stanley Jones (chapter 7). In the course of preparing my evaluation, I have found it necessary to re-examine some of the debated issues, as well as some of the data bearing on the alleged "market breakdown" and the remedies proposed for it in the new Kennedy plan. My analysis is presented in two parts. In the first part, I discuss the rationale for government action in light of what the authors of NHI bills seem to regard as the main arguments for it. In addition to a critical evaluation, I present data concerning the role of explicit and implicit public intervention in the private market for health care services and insurance. My conclusion is that much of the observed imperfections concerning the level and distribution of health care services seem to be attributable to the present system of inefficient and regressive subsidization of these services, rather than to the failure of the private health insurance system. In the second part, I examine in some detail the remedies proposed in Senator Kennedy's new program and especially its economic price tag. This discussion leads to a more general evaluation of the true welfare (resource) costs of a public insurance system of the type proposed by Senator Kennedy. I conclude with some brief thoughts on some critical targets of reform in the health services sector.

Market Failure

The basic theoretical rationale for government intervention, or a specific role for government in the marketplace, is the failure of private markets to bring about socially optimal outcomes in terms of the rate and direction of economic activity. Where did the private market for health insurance fail in this regard? Authors of national health insurance bills typically do not address this issue directly. One can identify the main perceived indicators of failure indirectly, however, by examining the list of goals underlying the Health Care for all Americans Act and other major NHI plans.[4] The three basic indicators by this list are:

1. Insufficient coverage in both breadth and intensity. Existing plans typically do not provide full insurance against all medical hazards. Different hazards are covered in varying degrees, and some medical hazards are not covered at all. The more ambitious national health insurance plans call for complete coverage of the main medical services: hospital care, physician services, and laboratory bills. They call for at least partial coverage of preventive services, nursing home care, mental health care, and prescription drugs.
2. Rising health care costs. The inflation of hospital and medical care costs, as well as the continuous increase in the share of health care costs in the gross national product over the last two decades (particularly since 1966, see table 9.1), are implicitly considered to be a major, if not the most important, indicator of the failure of the private health insurance system to contain costs. A central element of some national health insurance plans is cost containment through a national budgeting and planning system, or through direct quantity, quality, and price controls.
3. The failure of the private health insurance market to provide insur-

TABLE 9.1

Aggregate national health expenditures by source of funds
(1950–1978 with current projections to 1990)

Calendar year	Gross national product (in billions)	Total expenditures $ Amount (in billions)	Total expenditures Percent of GNP	Public (direct)[a] expenditures $ Amount (in billions)	Public (direct)[a] expenditures Percent of total
1950	284.8	12.7	4.5	3.4	27.2
1955	398.0	17.7	4.4	4.6	25.7
1960	503.7	26.9	5.3	6.6	24.7
1965	688.1	43.0	6.2	10.7	24.9
1970	982.4	74.7	7.6	27.3	36.5
1975	1,528.8	131.5	8.6	55.7	42.3
1978	2,107.6	192.4	9.1	78.1	40.6
1980[b]	2,572.0	244.6	9.5	100.6	41.1
1985[b]	4,168.7	438.2	10.5	184.0	42.0
1990[b]	6,562.5	757.9	11.5	325.8	43.0

a. Share of public expenditures in total health expenditures represents only explicit payments by the public sector. It omits implicit tax expenditures due to exemption of premiums and other deductible medical outlays from taxation.

b. Projections based on continuation of the present system of health care services without NHI.

Sources: For 1950–1978, Gibson (1979), table 1. Projections for 1980–1990, Freeland et al. (1980), table 1.

ance of medical services to all persons and, in particular, to people who cannot afford the market insurance premiums for large medical bills. In some plans, insufficient access to (or utilization of) medical care services in the case of specific population groups is listed as a separate, though related, indicator of market failure (see, for example, Cavalier 1979, p. 16). Let us examine each of these indicators more closely.

Incomplete Coverage

Partial and variable coverage of specific medical hazards could be regarded as an indication of market failure only on three rather implausible conditions:

a. Monetary payments provide a perfect replacement for the loss of consumption opportunities in the event of illness
b. The monetary prices of insurance charged individuals are actuarially fair
c. Literally every consumption unit in the economy is "risk averse."

a. Monetary compensations While the explicit transactions in insurance markets relate to contingent money claims (i.e., the opportunity to purchase a desired set of market goods and services), the implicit objects of choice underlying these transactions are contingent *consumption claims* (i.e., the opportunity to produce a set of basic consumption characteristics or activities) that directly increase consumer welfare.[5] Although market goods and services, including medical care services, are important inputs in the production of the desired consumption services, they are not the only relevant inputs, as personal time and energy also play an important role. Moreover, the marginal productivity of any given bundle of market (money) goods will generally be affected by the consumer's state of health. For these reasons, one can show that it might not be optimal for individuals to fully insure themselves against the detrimental consequences of specific health hazards (in the sense that all relevant losses be fully covered, or that only medical care outlays be fully covered) even if insurance premiums are actuarially fair. Indeed, the sufficient conditions for such full insurance to be optimal are rather stringent: they require either (1) that monetary compensations be a perfect substitute for all the basic consumption opportunities lost through illness or (2) that the onslaught of illness not affect the marginal productivity of the original bundle of market goods and services that were used in the state of good health, in producing consumption activities (and utility) in the state of ill health.[6]

This analysis provides one possible explanation for the perceived low market interest in so-called catastrophic insurance. Despite some studies showing that such insurance could be sold at seemingly low premiums (see Frech and Ginsburg 1978, p. 9), many families, including some in middle- and upper-income brackets, have been judged to lack adequate protection.[7] This evidence appears puzzling because the theory of rational insurance purchases predicts a stronger incentive to protect large rather than small financial losses, all other things equal. If, however, some illnesses of catastrophic proportions involved temporary or permanent physical impediments that reduced the marginal utility from the original bundle of market goods and services (other than remedial medical services) consumed, then full coverage of the resulting medical care outlays would not be optimal even if actuarially fair insurance could be obtained. An alternative explanation is that people contemplating insurance of medical needs of catastrophic proportions would prefer to depend on public welfare systems for this contingency rather than pay the market premium. The reason why even middle- and upper-income families might expect to take advantage of this option is that the huge financial burdens resulting from a prolonged catastrophic illness would deplete personal and family resources to an extent that would qualify them for public welfare assistance.

b. The real price of insurance An actuarially fair price of insurance is feasible only if insurance services can be provided free of charge. Needless to say, health insurance, like any other type of insurance, involves administrative, information-gathering, and monitoring costs, as well as "insurance-induced" claims, or "moral hazard" costs, that are particularly high in connection with medical risks that involve a large element of pure consumption. As has been argued elsewhere (see Ehrlich 1975 and Ehrlich and Becker 1972), the basic reason behind the prevalence of moral hazard in all insurance transactions is the economic inexpediency of a perfect adjustment of individual premiums by insurers to reflect the true personal odds of incurring medical ex-

penses, which causes consumers to substitute "covered" medical services for self-insurance and protection, including self-care. It does not
pay insurance to adjust individual premiums because of the large costs
of monitoring individual performance under the insurance plan. This,
indeed, is one of the main reasons for the popularity of group insurance
plans, based on the member's employment association; these plans replace the high cost of monitoring individual behavior or endowed risk
with the more economical cost of observing group performance, and
they minimize the self-selection problem of asymmetric information
discussed by Rothchild and Stiglitz (1977). The optimal degree of
moral hazard then is a reflection of a minimized but unavoidable cost
of doing business, and since that cost is particularly high for specific
hazards, complete coverage of these must be an exception rather than
the rule. Moreover, no NHI plan can eliminate or reduce these costs.
Therefore, full coverage of medical services cannot be socially optimal
under any system of insurance.

c. Tastes for risk It is, of course, inconceivable that all persons share
the same aversion to risk. Those who prefer risk, by definition, would
maximize their personal welfare by rejecting an actuarially fair insurance deal and might accept insurance only if premiums were heavily
subsidized. To the extent that the actual prices charged include a positive loading fee, persons with a lower aversion to risk would find it
optimal to demand a lesser insurance coverage than people with a high
degree of risk aversion. Clearly, any attempt to impose a uniform, let
alone "full," coverage on all persons would, by this argument, serve to
lower rather than raise social welfare.

The Rising Cost of Health Care

Health care costs have indeed been rising sharply in the United States
over the past two decades, but not primarily as a result of excessive
medical price inflation. The rise in the medical care price index,
which is not adjusted for changes in the quality of care, has not significantly exceeded that of food or housing; the latter increased about 130
percent between 1967 and September of 1979, as against the 110 percent increase in the consumer price index (CPI) for all items.[8] The
sharpest increases in the average medical care price index took place

in 1967, following the introduction of Medicare and Medicaid, and in 1974–75, following the abolition of general wage and price controls present from late 1971 to mid–1974. It appears then that the rising cost of health care is due chiefly to the increase in the quantity, quality, and complexity of the medical services that are being rendered to patients. Is this increase in the real amount of health care services consumed an indication of market failure? While the following discussion does not attempt to resolve this issue via a systematic econometric study of the health care sector,[9] it does point to dynamic changes in some key variables that could account for a good deal of its rapid growth in recent years.

Economic growth and technological medical advances There is, of course, no reason to expect stagnation in the volume or even the share of national resources going into any specific industry unless the economy itself is stagnant and there are no changes in the relevant relative prices. The steady growth in consumers' real income since World War II, coupled with significant advances in medical technology (especially in so far as general hospital and surgical services are concerned), undoubtedly have contributed to the steady growth in the demand for, and volume of, services rendered. Indeed, as impressive as the overall growth of the medical industry appears to be, the growth in hospital care has been even more dramatic: the share of national health expenditures devoted to hospital care services has increased from 18.2 percent in 1929 to approximately 40 percent in 1978 (see Gibson 1979, pp. 23–24). The growth in age-adjusted life expectancies and the associated aging of the population—itself possibly an outcome, in part, of advancing medical technology—may have precipitated the overall increase in the demand for health care services since a disproportionate amount of these services is consumed by older age groups.

The explicit role of government The increased share of direct public (federal and state) outlays on medical care, especially following the introduction of Medicare and Medicaid, has been by far the most important structural change in health care financing in the last fifteen years. The share of public expenditures in total health care costs, which was steady over the period of 1950 through 1965, jumped by over 170 percent from 1965 to 1978, reaching the point where roughly

TABLE 9.2

Percentage distribution of personal health care expenditures by type of coverage and source of funds (selected calendar years, 1950–1978[a])

Source of fund	Total personal health care					Hospital care			Physicians' services		
	Total Millions of $	% Public Total	Federal	% Private Direct	Insurance	Total Millions of $	% Private Direct	Insurance	Total Millions of $	% Private Direct	Insurance
Percent of total											
1950	10,885	22.4	10.4	65.5	9.1	3,851	29.9	17.7	2,747	83.2	11.4
1955	15,708	23.0	10.5	58.1	16.1	5,900	22.3	28.5	3,689	69.8	23.2
1960	23,680	21.8	9.3	54.9	21.1	9,092	19.8	36.3	5,684	65.4	28.0
1965	37,267	21.1	10.2	53.4	23.4	13,935	17.7	41.5	8,474	61.4	31.6
1970	65,723	34.1	22.2	40.4	24.0	27,799	10.4	36.0	14,340	44.2	34.2
1975	116,297	39.7	27.1	32.5	26.6	52,138	7.6	36.2	24,932	35.9	37.8
1978	167,911	38.7	27.7	32.9	27.0	76,025	9.9	35.2	35,250	34.1	39.1

a. Note that the combined shares of direct payments, private insurance, and public payments do not add up to one because I have not listed other private payments (mainly philanthropy) which have accounted (on average) for roughly 2 percent of the total.

Source: Gibson (1979), tables 7, 8.

39 percent of personal health care expenditures (see table 9.2) and an even larger percentage of national health expenditures are not financed through direct public payments.[10] Over the same two subperiods, the share of private insurance payments in total personal health care expenses exhibited just the opposite pattern: it rose dramatically over the fifteen-year period from 1950 to 1965 and remained roughly constant over the period of 1965 to 1978, except for a slight increase in the share of coverage for physicians' services. It is, however, the fifteen-year period since 1965 that saw a markedly faster rate of growth of total medical care outlays, both in absolute terms and as a percentage of GNP, relative to the preceding fifteen-year period. While this evidence is not sufficient, of course, to establish any strict causal relationships, it is at least indicative of the strong association existing in recent years between the enhanced role of public financing and the rising overall cost of health care services. For a more specific evaluation of the efficiency of the publicly financed Medicare and Medicaid programs and their contributions to the rising cost of health care, see, for example, Enthoven (1978) and Feldstein (1971).

Indirect subsidies The measured, on-budget public outlays do not fully reflect the extent of public financing of health care services, which also include indirect subsidies resulting from exemption from taxation of various medical expenditures. The sources of exemption are: (1) the exclusion of all contributions made by employers to employee group insurance plans ("employer exclusion") from taxable income and from the wage base for determining social security taxes; (2) the deduction of large out-of-pocket medical expenditures, including health insurance premiums from taxable income for those who itemize their deductions ("itemized medical expense deduction"); (3) the deduction of charitable contributions to nonprofit medical facilities ("charity deduction"); and (4) the issuance of tax-exempt bonds to finance capital projects at private hospitals ("tax-exempt bonds"). Table 9.3 presents my best estimates of the aggregate subsidies resulting only from the first two sources of exemption in 1970 and 1975 and my rough projection of the corresponding sums for 1980. These estimates must be evaluated with a great deal of caution: while the estimates for 1970 and 1975 are based on the relevant set of raw data or published estimates by others, some of the basic data underlying the latter have undergone a number of revisions over time. I have relied

TABLE 9.3

Indirect federal subsidies to health services through tax
exemptions, selected years[a] (billions of dollars)

Source of exemption	1970[b]	1975[b]	1980[c]
Employer exclusion	2.4	6.2	14.8
Itemized premium expenses	0.6	1.0	1.7
Other itemized medical expenses	1.5	1.9	2.4
Total	4.5	9.2	19.0

a. Excluding foregone social security tax revenues.
b. Calculations based on actual incidence of exemptions.
c. Author's projections.
For sources and computations, see chapter 9 appendix B.

upon the most recent material on the topic to resolve apparent inconsistencies and inaccuracies, and to make simple projections for 1980.[11]
In all, the calculations tend to be conservative estimates. Moreover,
the tax subsidy estimates relating to the employer exclusion include
only the foregone federal tax revenues; they omit all the foregone state
tax revenues and social security taxes. Despite these and the complete
omission of all tax subsidies due to the "charity deduction" and the
"tax exempt bonds" exclusion provisions, the projected total indirect
subsidies for 1980 is $19 billion, or approximately one-third of the di-
rect federal expenditures on personal health care services. A conservative estimate of the missing subsidies due to the omitted sources of
exemption and taxation could bring the total amount in 1980 to over
$23 billion. By these admittedly crude estimates, the total share of the
public sector in financing the national health care expenditures in
1980 may have already exceeded the 50 percent mark.

The effect of the subsidies on the net price of insurance The exemption from taxation of all premium payments by employees and the
more limited exemption of direct premium payments by individuals[12]
affect directly the net price of insurance for individuals, and hence
their incentive to buy insurance. The point has already been addressed
in the literature,[13] but the extent of the price reduction and its dynamics have not been fully fleshed out.

In table 9.3 I have estimated the aggregate "premium subsidy" due only to the exemption of payments from federal income taxes at $3 billion in 1970, $7.2 billion in 1975, and $16.5 billion in 1980. When estimated as a proportion of total premium payments for private health insurance, the average subsidy per premium amounts to 18 percent, 21 percent, and 23 percent for these three years, respectively.

A more meaningful description of these subsidies is in terms of their impact on the net real prices paid by individuals for their insurance purchases. An actuarially fair premium amounts to a zero real price of insurance from a social point of view (see Ehrlich and Becker 1972). In reality, premiums and prices must include a "loading factor" above the actuarially fair level to compensate insurers for all their relevant costs. A convenient measure for the loading rate or the real price of insurance for a particular insurance plan is given by the deviation from unity of the ratio of premiums to expected benefits[14] in that plan, or

$$\lambda^* = [P/E(B)] - 1.$$

In table 9.4, I have provided alternative estimates for λ^* depending upon the method of estimating expected benefits. Thus, λ_0 is an average loading rate estimated from the ratio of total premiums and benefit payments over the period 1960—1977. λ_1 is computed on the basis of current values of premiums and benefits, and $\hat{\lambda}_2$ and $\hat{\lambda}_3$ are based on the expected values of benefits, $\hat{E}(B)$, as derived from two simple regression models (see chapter 9 appendix B, part 2, for details). The different procedures yield different estimates of (gross) loading rates for any one year. The trend in the net real prices to consumers (i.e., gross loading net of the federal subsidy per premium), however, is found to be unambiguously downward, regardless of the estimate of λ^* used. It indicates that, on average, the net prices paid, which appear to be at most negligible in 1970, have become considerably more negative by 1975 to the point where they may be at least 5 percent lower than the actuarially fair prices.

This development within the short span of five years is predominately the result of general inflation. The reason is apparent from the mechanics of the tax subsidy, which are dictated by the marginal tax liabilities of the groups benefiting from the exemption of premiums

TABLE 9.4

The impact of the federal subsidy on the net price of
insurance, 1970 and 1975

Price data	1970		1975	
1. Total federal subsidy[a] (billions)	$ 3.0		$ 7.2	
2. Total premiums (billions)	$17.2		$33.8	
3. Average subsidy per premium	17.5%		21.0%	
4. Alternative loading rates[b] (% of premiums)		Net of		Net of
	Gross	subsidy	Gross	subsidy
λ_0 = average for 1960–1977	11.87	−5.63	11.87	− 9.13
λ_1 = based on current data	9.15	−8.35	5.93	−15.07
$\hat{\lambda}_2$ = based on "expected" benefits (1)	16.62	−0.88	16.30	− 4.70
$\hat{\lambda}_3$ = based on "expected" benefits (2)	12.32	−5.18	8.40	−12.60
5. Average premium per policy[b]	$241.3		$398.9	
6. Average premium per tax unit[b]	$287.5		$481.1	
7. Average subsidy per itemizing tax unit	$ 24.8		$ 60.0	
8. Average subsidy per tax unit benefiting from "employer exclusion"	NA		$122.0	

a. From table 9.3.

b. Author's estimates based on indirect data.

Sources and explanation: See chapter 9 appendix B, part 2.

from taxation. Since inflation pushes marginal tax brackets upward, and since the tax structure is nominally progressive, the value of the tax saving from the premium exemption is likely to rise faster with inflation than the cost of the premiums themselves. Put differently, here, as in the case of all other exclusions, the "inflation-tax" works in reverse. Furthermore, the increase in nominal premiums above the critical level of $300 (see note 12) and changes in the tax law which have encouraged the utilization of the standard general deduction in lieu of itemized deductions (see *Statistics of Income* 1975) apparently have increased the incentives of workers to negotiate wage agreements that make the share of employers' contributions to employee premiums higher.[15] Since the latter are fully exempted from taxation, this development has further contributed to the rise in the average subsidy per premium.

But not all individuals have benefited from these federal and corresponding state subsidies to insurance (and direct medical expenses). Not only is the magnitude of the subsidy increasingly higher for higher income tax units, but also the taxpayers who do not itemize deductions, and consequently cannot benefit from the personal expense deduction provision, tend to be of low and moderate income levels. The result has been a grossly inequitable and regressive subsidy system, whose regressiveness has increased even more in the last decade because of stepped-up inflation.[16]

The artificial and continuous decrease in the net prices of health insurance may have been the single most important factor behind the growth in the level of insurance purchases since the mid–1960s. Furthermore, the apparent "negative real prices" may help resolve a few outstanding puzzles in health insurance. For example, the high propensity of individuals to purchase first-dollar hospital insurance coverage is cited in the literature as an apparent irrational behavior,[17] since theory predicts that the degree of insurance coverage by risk-avoiding consumers would be an increasing function of the prospective financial losses. What may not have been sufficiently stressed, however, is that the latter prediction applies only if the real price of insurance is positive. With the net loading rate being negative or negligible, it would be rational for consumers to seek and for insurers to provide even a large degree of shallow as well as "major medical" insurance coverage. Indeed, since coverage of major medical or hospital insurance has traditionally been the highest (see table 9.2), the decline in the net prices of insurance in recent years should have resulted in a greater rate of growth of shallow, relative to "major" insurance coverage. By the same token, this trend in prices should have affected (and apparently has affected) a significant growth of catastrophic insurance coverage in recent years as well.[18]

Moral hazard? The conventional analysis of moral hazard in private health insurance markets links the increase in insurance coverage directly with the growth in the consumption of health care services by the argument that the coinsurance rate acts like the marginal price of medical care services at the time of care.[19] By this argument, the mere

availability of any reimbursement insurance protection with a coinsurance rate less than unity induces excessive purchases of care, or
moral hazard. I believe that the relationship between insurance and
excessive use of (insured) medical care services is more complex for
three basic reasons. First, the coinsurance rate does not automatically
reflect the marginal price of care, as perceived by the consumer. It
does so only if there is no explicit or implicit feedback linking the premium payments by the insured unit directly with its actual consumption of health care services. Some existing insurance plans do take
steps toward establishing such links via experience rating of members'
premiums. Theory predicts that if the latter were perfect, consumers
would perceive their effective medical care prices to be equivalent to
the true prices charged by providers.[20] Second, if health insurance
were provided through an indemnity rather than a reimbursement
plan, there would be no room for the price-induced type of moral hazard, because under indemnity insurance, contingent dollar benefits are
fixed as part of the contract. Some health insurance policies sold in
private markets are in fact modeled along the indemnity type of insurance.[21] Third, the introduction of insurance might indeed lead to a
greater use of covered medical services, even under an indemnity plan,
not because of a perceived drop in the price of services at the time of
care, but because of a substitution of insured medical services for relatively less efficient forms of individual "self-insurance" and "self-protection." By this argument, the market for insured medical services is
an alternative to other insurance setups involving resource pooling by
members of large households, and guaranteed home care services to be
provided by household members. As the real price of insurance falls, or
the shadow cost of "home insurance" rises (because of improved labor
market opportunities for females, for example), more market insurance coverage and less home care will be demanded. Note, however,
that the assessment of the welfare costs implicit in this type of shift
toward insured medical services is different from the assessment under
the hypothesis of price-induced excess consumption of care because the
shift from home insurance to market insurance may be largely efficient. Thus, estimates of the welfare cost of "excess health insurance"
that ignore this trade-off may be grossly overstated.[22]

There is no important reason why a competitive market could not
induce the least costly (hence "optimal") mix of market and home
insurance, reimbursement and indemnity insurance, or group insur-

ance and individually based policies, given that consumers would bear the full marginal costs associated with the provision of insurance services under each type of plan. What is undoubtedly true, however, is that an artificial public subsidization of market insurance would distort the optimal mix of different insurance plans, the optimal degree of coverage under each plan, and, as a result, the actual utilization of insured health care services (if only because of an inefficient shift from home care to market services). As my analysis in the previous subsection of this paper shows, a considerable amount of artificial subsidization of market insurance has taken place in recent decades and has undoubtedly caused a significant welfare loss. But this distortion, or true moral hazard, has been the result of public intervention in private insurance, not of a market breakdown. To correct this distortion and contain the rising costs of health services, it is necessary to correct the distorting subsidy system (both explicit and implicit), rather than impose a comprehensive NHI system with zero coinsurance rates and uniform, mandated benefits.

Failure to Cover all Persons

Few people would deny the strong public sentiment for government aid to the old, to disabled persons in acute need for medical care, and to others who are excluded from the health insurance market because of inability to pay. This parallels the sentiment for general public aid and assistance to persons in extreme financial distress. The percentage of Americans without any private or public insurance coverage, however, has been on a continuous decline over time. In 1977, 80 percent of the population under age 65 and 78 percent of the general population were covered by at least a private hospital insurance plan, and the number of persons receiving Medicare and Medicaid reached close to 40 million (over 17 percent of the population). Still, it is estimated that 8 percent of the total population remains without any private or public coverage, and that this group is comprised mainly of low-income persons below the age of 65.[23] The number of indigent persons lacking coverage may then be greater than the number actually covered, and perhaps the level of assistance is inadequate. The real issue is this: If it is care for people in extreme medical need that is being sought, why not attack this problem directly through a genuinely progressive system of guaranteed premium subsidies or other transfer payments? Why should the solution involve a mandatory comprehensive insurance package for all people and all types of medical expenses, which, coupled with direct supply controls to "contain" costs, would decrease the choices available to patients, providers, and insurers, and increase the real social costs of providing health services only because of the desire to extend medical assistance to a relatively small section of the population unable to afford coverage? As the analysis in the previous subsection indicates, a frontal attack on this problem need not cost more to finance, given the implicit NHI system of regressive and inefficient public subsidies that is presently used to support public and private outlays on insurance and health care.

Some Economic Aspects of the
Health Care for All Americans Act

The basic list of goals underlying Senator Kennedy's new—1980—(as old) NHI plan is summarized succinctly in Stanley Jones's paper (chapter 7). These are: (1) to assure that all residents of the country can afford to purchase all needed health care; (2) to assure that needed health care is accessible to all; (3) to assure that individuals pay for their insurance on an equitable basis; (4) to assure that the health care received by all is of comparable quality and desirability; and (5) to assure that long-term health care costs grow no faster than the rate of increase of GNP.

The first four goals seem almost irresistible. A closer examination, however, reveals a fundamental misconception: the implicit notion that an efficient allocative mechanism for health services can be established on "need" without concern for scarcity; put differently, that standards of medical services can be established on purely objective grounds without reference to economics. There exists no scientific consensus about what medical need implies in individual cases, except for the recognition of wide variability and uncertainty with respect to personal conditions and circumstances that affect choice among alternative forms of treatment, which are subject to different costs. What does "need" mean? If need is what the consumer believes that he deserves, the answer may be prohibitively costly. Economic reality dictates that need be defined in terms of what someone in charge feels that anybody else should have. An allocative system based on need inevitably leads to the necessity of physically rationing available medical resources through bureaucratic choices. This eventuality becomes even more apparent after examining the specific program proposed for implementing these goals (for details, see Jones's paper, chapter 7).

Can you both have the cake and eat it? The program seems to imply that you can, since it proposes to: (1) cover all U.S. residents in private health insurance plans certified by the government, for which the government assumes ultimate liability by agreeing to finance any and all deficits; (2) cover hospital, physician (inpatient and outpatient), and laboratory services on an unlimited basis; and (3) charge no deductibles, no coinsurance rates (indeed, no out-of-pocket payments for these services) and eliminate all experience-rating based premium payments by users.

The last provision contrasts rather sharply with the thrust of the analysis of a previous section ("Moral Hazard") because it amounts to a complete separation between personal utilization of medical care services and the actual payment by users. This spells the ultimate degree of moral hazard (or induced-demand). Jones defends this provision by saying that "it grows out of the long-standing conviction in the unions that deductibles and coinsurance unduly discourage low-income individuals from seeking needed care."

Surely, anyone would agree that there is no such thing as "free unlimited" medical care. Since at a zero market price the aggregate demand for health care services is bound to drastically exceed the available supplies, the only options available to keep the plan at balance would be severe nonprice-rationing of demand or an unrealistic increase in appropriations.

Add to these prospective costs the huge administrative cost of the proposed plan. To implement the new NHI system, no less than four separate bureaucracies are proposed:

1. National banks or "consortia" that would use the incoming revenues from wage-related and income-related premiums paid by employers, employees, and individuals to pay their member insurers adequate premiums for the persons they enroll, based on community-related premiums to be negotiated with government.

2. A federal group that will negotiate these community pay standards and monitor procedural requirements of insurers, providers, and purchasers of health care services.

3. A federal collection agency that will collect the premiums that the insurance companies will not be able to collect because of the mandated wage-based premiums.

4. Finally, the government is to assume a direct regulatory role that would set up limits on prices and fees and otherwise ration expenditures. This role is to be achieved by establishing a national planning and budgeting system and by offering resource development funds.

To what extent do the cost estimates of the proposed Kennedy plan reflect the "induced demand" outlays, resulting from lowering the effective marginal prices of the bulk of health care services to zero, and the costs of the bureaucratic labyrinth just described?

The official figures, which are attributed to Gordon Trapnell of Actuarial Research Corporation (see United States Senate Hearings, 1979, p. 491), put the added total spending in fiscal year 1983 at $40 billion in 1980 dollars. Of these, $29 billion are to be additional on-budget federal costs and $11 billion represent additional contributions by employers, employees, and self-employed individuals. Unfortunately, I have been told that no official documents or technical notes are presently available that fully describe the methodology and data used to arrive at these estimates. Thus, their accuracy could not be ascertained. My personal inquiries with Mr. Trapnell, however, reveal the following:

1. The cost estimates have not been designed to reflect fully the added expenditures necessary to meet the induced demand due to the artificial lowering of users' prices. The induction method actually used is a mix of a limited allowance for the projected change in demand (as can be predicted from estimates of the price elasticities of demand for medical care services) and direct supply controls.[24]

2. The estimates are constructed on the assumption that the average fees paid to all physicians would be 5 percent lower than the currently prevailing fees for Medicare.

3. They are also based on the assumption that a strong hospital cost-containment bill will be passed by Congress.

4. Not all the added federal and nonfederal administrative costs of the program appear to have been accounted for.[25]

It appears that the true economic costs of the Kennedy bill would be substantially higher than what the official estimates show. I say this not only because of the experience with similar cost projections of public outlays for Medicare and Medicaid,[26] but especially because the estimates ignore altogether the implicit dead-weight costs of nonprice rationing devices that are explicitly suggested in the program to avoid a potential explosion in the visible costs of the system.

What are the implicit costs of rationing? To illustrate the type and potential magnitude of the costs involved, assume that in order to contain costs in the face of a potentially exploding market demand for services at zero money prices, the government would in effect freeze the quantity of health care services by freezing the fees paid to providers at their current or any planned future level. Many medical services would then have to be rationed on a first-come, first-served basis. Assume the rationing mechanism would be waiting time. Thus, queues, or related waiting costs, would replace out-of-pocket or premium-related payments as implicit, or shadow prices. (These would add substantially to the normal amount of waiting time patients must spend even in an unregulated market for care because of the stochastic nature of demand.) But queues (explicit or implicit), unlike money prices, absorb real resources and are not simply transfer payments. These resource costs are the foregone value of patients' time and full productive capacity that could be utilized for market or home production. Furthermore, it can be shown on the basis of some simplifying assumptions that the shadow queuing prices that must equilibrate the new system would, as a first approximation, equal the original level of the marginal (money) prices paid by consumers for health care services under the private health insurance system. Hence, the aggregate resource costs of the new NHI system could exceed those of the private system by as much as the original volume of direct payments by users. (See chapter 9, appendix C.) This amount was equal to $55.3 billion in 1978. The corresponding projected amounts in 1980 and 1985 are $65 billion and $117 billion, respectively, and are based on the anticipated levels of supply of personal health care services in these years (see Freeland et al. 1980, p. 17) and a conservative estimate of the current average rate of direct payments by consumers (30 percent of the total).

Similar arguments would apply in those cases where medical services would be rationed through implicit, rather than explicit, queues.

In the experience of the British National Health Service System, waiting lists for some types of hospitalization have reached six years (see Davis 1975, p. 26). Under such circumstances, denial of services and a deterioration of the quality of care delivered are bound to happen and cause analogous resource costs to society (see Newhouse et al. 1974). The basic point of this analysis is that, under realistic assumptions regarding the mechanism for allocating medical resources in a regulated NHI system of the kind proposed by Senator Kennedy, the real costs of the system could drastically exceed the official estimates for 1983.

Concluding Remarks

Whether government has a special role to play in health insurance and the health services sector in general depends not only on the interpretation of alleged indicators of market failure, but also on whether what is considered to be an imperfection in the private markets can be remedied by a specific NHI prescription. My limited analysis suggests that the answer to the second question may be easier than that to the first. It appears that the basic justification for a mandatory and comprehensive NHI system of the type proposed by Senator Kennedy lies not in the achievement of greater efficiency in the allocation of resources to health care services, but in the promotion of a visibly more "equal" (though not necessarily equitable) distribution of health care services by income. Even here the merit of the plan is not unambiguous. Although the proposal makes premium payments proportional to wages, it does not call for the abolition of the current regressive system of implicit tax subsidies. Moreover, the notion that the plan guarantees that employers will be responsible for at least 65 percent of the total premium payments, as formally mandated, is without basis. In the long run, the actual share borne by employees will be dictated by the ability of employers to shift the burden of the proposed "employment tax" to employees through a trade-off between premium payments and (future) wage increases. The latter is dictated by the relative elasticities of the demand and supply curves for labor services, rather than by the mandated split of premium payments. In the short run, the mandated increase in employers' total wage and benefit payments is likely to result in a significant drop in total employment, especially of low wage earners.

There are, however, reasons to believe that the government does have a special role to play in the present mixed system of private enterprise and governmental subsidies because of the unusual power and authority given by law to the American Medical Association and, to a lesser degree, to other providers' organizations (see Kessel 1970). To the extent that the special providers' privileges lead to artificial barriers on the entry into medicine of primary and auxiliary manpower and other resources, and to barriers on competition among providers in terms of the type and organization of medical services offered and the information disseminated to consumers (through advertising restrictions), the private market system would indeed fail to achieve allocative efficiency. Similarly, the mix of insurance plans provided may be distorted through pressures from providers (see Enthoven 1978, and Frech and Ginsburg 1975, p. 47). A stronger role for the government can be justified to assure greater competition.

Not less important would be the transformation of the current system of distortive and regressive implicit tax subsidies to a genuine system of progressive credits for health insurance premiums with special attention to the poor and the medically indigent.

Chapter 9 Appendix A: On Optimal Health Insurance—A Household Production Model

As the discussion in the text of this paper suggests, the direct objects of choice entering a consumer's utility function in any state of health are not contingent financial claims, but contingent consumption activities that are functions of those claims and the consumer's state of health.

$$z_h = g(x_h, m_h, h) \tag{1}$$

In equation (1) m_h represents remedial medical care services; x_h stands for all other goods and services, and the consumer's state of health, h, is introduced as a distinct argument. The production function z is assumed to be strictly concave.

To achieve a simple illustration of the basic theoretical arguments developed, I shall adopt a number of simplifying assumptions, none of which affect the generality of these arguments:

1. There are only two states of health: sick (s) with probability p, and well (w) with probability $1-p$.

2. The prices of x and m are constant. Both are normalized at unity through the proper choice of units.
3. The consumer is an expected utility maximizer, and the utility function itself is state-independent.
4. The quantities of remedial care consumed are exogenously determined by the state of health. In particular,

$$m_s^0 > m_w^0 = 0.$$

5. The expenditures on remedial care are the only financial loss from illness; for example,

$$x_h + m_h^0 = y^0 \tag{2}$$

where y^0 represents an endowment of market income, defined in terms of units of x. (Alternatively, y^0 can be defined as the endowment of potential market income, and m^0 as the full financial loss from illness, including foregone earnings.) In the absence of health insurance, the "endowed" consumption of x_h is thus given by

$$x_h^0 = \begin{cases} y^0 & \text{(if } h = w) \\ y^0 - m^0 & \text{(if } h = s) \end{cases}$$

and equation (1) can be rewritten in the reduced form

$$z_h = z(x_h^0, h).$$

The availability of health insurance enables a trade-off between x_w^0 and x_s^0. Let the market price of insurance be given by

$$\frac{dx_w}{dx_s} \equiv \pi = (1+\lambda)p/(1-p) \tag{3}$$

where λ represents the net loading term. The consumption possibilities for x_h are given by

$$x_h = \begin{cases} y^0 - n\pi & \text{(if } h = w) \\ y^0 - m_s^0 + n & \text{(if } h = s) \end{cases} \tag{4}$$

with n representing the purchased amount of "insurance" (coverage net of the premium) which the consumer can use toward the purchase of x in the sick state of health. The optimal amount of insurance can be determined by maximizing the expected utility function

$$U^* = (1 - p)U[z(x_w, w)] + pU[z(x_s, s)] \tag{5}$$

with respect to n, subject to equations (3) and (4). The first-order optimality condition is given by

$$\frac{U'(z_s^*)z'(x_s^*, s)}{U'(z_w^*)z'(x_w^*, w)} = 1 + \lambda \tag{6}$$

and the second-order condition for a local optimum requires that U be a concave function of the solution-bundle x_h^*. The latter condition may be satisfied just if the production function z_h is sufficiently concave in x_h. It may therefore be satisfied even if U is a linear function of z_h.

Equation (6) indicates that the optimal degree of coverage of financial medical losses depends not only on the "real" price of insurance, λ, but also on the relative marginal efficiency of x in producing z in the poor state of health. Let the market price of insurance be actuarially fair. Then full coverage (i.e., $x_s^* = x_w^*$) would be optimal only if the marginal and average products of x, $z'(x_h)$ and $z(x_h)/x_h$, respectively, were independent of both the consumption of remedial care services and the state of health: for example, if $z_h = x_h + m_h$ (monetary compensations were a perfect substitute for lost consumption opportunities) or if $z_h = f(x_h) + g(m_h)$.

In the more general case, it is conceivable that the onslaught of illness generally lowers the relative efficiency of any given amount of x in producing z_s, or $z'(\bar{x}_s, s)/z'(\bar{x}_w, w) < 1$ for any $x_s = x_w = \bar{x}$. Then, if the marginal utility of z_h, $U'(z_h)$ is constant, or if $U''(z_h)$ is not sufficiently negative, equation (6) implies that the optimal bundle must be such that $x_w^* > x_s^*$. It will not pay consumers to insure their medical care costs fully even if the price is actuarially fair. Indeed, even zero coverage might be optimal in specific cases.

Of course, if $\lambda = 0$ and U were sufficiently concave in z, it is possible that full coverage or even more than full coverage would be optimal ($x_s^* \geq x_w^*$) because the reduced efficiency of x in producing z_s also implies that the ratio z_s/z_w becomes less than unity at any given amount of $\bar{x} = \bar{x}_s = \bar{x}_w$. With $U''(z) < 0$, the ratio $U'(z_s)/U'(z_w)$ might then become considerably higher than unity. Note, however, that even in that case the optimal bundle of consumption activities would necessarily be such that $z_w^* > z_s^*$. Put differently, there will not be "full insurance" in terms of basic consumption opportunities, and the consumer could not be indifferent as to which state of health occurred.

Chapter 9 Appendix B: Statistical Computations

Indirect Federal Subsidies to Health Services Through Tax Exemptions (Table 9.3)

The employer exclusion The estimates for 1970 and 1975 are based on the revised data summarized in Phelps (1980, table 3). Employer-paid premiums in 1970 and 1975 are estimated at $9.1 and $19.4 billion, respectively, and the average marginal tax rate for the employee tax units benefiting from the exemption is calculated at 31.82 percent in Mitchell and Phelps (1975, table 15). To arrive at the projected employer-paid premiums in 1980, I first projected the growth of total premiums through 1980 at the 1976–77 rate (see Caroll and Arnett 1979) and then multiplied this total by the average proportion of employer group-premiums ($\sim$ .80 throughout the 1970s) and the proportion of the latter paid by employers (.81 as estimated by Phelps 1980, table 3).

My estimated subsidy in 1980 due to the employer exclusion appears to be considerably higher than the estimate reported in Steurele and Hoffman (1979). However, the latter has been found to be inaccurate, and the revised estimate provided by Mr. Steurele puts the figure much closer to the estimate reported in table 9.3. The true estimate must be based, of course, on the average marginal tax rate applying to tax units benefiting from the employer exclusion in 1980. This rate is likely to be higher than the average marginal tax rate for all tax units. It is possible that the treasury estimates are based on the latter rather than the former.

Itemized premium and other medical expenses My calculations for 1970 and 1975 are based on actual IRS data (United States Internal Revenue Service, 1970, 1975) (which report the distributions of itemized deductions by income groups) and the effective average marginal tax rates for the same groups in each year. The methodology is the same as that used in Mitchell and Vogel (1975), except that my calculations are based on the published IRS returns, rather than the projections used by these authors. My projections for 1980 are based on the assumption that the rate of increase in the subsidies between 1970 and 1975 would persist through 1980.

The Impact of the Federal Subsidy
on the Net Price of Insurance (Table 9.4)

The basic data on premiums and benefit payments for private insurance are from Caroll and Arnett (1979, p. 11). The first two estimates of the insurance loading rates, λ_0 and λ_1, are based on the current figures; i.e., $\lambda_0 = \Sigma P/\Sigma B - 1$, and $\lambda_1 = P/B - 1$, respectively. The latter two estimates, $\hat{\lambda}_2$ and $\hat{\lambda}_3$, are derived from the formula $\hat{\lambda}_i = [P/\hat{E}(B)]_i - 1$, $i = 2,3$. Here $\hat{E}(B)_i$ was computed through a regression analysis using the Cochrane-Orcutt method to account for first-order autoregressiveness in the residuals. The corresponding regression results were (t-values in parentheses):

$$\frac{\hat{E}(B)_2}{\text{CPI}} = -19624.7 + 55.4650\ C \qquad\qquad R^2 = 0.9765$$
$$(-2.85) \qquad (9.11) \qquad\qquad\qquad \hat{\rho} = 0.7865$$

$$\hat{E}(B)_3 = -23215.6 + 18.5286\ C + 298.087\ \text{CPI} \qquad R^2 = 0.9946$$
$$(-3.62) \qquad (1.49) \qquad (1.99) \qquad\qquad \hat{\rho} = 0.6301$$

where C denotes aggregate consumption expenditures, CPI the implicit deflator for consumption expenditures, and $\hat{\rho}$ the estimated serial correlation coefficient. The data sources for C and CPI are from the *Survey of Current Business* 57 (8), August 1977, p. 62, (Table A) and 58 (7), July 1978, p. 26 (Table 1.2) and p. 61 (Table 7.1).

The average premium per insurance policy was estimated as the ratio of total premium income (based on Caroll and Arnett 1979) to the total number of policies. The latter statistic was computed on the basis of the reported number of persons covered by hospital insurance plans (Caroll and Arnett 1979, p. 8) and the proportions of the population living in single- and multiple-person households (the latter weighted by the average family size). The formulae used are based on the following identities:

$$N_{\text{plan}} = \text{Av.} \times N_m + N_s \tag{1}$$

where N_{plan} denotes the number of persons enrolled in insurance plans; N_s and N_m denote the total number of policies purchased by single- and multiple-person families; and Av. represents average family size. The total number of policies $N_T = N_m + N_s$ can then be solved from

$$N_T = \frac{1}{Av \times \left(\dfrac{N_m}{N_T}\right) + \left(\dfrac{N_s}{N_T}\right)} N_{plan}. \qquad (2)$$

I have approximated the ratios N_m/N_T and N_s/N_T as the proportions of multiple- and single-person families in the total population as reported in United States Internal Revenue Service (1970, 1975). The average family size was taken from the U.S. Bureau of the Census' *Statistical Abstract of the U.S.* 1977, p. 41.

The average premium per tax unit (row 6 of table 9.4) was estimated by multiplying the average premium per policy by the average number of policies carried per tax unit. The latter statistic was estimated from data on the percentage of gross enrollments with multiple policies, i.e.,

$$\frac{\text{No. of Gross Enrollments } - \text{ No. of Net Enrollments}}{\text{No. of Gross Enrollments}}$$

as reported in Caroll and Arnett (1979), tables 2 and 5.

The average subsidy per itemizing tax unit benefiting from the medical expense exclusion is calculated from the same IRS data used in table 3. The average subsidy per tax unit benefiting from the employer exclusion is from Mitchell and Phelps (1975), table 15.

Chapter 9 Appendix C:
On the Welfare Cost of National Health Insurance

In the second part of this paper ("Some Economic Aspects of the Health Care for All Americans Act") it was argued that if an NHI plan is based on a simultaneous abolition of any direct costs to the patient at the time of care and the introduction of supply controls through price ceilings and other cost containments (so that queues and other forms of waiting time are the mechanism through which the system is equilibrated), then the deadweight costs of the system could be approximated by the magnitude of the direct expenditures by consumers on personal health care services at the initial market price.

The argument is illustrated in figure 9.1. The initial market supply and demand curves for health services under the private insurance system are denoted by $S_0(p)$ and $D_0(c^*p)$, respectively. It is implicitly assumed that all private insurance is of the reimbursement form. Thus, while supply is depicted as a function of the fee received by providers, p, private demand is depicted as a function of only a fraction of that fee, c^*p, where c^* is the consumer's perception of the share of the market price he is held accountable for. Only in the event that insurance premiums are perceived to be entirely independent of personal utilization of health services at the time of care would c^* be equivalent to the consumer's effective marginal coinsurance rate. The auxil-

FIGURE 9.1

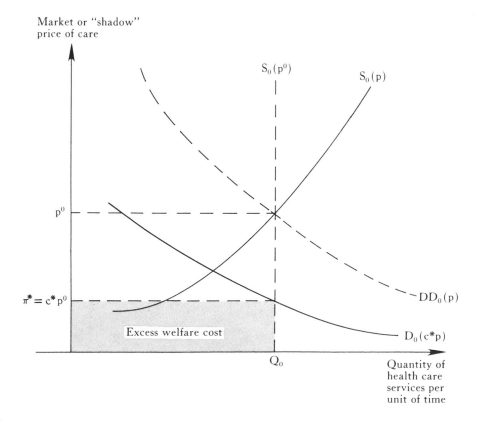

iary "market demand" schedule $DD_0(p)$ (which is specified as a function of the fees received by providers) is derived from the underlying consumer demand schedule $D_0(c^*p)$, with $DD_0(p) \equiv D(c^*p)$. The equilibrium price and quantity of health care services, P^0 and Q_0, are determined from the necessary condition for equilibrium:

$$DD_0(P^0) \equiv D_0(c^*p^0) = S_0(P^0) = Q_0. \qquad (1)$$

I shall assume, for methodological convenience, that the introduction of NHI does not cause a shift in the initial market demand schedule at identical shadow prices. (This assumption is open to criticism both because NHI is expected to change the level and distribution of aggregate income and because the shadow price of queuing, being an increasing function of a person's opportunity cost of time, "discriminates" in favor of low-wage earners and increases their relative demand. It is not clear, however, what would be the net effects of these distributional changes on aggregate demand.) Since, by assumption, the supply price, hence quantity, of health services is fixed by the government at their initial level, $Q^0 = S(p^0)$, the only way equilibrium can be restored is for the shadow market price of queuing (π^*) to rise sufficiently so as to equate the quantity demanded with the available, or "planned," supply. That is,

$$D_0(\pi^*) = Q_0 \qquad (2)$$

Equations (1) and (2) and the assumed constancy of the D_0 schedules imply that

$$\pi^* = cp^0. \qquad (3)$$

The shadow price of queuing can be thought of simply as a product of the average consumer's opportunity cost of time, $\bar{w}$, and the average size of the queue, l, on the assumption that queuing involves a direct loss of time. Alternatively, if treatment is denied for a duration of l units of time and there is no explicit physical queue, $\bar{w}$ can be thought of as the reduction in a person's average productivity over that period. In either case, the assumption is that explicit or implicit queuing causes a real cost to consumers in terms of foregone production in the market or nonmarket sectors. This cost to the consumer is also a real loss from a social point of view.

In the following calculation I shall ignore the social costs of travel and "normal" waiting time under the private system because these costs persist under the NHI system as well. The full social or resource costs of providing health care under the NHI system in question, then, is the sum of the values of providers' inputs and the (differential) opportunity costs of queuing to consumers, $Q_0 p^0 (1+c^*)$. It exceeds the resource costs under the private system of price rationing by the amount $Q_0 p^0 c^*$, which would be the actual out-of-pocket payments for medical care by consumers under the assumption that c^* equals the average coinsurance rate. It is interesting to note that this measurement of the excess welfare costs of NHI does not require knowledge of the true price elasticity of demand for health care services.

Chapter 9 Notes

1. See Frech and Ginsburg (1978), p. 1. For a detailed comparison of key proposals, see Davis (1975).

2. For a systematic distinction between health and medical care services, see Grossman (1972).

3. See Pauly (1971a, 1971b), Davis (1975), Frech and Ginsburg (1978), and Lindsay (1976) for detailed references and specific arguments.

4. See United States Senate Hearings (1979) and Cavalier (1979).

5. This approach is outlined in the introductory section of Ehrlich and Becker (1972). The distinction between market goods and final consumption activities, or characteristics, has been emphasized in Becker (1965) and Lancaster (1966).

6. For a formal illustration of these arguments, see chapter 9 appendix A.

7. As my discussion under the heading "The Real Price of Insurance" indicates, this situation is changing. There is also some question regarding the precise dollar amount of protection that falls in the category of catastrophic insurance.

8. See *Health Care Financing Trend*, Winter 1980, p. 10. The measured price index of a hospital room, again unadjusted for many changes in quality, has exhibited a whopping 260 percent increase over the same period.

9. For some published attempts along these lines, see, for example, Feldstein (1970) and Fuchs and Kramer (1972).

10. By far the dominant source of increase in public spending has been

Medicare and Medicaid. In the eleven-year period between 1967 and 1978, federal outlays on Medicare increased from $3.4 billion to $24.9 billion, and federal and state expenditures on Medicaid increased from $2.5 billion to $18.4 billion. Both outlays have thus increased by roughly 630 percent (see *Statistical Abstract of the United States,* various years and Gibson [1979], p. 29, for the most recent period). Today they constitute two-thirds of all public expenditures on personal health care services.

11. See the first part of chapter 9 appendix B for the detailed calculations. The sources I have relied upon include: United States Internal Revenue Service Statistics of Income: Individual Tax Returns (1970 and 1975), Mitchell and Vogel (1975), Mitchell and Phelps (1975), Phelps (1980), Caroll and Arnett (1979), Steurele and Hoffman (1979), Congressional Budget Office (1980), and corrections to the estimates appearing in the last two sources, as provided to me by Steurele.

12. In calculating the taxable income, an itemizing tax unit may deduct 50 percent of its direct payments for health insurance premiums up to a maximum deduction of $150 and then deduct the remainder of the premiums only if its out-of-pocket payments for all medical and dental expenses exceed 3 percent of its adjusted gross income (see United States Internal Revenue Service, *Statistics of Income*, 1975, pp. 172–73).

13. See, in particular, Congressional Budget Office (1980), Feldstein and Friedman (1977), Mitchell and Vogel (1975), Frech and Ginsburg (1978), and Steurele and Hoffman (1979).

14. Expected, rather than actual, benefits are the relevant data because benefit payments by an insurer are subject to random fluctuations from one year to another due to the randomness in the occurrence of insured hazards. For a more sophisticated definition of the loading rate as a measure of the real price of insurance, see Ehrlich and Becker (1972).

15. Table 9.3 indicates that the share of the subsidy to employer-paid premiums in the overall federal subsidy to insurance premiums has increased from 80 percent in 1970 to 86 percent in 1975 and to a projected 90 percent in 1980.

16. An indication of the extent of variability in the net prices paid by different families is given by the fact that while those families enjoying both the average "employer exclusion subsidy" and the "itemized deduction subsidy" (rows 7 and 8 in table 9.4) received a subsidy rate of approximately 46 percent of the average family premium in 1975, the average subsidy per premium for all tax units in that year was only 21 percent.

17. See, for example, Fuchs (1976).

18. See Frech and Ginsburg (1978), p. 8 and *Source Book of Health Insurance Data* (1977–78), p. 30. According to the latter source, which defines

"catastrophic-type coverage" to be any coverage with maximum benefit levels of $10,000 or more, three in four Americans under the age of 65 were already protected by some form of catastrophic insurance in 1976.

19. See, for example, Pauly (1968), Arrow (1976), Feldstein and Friedman (1977).

20. This is an application of a more general "moral hazard" proposition derived in Ehrlich and Becker (1972).

21. For example, Blue Cross Physician insurance, most commercial hospital insurance plans, and a minority of Blue Cross hospital packages.

22. See, for example, Feldstein (1973), Feldstein and Friedman (1977), and Arrow (1976). For a critical evaluation of some of this work, see Ehrlich (1976). Also note that the considerably faster rate of growth of hospital care services relative to other medical services in recent years is not quite consistent with the price-induced, excess-consumption hypothesis, since empirical estimates indicate that the price elasticity of demand for hospital care services is lower than that for other medical services.

23. See Caroll and Arnett (1979), p. 16, for the statistics on private insurance and United States Senate Hearings (1979), pp. 62–64 for official data on people receiving Medicare and Medicaid and those without coverage.

24. The magnitude of the increase cannot be judged solely from current estimates of the own-price elasticities of demand for medical services, since these are derived from observed changes in coinsurance rates under the private insurance system. As my analysis under the head "Moral Hazard?" indicates, these need not be accurate measures of the true changes in the perceived prices. Also, the effective market price elasticity about zero may be much higher than that estimated at positive prices. In any event, Trapnell's induction method translates to only a portion of the induced-demand changes that can be anticipated on the basis of the available price-elasticity estimates for both hospital care and physician's services.

25. The cost estimates are said to include a budget for negotiated fee schedules.

26. The original estimates of the cost of medicare Part A in 1990 was to be $9.4 billion. It has been, in fact, $17.8 billion in 1978. The discrepancy appears to be even greater in the case of Medicaid (see *Hearings* 1979, pp. 359–60).

Chapter 9 References

Arrow, Kenneth J., 1976. "Welfare Analysis of Changes in Health Insurance Rates." In *The Role of Health Insurance in the Health Services Sector*, ed. R. Rosett, pp. 3–24. New York: National Bureau of Economic Research.

Becker, G. S. 1965. "A Theory of the Allocation of Time." *Economic Journal* 75 (September 1965): 493–517.

Cavalier, Kay. 1979. "National Health Insurance." Revised document of the Health Section of the Education and Public Welfare Division, report no. 79–92, Education and Public Welfare, Congressional Research Service, March 1979.

Caroll, Marjorie Smith, and Arnett, Ross H. 1979. "Private Health Insurance Plans in 1977: Coverage, Enrollment and Financial Experience." *Health Care Financing Review* Fall 1979: 3–22.

Congressional Budget Office (CBO). 1980. *Tax Subsidies for Medical Care: Current Policies and Possible Alternatives.* Washington, D.C.: U.S. Government Printing Office.

Davis, Karen. 1975. *National Health Insurance: Benefits, Costs and Consequences.* Washington, D.C.: The Brookings Institute.

Ehrlich, Isaac. 1976. "Welfare Analysis of Changes in Health Insurance Rates—A Comment." In *The Role of Health Insurance in the Health Services Sector,* ed. R. Rosett, pp. 28–33. New York: National Bureau of Economic Research.

Ehrlich, Isaac, and Becker, Gary S. 1972. "Market Insurance, Self-Insurance and Self-Protection." *Journal of Political Economy* 80 (no. 4): 623–48.

Enthoven, Alain C. 1978a. "Consumer-Choice Health Plan." (First of two parts.) *New England Journal of Medicine* 298: 650–58.

Feldstein, Martin S. 1970. "The Rising Price of Physicians' Services." *Review of Economics and Statistics* 52 (no. 2): 121–33.

———. 1973. "The Welfare Loss of Excess Health Insurance. *Journal of Political Economy* 81(2), part I: 251–80.

———. 1971. "Hospital Cost Inflation: A Study of Nonprofit Price Dynamics." *American Economic Review* 61(5): 853–72.

Feldstein, M. S., and Friedman, Bernard. 1977. "Tax Subsidies, The Rational Demand for Insurance and the Health Care Crisis." *Journal of Public Economics* 7: 155–78.

Frech, H. E. III, and Ginsburg, Paul B. 1978. *Public Insurance in Private Markets.* Washington, D.C.: American Enterprise Institute.

Freeland, Mark; Calab, George; and Ellen, Carol. 1980. "Projections of National Health Expenditures, 1980, 1985, and 1990." *Health Care Financing Review* Winter 1980: 1–27.

Fuchs, Victor R. 1976. "From Bismark to Woodcock: The 'Irrational' Pursuit of National Health Insurance." *Journal of Law and Economics* 19.

Fuchs, Victor R., and Kramer, Marcia J. 1972. *Determinants of Expenditures for Physician Services in the United States, 1948–1968.* New York: National Bureau of Economic Research.

Gibson, Robert M. 1979. "National Health Expenditures, 1978." *Health Care Financing Review* Summer 1979: 1–36.

Grossman, Michael. 1972. *The Demand for Health: A Theoretical and Empirical Investigation.* New York: National Bureau of Economic Research.

Jones, Stanley B. 1982. "Labor's New Approach to National Health Insurance." In Ehrlich, Isaac, ed. *National Health Policy: What Role for Government?*, ch. 7. Stanford: Hoover Institution Press.

Kessel, Reuben A. 1970. "The AMA and the Supply of Physicians." *Law and Contemporary Problems* 38 (Autumn 1970): 267–83.

Lancaster, Kelvin. 1966. "A New Approach to Consumer Theory." *Journal of Political Economy* 70 (April 1966): 132–57.

Lindsay, Cotton M. ed. 1976. *New Directions in Public Health Care, An Evaluation of Proposals for National Health Insurance.* San Francisco: The Institute for Contemporary Studies.

Mitchell, Bridger M., and Phelps, Charles E. 1975. *Employer-Paid Group Health Insurance and the Costs of Mandated National Coverage.* Santa Monica, California: The Rand Corporation.

Mitchell, B. M., and Vogel, Ronald J. 1975. "Health and Taxes: An Assessment of the Medical Deduction." *Southern Economic Review* 41 (April 1975): 660–72.

Newhouse, Joseph P.; Phelps, Charles E.; and Schwartz, William B. 1979. "Policy Options and the Impact of National Health Insurance." *New England Journal of Medicine* June 1979: 1340–59.

Pauly, Mark V. 1968. "The Economics of Moral Hazard." *American Economic Review* 58(3): 531–37.

———. 1971a. *Medical Care at Public Expense.* New York: Praeger.

———. 1971b. *National Health Insurance: An Analysis.* Washington, D.C.: American Enterprise Institute.

Phelps, Charles E. 1980. *National Health Insurance by Regulation: Mandated Employee Benefits.* Rand/P-6391, April 1980, Santa Monica, California: The Rand Corporation.

Rothchild, Michael, and Stiglitz, Joseph E. 1976. "Equilibrium in Competitive Insurance Markets: An Essay on the Economics of Imperfect Information." *Quarterly Journal of Economics* 90(4): 629–49.

Source Book of Health Insurance Data, 1977-78. Washington, D.C.: Health Insurance Institute.

Steurele, Eugene, and Hoffman, Ronald. 1979. "Tax Expenditures for Health Care." *National Tax Journal* June 1979: 101-14.

United States Internal Revenue Service. *Statistics of Income, 1970* and *1975.* Individual Income Tax Returns. Washington, D.C.: U.S. Government Printing Office.

United States Senate, Hearings Before the Committee on Finance, Ninety-sixth Congress. 1979. *Presentation of Major Health Insurance Proposals.* Washington, D.C.: U.S. Government Printing Office.

Waldo, D.R. 1980. *Health Care Financing Trends*, 1, no. 2 (Winter, 1980).

Discussants' Comments on Section II

Harold S. Luft

Charles Phelps

Paul Feldstein

Harold S. Luft[1]

The paper by Lu Ann Aday continues the important work she and Ronald Andersen have been pursuing for almost a decade at the Center for Health Administration Studies at the University of Chicago (CHAS). Moreover, it is linked to earlier CHAS studies to provide a continuing series of snapshots of the U.S. health care system over the past quarter century. These surveys have changed in focus over time, reflecting an awareness of the then-current policy issues. Thus, the first surveys in the 1950s and early 1960s focused primarily on the growth of voluntary (nongovernment) health insurance and its impact on family expenditures for medical care. As the growth in private health insurance leveled off and the major public programs of Medicare- and Medicaid-provided coverage for many of the elderly and poor, the CHAS surveys shifted to focus on problems of access.

Aday defines access as "those dimensions which describe the potential and actual entry of a given population group to the health care delivery system. . . . The greatest 'equity' of access is said to exist when need, rather than structural or individual characteristics, determines who gains entry to the health care system. ..." (See chapter six.) Using these concepts, Aday finds that, in general, access has become more equitable between 1970 and 1976, but there are still some population subgroups who are disadvantaged. A major purpose of her paper is to identify those subgroups, determine what factors most significantly stand in the way of their access to the system, and then suggest policies to remedy those problems.

The methodology used in this paper is simple, yet powerful. Various access measures, such as "percent who wait more than 30 minutes to see doctor," are examined for subgroups of the population, such as urban blacks or Spanish-heritage people in the Southwest, with cross-tabulations by policy variables, such as poverty level, physician to population ratio, and type of regular source of care. Thus, one can see that in all population subgroups, those who use a hospital out-patient department (OPD) or emergency room (ER) are substantially more likely to have long waits than those with a private MD. However, controlling for usual source of care, the likelihood of a long wait is relatively similar for all groups except Southern rural blacks. The same analyses were undertaken controlling for various measures of need, such as age, sex, perceived health level, and number of disability days, but the adjustments make little difference.

One may contrast this approach with the common multiple regression technique. If all the relevant interactions are included in the regression, the results will be similar. The regression approach is to be preferred if there are many variables to examine or if it is difficult to express the variables in terms of a small number of categories. The cross-tab approach allows one to zero in more easily on factors that influence subgroups in different ways. It also is a technique more readily understood by policymakers. Both approaches, however, can lead to incorrect interpretations unless one has a clear understanding of the causal relationships. Likewise, complex relationships may be examined either with regressions or well constructed cross-tabs.

At this point I will take advantage of the broad latitude given discussants at this conference and use Aday's paper as a starting point for an outline of the issues I would like her to address in future analyses. This approach is made possible by the wealth of data in the CHAS survey and the extensive information included in the current paper. My remarks will fall into three major categories: (1) the definition of equity and access, and the design of policy-relevant questions; (2) questions raised by some of the data presented in the paper; and (3) policy issues and alternatives.

Equity, Access, and Policy

It is unfortunate that people with different disciplinary backgrounds will use different terminology to describe the same phenomenon. If the labels are different but the concepts identical, then a simple translation is in order. If the concepts differ, then something may be lost in the translation, and one must think carefully about which language best captures the essence of the situation. "Best," of course, is in the mind of the beholder, but in some situations there may be an external measure against which concepts can be evaluated. In this instance, we might ask which conceptual framework is the most useful for setting policy.

As an economist, I automatically look at Aday's figure 6.1, "Framework for the study of access," and figure 6.2, "Operational indicators of the access framework," and attempt to translate it into concepts of supply and demand. In these figures, the "Potential Access–Structural Indicators," such as the availability of providers and their organization, seem to approximate the economist's notion of supply. Some of these factors, such as the convenience of the regular source of care in terms of travel time and waiting time, are price variables. Similarly, the major role of health insurance coverage is to lower the money price faced by a potential consumer of services. The second group of variables in the figures, "Potential Access–Process Indicators," include variables that are appropriate to the demand side of the equation. Clearly, a major determinant of demand is medical need and how this is perceived by the potential consumer. We must recognize, however, that policies may be undertaken to alter people's perceptions of their health problems. Not the least of these factors is prior experiences with the medical system—both in terms of supplier-induced demand and the consumer's own evaluation of the efficacy of certain types of treatment.

We next come to measures of realized access, for which there are both objective and subjective indicators. The objective indicators include utilization variables such as the number, type, and location of medical care visits. This is the analogue to the economist's measure of actual consumption, as determined by the intersection of supply and demand. The subjective indicators measure consumer satisfaction with various aspects of utilization. This dimension has no direct analogue in the economist's lexicon, yet it provides important insights as to how one should evaluate certain situations.

Does this reconceptualization help in understanding Aday's paper? I think so, because it helps identify certain potential problems in her analysis—problems which arise because the causality of certain relationships are unclear or because the concept of equity itself is not sufficiently well defined for policy purposes. Aday states:

> To the extent that having a family doctor, insurance coverage or actual utilization is a function of the person's general physical health or of particular presenting complaints then an "equitable" system of health resource allocation is said to exist. Inequity is suggested, however, if services are distributed on the basis of demographic variables such as race, family income or place of residence rather than need.

Two problems arise with this definition. The first is that an equitable distribution of resources is said to exist if utilization is equal, controlling for health status. But, the definition does not distinguish among types of medical services. Access to trauma care is clearly different from access to cosmetic surgery. The policy implications of unequal access for the two types of treatment are very different. Second, Aday's definition of equity places medical care in a unique position. Poor people consume less food, clothing, and shelter than the rich, but they are supposed to consume the same amount of medical care. By itself, that may not be an unreasonable goal, but how should one reconcile it with the notion that some visits are not medically necessary. Moreover, one may question whether it is appropriate to use white, middle-class values in evaluating the medical utilization of other subgroups. For instance, some of the low use of physician services by people of Spanish heritage in the Southwest may be a reflection of their use of *curanderos,* or other nonphysician providers. Thus, might not an alternative measure of equity be derived from the consumers' evaluation of their own experiences?[2]

Causality and Differential Access

A key aspect of Aday's policy recommendations is that when differences in various access measures are identified for certain population subgroups, policies should be undertaken to reduce the barriers. Before one can address the policy issues, however, one must identify clearly the causes of the observed differences. For instance, two important relationships appear in both Aday's study and other surveys. One is that people without health insurance are much more likely than those with coverage to be without a usual source of medical care. The second is that people without a regular source of medical care are much less likely to see a physician. People without health insurance coverage seem to fall into several categories: those who have access to Medicaid but have not used medical services and thus report no Medicaid coverage; low income people ineligible for coverage; and young people just entering the labor force. On the question of regular source of care, the primary reason given for not having a usual source of care is that none was needed. What we do not know is how many of the people without private insurance are also without a regular physician and, more importantly, are not particularly bothered by the situation. Knowing that physicians may think such people underutilize services does not tell us that access barriers are the problem.[3] Yet this is the type of information we need in order to design appropriate policies. Moreover, recasting the analysis in terms of supply and demand (or even a more rigorous application of the predisposing-need-enabling paradigm) makes it clear that one linkage is from symptoms to their recognition, to a desire for treatment, to a demand function that incorporates money and time prices along with social and other barriers such as language. A second linkage recognizes that, to some extent, insurance coverage is a reflection of a person's perception of what such coverage is worth. The same holds for an established relationship with a usual source of care.

Recasting the analysis may also help explain certain apparent inconsistencies in the data. For instance, very high proportions of the elderly and rural farm residents wait more than 30 minutes to see their regular source of care, yet these people are among the least dissatisfied with their waiting time. One explanation is that a visit to a physician's office is an important form of social contact. A second explanation is that people make trade-offs between time and money in their choice of providers. They may also make trade-offs between scheduled and non-scheduled use. (This may also be the case in comparisons between people who join prepaid group practices versus independent practitioners.) For instance, table 6.4 in Aday's paper indicates a much higher likelihood of long office waits for people who just walk in, yet in table 6.10 there is much less difference in satisfaction with waiting time between those who walk in and those who make appointments. For some people, hospital emergency rooms with long waits and high fees are the only available source of care; others may choose such seemingly undesirable sources (from a middle-class perspective) for a variety of social and psychological, as well as economic, reasons. We must beware of attacking noneconomic problems with primarily economic policy tools such as increased insurance coverage and physician supply.[4] Even the economic barriers do not seem to yield to simple solutions—there is relatively little difference between those with and without doctor office insurance in the proportion dissatisfied with the cost of the most recent visit.

Policy Issues and Alternatives

Aday's general policy statement is that the major financing initiatives (Medicare and Medicaid) have reduced many of the historic racial and income-related differences, but certain groups still "fall through the cracks." Given the existence of such broad strategies, one should now focus attention on those subgroups with specific types of access barriers. Aday points out, and I heartily agree, that future policies must be highly targeted. More analyses of her data may help identify more precisely the policies appropriate for specific areas.

Southern rural blacks stand out as a group with particular difficulties in obtaining care. However, is the crucial factor that they are black, rural, or Southern? For instance, do Southern rural whites have similar problems? Do these people wait in the doctor's office because appointments are not available, because travel problems make scheduling difficult, or because they do not have telephones? While health maintenance organizations are good for many things, there is little reason to believe they will fit well within the social and economic environment of such communities. A more appropriate policy might try to address the low physician to population ratios in such areas, but

Aday's data suggest that access is sometimes negatively related to supply.

Hispanics in the Southwest also have access problems. But again, we need to identify precisely the type of problems. Do some use traditional (non–Anglo) providers by preference? What is the role of language rather than economic barriers? How important is the fear of "undocumented aliens" that contact with the medical care system will lead to deportation? The answers to such questions will help determine whether policies should be of a conventional medical nature, such as an expansion of health insurance coverage or an increase in Spanish-speaking providers, or of a nonmedical nature, such as expanded educational programs or changes in immigration laws.

Fortunately, the CHAS data set includes much of the data necessary to answer these and other questions. Aday's paper has helped define more clearly the areas in which access may be a problem. Hopefully, future studies will provide the specific answers we need to design the appropriate policies.

Charles Phelps

I'll concentrate my remarks primarily on Larry Seidman's paper. Let me read two sentences from his paper summarizing his position—a position with which I think most economists will be very sympathetic, myself included. "Extensive insurance induced by federal tax policy has undermined the market mechanism by removing a crucial ingredient: consumer cost-sharing. The sensible inference is that removal of the tax subsidy is likely to restore the potency of the market mechanism." This and several ancillary provisions that he has dealt with, such as tax credits, form the basis for what sounds like an extremely useful and simple to administer policy of national health insurance. I think Larry may well be right, but I don't think he has proven the point. In fact, I can identify seven hypotheses that lie behind that proposal, all of which are empirically testable and one of which, in fact, has been tested. Let me state the hypotheses.

1. There exists shallow "first-dollar" coverage.
2. If loading fees or taxes on insurance increase, then shallow coverage will diminish or vanish.

3. Without shallow coverage, competition in the medical marketplace would control prices.

4. It is in fact feasible to operate a family, income-oriented health insurance plan through the tax system.

5. Some doctors price services on the basis of community insurance norms. (This hypothesis is stated implicitly in the paper but is not discussed.)

6. There is basically only one form of regulation that is feasible, and that is to have a panel of experts choose among competing claims on health resources.

7. The demand-curve of the consumer for medical care is downward sloping.

The first question is whether shallow coverage does exist. I would beg you to consider that the evidence supporting this has primarily been misinterpreted. The evidence supporting shallow first-dollar coverage, including that from Larry Seidman, is invariably related to first-dollar coverage in hospitalization. Now when you and I get sick, we don't just appear at the hospital, go into the hospital, and vanish. The episode of illness is the pertinent feature here. In episodes of illness, people do not have shallow first-dollar coverage. In fact, the coverage that people have looks very much like what rational theory of insurance suggests. Let me bring some data to bear on this from a 1970 health survey by Ron Andersen of Chicago. These numbers are in 1970 dollars, so you'll pardon if they sound a bit low. For individuals with annual expenditures under $150, health insurance paid 7 percent of those expenditures—almost nothing. When the annual expense of an individual increased to between $150 and $300, insurance covered 16 percent; in the range of $300 to $750 expenditures annually, health insurance covered 38 percent; in the range of $750 to $1,500, health insurance paid 57 percent; and in the range of $1,500 and upward, health insurance paid 76 percent. That does not look like shallow coverage to me. You can look at hospital policies that pay first-dollar at the door, but I don't think it is a fact at all.

The second question is a hypothesis relating to the demand for insurance. That hypothesis suggests that it is in fact the federal subsidy which has led to shallow coverage insurance. I will accept for a moment the belief that there is shallow coverage insurance, although I don't believe it. But setting this aside for a moment, let us ask what we need to know in order to accept the belief that it is the tax subsidy that caused this. In order to accept this, we have to believe that in fact there is a very particular dimension of the insurance policy that is sensitive to the subsidy from the tax system, that being the deductible. To characterize health insurance policies purchased in the United States requires something on the order of 50 to 100, or possibly 200, variables: copayments, deductibles, payment schedules, internal limits for hospitalization, internal limits for laboratory services, fee schedules for physician payments for surgery, office visits, and a scope of benefits. Is there coverage for psychiatric care and dental work? There is an enormous array of devices, all of which are potential mechanisms for adjustment of the coverage of the insurance policy, when one considers an episode of illness. Saying that the tax credit would increase the size of the deductible people have—which is really what is being sought here—is equivalent to saying that an ad valorem tax on automobiles would have its effect on one particular dimension of automobile purchase; for example, air conditioners, the cushiness of seats, or the quality of the radio in the car. We just don't know. That is an untested hypothesis.

I'm the first person to analyze empirically the demand for health insurance by looking at parameters of an insurance policy—deductibles, size of maximum payment. I would be very loath to tell you what would happen if the loading fee were changed or if the tax subsidy were reduced on health insurance. I just don't think we can tell, so that is another untested assumption.

The third assumption that has been made here is that if we did have higher copayments in some fashion, waiving aside how they would emerge for a minute, then competition would in fact reduce prices and lead to at least a more appropriate level of consumption of medical services. I think that is an untested assumption about the hospital sector because we don't understand the behavior of hospitals. Hospitals in the United States are mostly nonprofit corporations. They legally have no residual claimants. If their average cost is lower than their marginal cost, they must either reduce their prices or spend the money in some way in order to use up the producer surplus within the organization. Most hospitals, I would guess, would tend to increase the quality of services they are providing in some fashion. But this dimension of adjustment is completely untested, and I don't think there is any obvious presumption to be made that competition in the United States under today's market of hospitals would in fact lead to what we think of as competitively controlled prices especially in the hospital sector.

The fourth hypothesis is that it is feasible to income-relate health insurance plans. Let me state it a bit more precisely in economic terms: the hypothesis is that the benefits of attempting to relate health insurance plans to income exceed the costs. I was once a strong proponent of income-related health plans. Then we started to run one at the Rand Corporation as a part of the health insurance studies that we are conducting experimentally for the Department of HEW. (We have been running a health insurance company at Rand for about six years now.) We do in fact income-relate the provisions of that plan, and we have an enormous expenditure of resources per capita—I would guess on the order of $50 to $100 per capita—just to keep track of the families. (Families reconfigure at the drop of a hat: they split up, they divorce, they get remarried, the kids leave, they come back, they have babies, people die. You just can't believe how fast families reconfigure until you try to track them.)

The proposal that Larry Seidman has set forth to deal with that is to accept the tax definition of the family unit, and that is a very simple method of defining families. Unfortunately, it is very likely to destroy any semblance of price competition that one is looking for. The reason is that the income tax system allows people to choose whether to file separately or jointly. Consider a household with a husband working, a wife working as a housewife, and two children or N children. If any of them gets sick, except the employed, the family has the choice of filing the sick person as his or her own tax unit. And since their income is zero, their out-of-pocket expenses will be zero. You can subvert that by requiring families to file jointly and not allowing children to file separately. But once you get into that particular response, you run afoul of all sorts of other reasons why the tax system allows individuals to choose whether to file separately or jointly. And here I pose the question: What are the costs associated with trying to administer that sort of tax plan? I don't know the answer, but the untested hypothesis here is that the benefits of income-relating on insurance plans exceed the costs, and the costs have not been discussed at all.

The fifth hypothesis is that some doctors price by norms; that is, they look at the modal average of the patients facing them and set their pricing according to that. Larry proposes that a tax on full coverage insurance is justified on this basis since it causes an externality: the prices go up for other patients. This in fact has been empirically tested. Two colleagues of mine, Joe Newhouse and Susan Marquise, tested this in a paper published in *The Journal of Human Resources*[5] supplement several years ago, and the norms hypothesis was not supported empirically.

The sixth hypothesis is that there is basically only one form of regulation that can be considered, and I think this is a very naive assumption. I am not proposing that we implement regulation; I don't know what regulations are best or whether any are justified, but we have a very simplified discussion of regulation here. The primary focus of the paper here is that the lack of a market signal makes the regulatory job impossible, that everyone will clamor for access to service, and that the regulator has no basis of sorting out who has the highest demand-curve for the service, if you will, because there is no revealed preference. And that is indeed a perplexing problem. To pose that this is not in fact an unusual problem, I want to refer to a very old article by Ronald Coase entitled "The Nature of the Firm."[6] Business managers every day in every way make decisions without market signals. This, according to Coase, is the logic for the existence of the firm: it avoids transaction costs in the market through nonmarket decisions. One immediately asks: What are the incentives posed to managers, or, what are the incentives posed to the "regulators" (if we could call the managers this) inside the firm to make correct decisions? They have all sorts of incentives; they are judged on criteria such as profitability. It is not impossible to set up incentives for regulators to make better decisions than those they make with no incentives. I don't know if a set of incentives exists that is ultimately socially desirable, but I don't want to rule it out. Health maintenance organizations make and set up a lot of incentives to make better decisions; HMOs without walls and independent practice associations do it. Jeff Harris, MD, Ph.D., at MIT has proposed an organizational form of the medical sector which provides incentives for physicians to make decisions that conserve resources. There are all sorts of ways to do this that haven't been explored very much in the context of this paper; and it is possible that the optimal way to run the health care sector, including transaction costs, is regulatory. I am not saying that this is or is not the optimal way, but only that it is an untested hypothesis here. The only hypothesis that is tested as far as I am concerned is the notion that the demand-curve of the consumer is downward sloping. I have contributed at least to the quantity, if not to the quality, of that literature myself, and I believe that the downward slopingness of the demand for medical care can be accepted as an empirical fact; the other six hypotheses that I have related to are either completely untested or partly refuted.

I have two comments about Stan Jones's paper. I want to pose primarily a methodological issue relating to this paper, (and, in fact, also to a paper by Reinhardt that is included in the first part of this volume). There is a statement in Stan's paper that the reason the labor movement has taken this new position that he describes is strictly for political compromise. What I would like to suggest is that we have not in fact explored the political economy of national health insurance at all. If one starts with the premise that the actors on the political scene are self-interest motivated, I think one is likely to learn something from it. The tastes of individuals are treated as exogenous by the economist, but the tastes of the political sector should be considered endogenous. Now, I'm submitting as a hypothesis—though currently untested—that the labor movement could have changed its position from social security financing to the current proposals they espouse because tax laws have changed, the maximum social security income has changed, et cetera, so that what was previously a favorable form of financing no longer is.

Reinhardt has set forth a notion in his paper (chapter 2) that tastes of individuals in fact form the legal structure of society in some fashion. In Germany, it is the utility value of solidarity and the utility function of Germans that is said to account for the form of national health insurance (NHI). It strikes me as plausible that in fact there are some very fundamental forces in the organization of the political structure of society that help determine issues like the structure of NHI. Does Congress work through committees? How many houses are there in the Congress? These factors could well determine the way individual interest groups are able to manipulate the political process in order to achieve their own gains. We have not come close to touching that sort of analysis in health insurance, and I think it might be useful.

Paul Feldstein

I would like to comment primarily on Stan Jones's paper, and then briefly on Larry's (Mr. Seidman's) paper. In examining both proposals, it is difficult to understand fully how they would be carried out, because when a proposal is written into bill form, a great many details have to be spelled out. At this stage, it is not clear how a number of things would work, particularly with regard to Stan Jones's proposal.

To begin with, most of the goals in his proposal could be subscribed to by most people and could be used for any national insurance plan. The fifth goal, however, would give a number of people trouble—the goal that states that growth in health expenditures should be tied to the increase in GNP, that there be a lid, basically, on how fast health expenditures could increase. When you look at the characteristics of the plan and compare it to the original Health Security Act, I think there are quite a few similarities; for example, the first part, which proposes a zero price and mandates comprehensive benefits. The big difference between the old and new proposal is that it is sold by private insurance companies and HMOs. I believe this was included for political reasons to make the proposal acceptable. Financing the plan primarily through payroll taxes, with some help from nonearned income, is again fairly similar to the original Health Security Act plan. What is also quite similar is the idea of pooling all of the money. In the original plan, the money was to go to the government and the government would then operate the pool. In the new plan, the pool is supposed to be operated by a consortium of banks, insurance companies, and HMOs. But the idea is basically the same: there is a pool and an expenditure lid that could be established on this pool of dollars. Because the details haven't been spelled out on how providers are to be paid, I am not sure how similar this is to the previous plan. There is the idea that there could be competition, but there is also a strong flavor of negotiations, regulation, budgeting, and planning.

I would like to discuss a few of these points in more detail. With respect to the zero price, it is obvious why a lid has to be placed on health expenditures. With a zero price, the government would want to limit how much medical prices and total expenditures could increase and also to be able to limit the commitment by both business and government. It is not clear whether the providers would have to participate in the plan. The plan states that there would be negotiations with providers on fee schedules. If these negotiations are not compulsory, then providers might opt out. I have a feeling that what would happen is that it would be like the British National Health Service or like public schools in this country. The service is free to the consumer if he or she participates; if not, the consumer must pay the full price for the service when purchased from providers outside the system. Again, these aspects of the proposal would have to be spelled out. I have the feeling that the "negotiation with providers" is a euphemism for a stronger word that would be used because I'm not sure what choice the providers would have. As some people have already mentioned, the consequences of the demand exceeding supply, which would occur under a zero price, would be rationing. This rationing would be either by time prices (people would either have to wait, and those who would get care would be those who could afford to wait), or it may be rationed by the providers on the basis of the seriousness of illness. In this case, there would not be a great deal of preventive care being provided, that some people would like to see in an NHI plan.

There is also a hope among some that the health system might be made more efficient, and therefore a lot more care would be provided by a reorganized free system than under the current system. I think there is a great potential for increasing productivity in the current system; there are many state practice acts that restrict tasks that people can perform and prohibit much that can be delegated. A great deal of substitution from inpatient to outpatient care could occur. The problem with all of this is that if there is a limit on total expenditures, then the limit would have to be increased to allow for large productivity increases. If there is an expenditure limit, I believe little productivity increase will occur because existing providers will all want to receive their revenues. It will be very difficult to eliminate existing physicians or hospitals to make room for productivity increases. Therefore, I don't believe large productivity increases will occur.

Another issue is what kind of incentives would result when you have a pool and you allow competition to occur between insurance companies and HMOs. Since these details are not spelled out, I believe that what the union has in mind can be illustrated by an example in Michigan, where the United Auto Workers union (UAW) is for strong restrictions. They have favored a bed-reduction act, the purpose of which is to cut costs by reducing the number of beds and placing restrictions on the system rather than relying on any kind of market mechanism. I believe the range in which competition is permitted will be sharply restricted.

Another aspect of the use of an expenditure lid is that promising free care to the population and then leaving it up to the provider to supply that free care places the onus of waiting, and the dissatisfaction that would occur, on the provider rather than on the government. This would be different if the government reimbursed the patient and the patient purchased the care; then, if the government did not pay the patient enough, he would be able to see that the government has not put up enough money. Under the proposed plan, the inability to receive as much care as patients want would result in the blame being placed on the provider rather than on the government.

With regard to the financing of the plan, it sounds very much like a payroll tax up to a maximum limit. This will raise the cost of low wage labor and will result in a decrease in their demand. It would, however, place an upper limit on how much employees, or employers on their behalf, would have to contribute, because a lid would be placed on health expenditures. Most national health insurance plans propose to shift the costs from the government to business, in order to make it more politically feasible. So this aspect of the plan is not different from other plans that attempt to remove health expenditures from the government budget and shift it to industry.

One of the more intriguing aspects of the proposed plan is how the pool will work. All this money comes into a central place controlled by banks, insurance companies, and HMOs; although this is similar to the old plan, at least it is not run by a monopolist, which would be the federal government or social security administration as in the previous plan (Health Security Act plan). In the proposed plan there presumably would be competition among a few more interest groups. Again, though, I have a feeling that with such a large pot of money, it would be very difficult for any politician or interest group to resist using these funds for their own objectives or interests. I believe that what would happen is that cross-subsidies would be established and different kinds of schemes devised to divide up the pool. The allocation process would be quite different than if it were left up to the market.

Another problem with the pool is that since there would be a limited amount of money for existing providers, it would be difficult for new providers to enter the market. This is because the money would have to be divided among the existing providers; they would have to negotiate budgets with the insurance companies, and so on, and I believe it would be very difficult for a new provider to receive part of that money.

The basic values underlying the union approach differ quite a bit from the Seidman proposal. The union proposal uses the idea of a lid, while the Seidman proposal bases total expenditures on consumer preferences to determine how much is to be spent and how. Another difference in value judgments between the union and Seidman proposals is a mistrust of competition in the union proposal for allocating resources, a belief that the government has to be included in the negotiations, and the use of regulation (rather than relying on competitive forces).

It appears that proposals for national health insurance have changed over time. Originally they were supposed to increase the use of medical services by those who could not afford them. Now national health insurance is suggested as a means to implement cost control, which obviously will not achieve the first objective.

I want to make a few comments on Seidman's paper. There are a number of aspects that I favor, such as the repeal of tax subsidies (relating government subsidies to income), the universality of catastrophic insurance, and Seidman's comments on regulation and how insensitive it would be. The concerns I have with the paper are that I think there are very high administrative costs on the government side, for the government to evaluate different insurance policies and to relate them to people's income. There are also very high information costs on the part of the patient for evaluating the different proposals to determine which ones can be matched with their income and their ceilings.

My last comment concerns the type of plan that I would favor. Such a plan would relate family income to a subsidy for insurance, such as a tax credit for an insurance voucher. Everyone could have the same type of coverage, such as catastrophic, or there could be several standard types of plans. By using a voucher system, there would be competition among suppliers, such as HMOs, for that voucher. Competition among suppliers for a voucher would place the emphasis of cost constraint on the supplier rather than on the patient through cost sharing, such as copayments. Thus if there are several standard packages upon which suppliers compete, they would have an incentive to provide those packages at lower cost.

Chapter 10 Notes

1. Associate Professor of Health Economics, Health Policy Program, University of California, San Francisco. Preparation of the paper was supported

by the National Center for Health Services Research Grant No. HS02975-02 for the Health Services Policy Analysis Center.

2. Two closely related aspects of these comments were brought into sharper focus by the discussion at the conference. The first is Reinhardt's distinction between the European "solidarity principle" and the generally accepted view in the United States that there should be an acceptable minimum package, but all else is optional. The second point deals with the use of language and was underscored by Blumstein. Aday's data clearly show differences in use of services. Whether these differences are inequitable depends both on the reasons for the differences and one's values.

3. For instance, Zubkoff's presentation suggests very wide variations among physicians in what they think is necessary.

4. For instance, income, education, and occupation are the primary determinants of insurance coverage. Yet even those Hispanics who are nonpoor, have 13 or more years of schooling, or are in professional and managerial positions have twice the rate of noninsurance as any other population subgroup, including rural Southern or urban blacks (table 6.5 in Aday's paper).

5. Joseph F. Newhouse and M. Susan Marquise, "The Norms Hypothesis and the Demand for Medical Care," *Journal of Human Resources* 13, supplement, (1978).

6. Ronald H. Coase, "The Nature of the Firm," reprinted in George Stigler and Kenneth E. Boulding, eds., *Reading in Price Theory* (Chicago: Richard D. Irwin, Inc., 1978).

General Discussion of Section II

Lu Ann Aday's Paper

Aday

First, with respect to the concerns expressed by Harold Luft about our approach to measuring equity, I think this goes back to some of the comments that were made in the first session about the commodity that we are dealing with—health care and the values that are associated with it. I suggest that need, and the use of services relative to need, are an important starting point for considering equitable distribution of the health care resource. A second point deals with the variance in the types of illnesses. Our indicators attempt to control differences in varied illnesses, the symptoms–response ratio in particular, which comes from information provided by physicians with respect to the probable severity of that type of complaint. A third point is with respect to variability in medical opinion: indeed, different providers may well provide different assessments of what is an appropriate response. We ourselves have collected information from two different sets of providers, who have collected information from university-based specialists and have constructed some norms of appropriate access on this basis. We have also collected information on appropriate access from community physicians, and the community physicians' norms were the ones we reported here. The evaluations of utilization varied across different classes of provider's norms—more under the community physicians' norms than the university-based norms. I think the point is that medical opinions may vary. Physicians apply different norms, and yet the relative position of subgroups does not differ.

Turning to the causality argument, which is in terms of the one indicator relationship between regular service care and physician use, we have pursued this particular question in more detail in some of our other work and did some tap analysis modeling which makes certain assumptions about the cause and relationship of certain variables. Our analysis suggests the availability of the resources would make an impact directly on utilization patterns.

Hal has suggested a number of useful hypotheses which I think are relevant. The data as presented here do suggest a correlation of important potential and realized access indicators, and he has outlined a scope of work for digging perhaps more deeply into these issues. Other issues mentioned here are different health policies that we need to be aware of and certain groups for whom inequities do exist; and perhaps this should be the focus of our resources and our attention at this time.

Audience

I just wanted to follow up on a point that Luft was making about vocabulary. It is my sense that the political debate that we were discussing this morning with Reinhardt's paper is shaped by the use of language. The example used was "maldistribution" or "equity of access," which I think are evaluating terms, and they have the effect of submerging the value of the question. The data set forth that there is a disparity between one group and another, and I would think that this is a neutral term. The question of whether this disparity should make a difference in terms of policy, or to what extent it should make a difference, calls for a value judgment that goes back to the question of solidarity versus a decent minimum. I was very glad that Luft brought out that point, because I think many times by using evaluating terms like maldistribution or inequity of access, we submerge the basic or prior order questions about what is fair and equitable. This goes on often in the health area and is not limited to the equity or maldistribution question.

My favorite example is to talk about physician "reimbursements," which is a nonsensical term. The view that money shouldn't matter in the health arena shapes our perception that somehow it is not dignified to talk about dollars or income. Physicians are really compensated. If we talk about physician compensation instead of physician reimbursement, we begin to think about a different type of issue: payment and fees.

Again, to the extent that we clean up the language to make it descriptive rather than make it to hide the underlying value of conflicts, we'll be able to talk more objectively.

Luft

The definition of inequality and access were Aday's, not mine, but one point on this. While we are on language, let us try to make a clear distinction, although I don't know where to draw the line, between necessary and discretionary services. The latter may have some value, but there are differences of opinion on the benefits.

Ingbar

I would like to pursue this a little further because we have an expert with some fascinating new data. Dorothy Rice's data from the National Ambulatory Medical Care Service (NAMCS) are highly relevant to this point. Approximately 50 percent of all visits to physicians' offices last less than ten minutes; 40 percent involve a drug of some kind or therapy procedure; less than 2 percent of all visits are deemed to be significant in the sense that, in the absence of that visit, the patient would have suffered in the view of the physician; and 80 percent are not significant.

Given this pattern of why people go to the offices of private physicians, it seems to me, the problem of how to get good statistics on whether people are getting needed access becomes even more complicated. I don't quite know how one deals with it, but the NAMCS data seem highly relevant in connection with this problem.

Rice

NAMCS, a survey of physicians in private practice, classifies the patient's reason for the visit as serious or not very serious, and it is clear that the vast proportion of visits are classified by the physician as not very serious. This does raise questions about needed versus not needed care, and who is to determine need. In the survey, it is defined to be the doctor.

Audience

The physician may decide that what the patient has is a scratch. The physician is undoubtedly right, and he may say the visit is not serious, but the patient's view is that he has just been cured of cancer.

Rice

This is clearly an issue. Our initial contacting of physicians to enlist their assistance in this enormous collection process points out that they had great difficulty themselves in coming up with a way to approach this, because they indicated that they want a lot of patients to come through for reassurance; and shouldn't everyone have a chance to come to them for that? Basically, our instruction on the severity criterion that they were to construct, was to think of what percentage would need to come see a physician for this particular service or otherwise suffer serious medical complications resulting from, say, the delay. I think the point raised here is that there are two perspectives, two approaches or sets of values that are being applied to this situation, but these are sets of values that certainly interact when care is being sought and delivered. The argument could be made that both are equally important to consider. The pattern does vary for different groups, and we should try to examine why that exists.

Phelps

I would like to raise another level of complication—the question of having or using expert assessment in determining severity of care. I think there is a large number of medical situations where the patient and the physician agree as to the seriousness of the illness and the treatment, but that does not determine how serious this event is to society. Allergic dermatitis for somebody digging trenches with a shovel is not as serious a problem as it would be for a person piloting a 747 aircraft, because he may crash the airplane while he's trying to scratch an itch. A broken foot is not a serious problem for the President of the United States, but it is a very serious problem for a professional athlete. This is one of the reasons why revealed preferences are appreciated by economists. I am fundamentally dubious of the ability of any group, either providers or any other, to assess the importance of providing medical care to a given class of illnesses, or a given set of persons, because you can't really tell the importance of receiving medical care personally. These differences can be obstructed completely from the willingness or the ability of the person to pay. That is, I could hold income constant and make the same sort of complaints about these measures as if I allow income to vary. I'm pessimistic about Aday's ability to continue to use such measures.

Goldbeck

It is interesting that one should decide that what constitutes equity is how close we get to something which, by happenstance, is what we have now as a national average of access and utilization. That makes a rather gigantic leap from what actually happens to what we ought to be doing. If we have five visits per person per year, all of the sudden that is the common symbol of equity. Then suppose we get everybody up to that national average for which there is no logical reason. Does that mean that we have solved the problem for those people who had previously been cut out of the system? I think it is an interesting and serious problem for those who make public policy; that is, the idea of closing gaps and finding some measure of whether we have successfully closed those gaps. How do we decide if access is up to an acceptable level, and what norms are deemed acceptable? Furthermore, we fail to take into consideration such questions as how many visits to regular physicians are made for specific kinds of problems that these physicians are not qualified to treat, such as emotional problems.

The kinds of statistics that Aday was using also point to a very basic question for those who want to change health policy. The basic poverty statistics that are related to income, employment, and housing would not address many of the causal factors that are relevant for NHI.

Aday

With respect to the observation that the national norms, as they exist, are somehow a goal to meet, let me respond. We are looking at individuals relative to some standard of comparison. Some comparisons are made between subgroup experiences and the national average. That's one of several modes of comparison which are available even in the small numbers of tables that I have submitted today. A second comparison is among groups themselves—the poor compared to the non-poor, majority whites as compared to people of Spanish heritage. This is another way of approaching the problem. There appear to be differences here. What may be accounting for these differences? A third option is using some sort of professional norms. As I mentioned, information was collected by and from providers. As Phelps is suggesting, perhaps this, even in terms of individual value judgments, may have serious problems. Another approach that we've used is individual subjective perceptions of the experience or satisfaction levels, for instance, what patients think about the care that they obtain. Examining their experiences relative to how they evaluate those experiences gives us another view. There are a number of different ways of approaching these comparisons; all have some merit and warrant some attention.

Stanley Jones's and Laurence Seidman's Papers

Jones

Let me start on the question of cost, because part of what Ehrlich has said[1] is speculative and part of it relates to what in fact these numbers mean. The forty billion dollars are in fact additional national expenditures; of that, thirty billion are additional on-budget federal expenditures. The numbers, in fact, were produced separately by HEW and the labor unions, and given the political competition between the two, are amazingly close. Both include estimates of increased demand as a result of no deductibles and coinsurance that are very substantial, and in fact they were based on early reports of the Rand work. There is a heavy burden in those numbers of induced demand. It might be argued that the estimate is inadequate, but in fact it is based on the best data available.

Ehrlich

A quick rebuttal on that. That was not my point. The cost estimates that you mention may already take into account excessive demand.

But my point was not about excessive demand. My point was about the new pricing system that would have to substitute for the current pricing system. Inefficient and imperfect as it may be because of all kinds of tax subsidies, we still have some sort of a pricing mechanism that equilibrates the system. The benefit of a money price system is that money prices are transfer payments. They do not consume real resources. But if I pay the price by standing in line waiting for whatever level of service you provide for me nationally, then there is another cost. It is not an explicit one, so politicians don't worry about it; but it is a real cost of foregone opportunities that I pay by spending my time waiting in line—time that could be valuable for the economy either through my participation in the production process or in consumptive activities.

Jones

The opportunity costs and how much queuing there will be as a result of this, is something yet to be determined. In fact, the cost estimates do include a good deal of estimates of increased demand as well as estimates of queuing. Unfortunately, these are much higher than the unions would like to include, based on the experience that Rand is having in this regard. The induced demand is fairly substantial and considerably more than anyone had suspected prior to the Rand experiments.

Let me make some other comments. Phelps suggested that the political question, why labor has done what it has done, might take some closer looking at, and I agree with that. There are many factors at work in the political environment that come back to economic realities, which in fact account for some of labor's flexibility today that wasn't there a number of years ago. It is a complicated picture because the labor movement is very diverse; there are some elements of the movement that have an enormous amount to gain out of this kind of legislation and others that have less.

On the point of competition and whether or not the bill provides for it (or whether in fact it is more regulatory than competition-inspiring), I would only suggest that labor unions have a real ambivalence on this point. I believe they would argue they've gone out of their way to try to make it as easy for HMOs to flourish as they can within this bill, by giving the HMOs every possible advantage in the market to attract enrollees. The other side of the coin is that the unions do insist on things like the Federal Reduction programs in Michigan, and they will continue to press for that kind of top down regulatory effect. How you interface that kind of concern with pro-competitive provisions is a real dilemma in Washington today; and if you had to pick the one area that is the frontier of policy formation, that is it. Work is needed in this area badly. It is not enough to say: "regulation is bad and competition is good"; the policy scene in Washington is such that there's going to be both. The question is how to interface them well, and I'd encourage you to get into that particular business.

One last point. Labor is coming from a certain value set when talking about health care. They (labor unions) don't feel they have to prove that the market has failed before they advocate that government, in the old Health Security sense, become the health insurer for the nation. They feel it is quite rational to say: "Here is a way of redistributing income that we find to be valued; and we should use that mechanism even if every possibility for making the market mechanism work has not been explored." The justification they are looking for is a desire by many people in our society for more of the kind of medical care that classically is being offered in the country. They don't want dollars and cents to get in the way of purchasing it. Many substantial issues can be raised about whether that is the best for them in the long run, but if you are asking what labor wants, alas, I'm afraid it is more medical care and more insurance of the customary sort to cover that medical care.

Seidman

I will try to respond to some of the points that Phelps made and then add two quick points on what Feldstein and Ehrlich said. The first point that Phelps raised was, "Is there really shallow coverage today?" Let me make sure I understand you (Phelps) right. You are not disputing that for the payment of hospital service itself there is first-dollar coverage. Your point is rather that there is a hospital episode, a whole package, and that includes paying for physicians, possibly nursing care, et cetera. It is not true, then, that when a person is going to have a hospital episode, he thinks it is free starting from dollar one. It is not, you're correct, but there still is a crucial distortion when one major component of that is free from the first dollar. In other words, it may be true that an individual patient would say: "It's not going to be costless to me if I go into the hospital; I'm going to have to pay part of the physician bill and so forth." But the choice of hospital, how many days to stay, and the set of tests you get as an inpatient are all factors which will cause serious distortions in the incentive structure.

The second point was: if we end the tax subsidy, will it in fact reduce such shallow coverage? Certainly, Phelps is an expert on what you can glean from the data and from the econometric approach. I would suggest several points, though. While we can't be sure, I think it depends very much on the whole package that goes with the system. I call attention to my description of the medical loan program to go with this. I think one reason why people may want to have shallow coverage is the cash flow motive. If they feel they have to come up with cash immediately, then insurance fulfills both an insurance and loan function. If you guarantee loan availability to people, that helps create a climate, coupled with the elimination of the tax incentive, where many people may well decide they don't need complete coverage. But I admit we'll never know for sure until we try. I would also make a point that Mark Pauly, in particular, has already emphasized; namely, suppose somebody does continue to prefer complete insurance, even if the tax subsidy were removed. Well, if it is true that complete coverage tends to inflate the use of services, then the premium charged by a private insurer is going to have to include that additional cost. If the individual is really willing to pay the higher premium and, on average, pay a larger amount out of his income each year for medical care (because he is so risk-averse that even without the subsidy he wants complete insurance), then the question is on what grounds should we object to that? The one grounds I did think might have some validity is the externality argument. If it is true that when one group becomes insured, physicians tend to prescribe more services for the uninsured as well as the insured, then a person becoming excessively insured is imposing costs on others. Whether or not this is true, I'm not sure. But that seems to me the only grounds to worry about with regard to complete insurance with no subsidy. Go back to why the subsidy was put into place originally: people like having cash as well as insurance. If an employer pays more for insurance, then he has less to give in compensation in the form of wages. Again, I think we can't be sure until it has been tried, but I'd be very surprised if we didn't have a significant movement away from complete insurance.

Ricardo-Campbell

The reason health insurance in this country grew so rapidly was because the wage controls of World War II resulted in employers developing rewards other than wage increases in order to hold their employees. Employers dreamed up many kinds of fringe benefits, including vitamin pills and time off for shopping, but the one relatively new fringe benefit that took hold was health benefits. It is a very attractive fringe benefit because the employee does not pay any income tax on the premium paid by the employer even though the premium amount is in lieu of wages. The employer expenses the premiums. The great growth in private health insurance was largely the result of wage control during World War II.

Seidman

All I'm saying is, don't you think that contributing to the reasons for having the tax subsidy was the concern that if you didn't encourage people to get private insurance, they would then be vulnerable because they have a tendency to prefer cash and not plan ahead? Wasn't that one concern?

Ricardo-Campbell

True. There is another facet of the problem that nobody here has raised. Only recently have any unions been willing to consider a trade-off between additional wages and less insurance. This trade-off has been a big part of collective bargaining negotiations by the United Mine Workers and some auto unions. We have been ignoring what is taking place in the corporate sector. Additionally, in an attempt to get more catastrophic insurance from the employer, a few unions are accepting lesser amounts of first-dollar coverage.

Seidman

On the feasibility of income relating, and this relates to the point that Ehrlich made: it is certainly true that if you don't try to income-relate, it is much simpler. But the question is whether it is satisfactory on an equity score. If you go for cost sharing but no income relating, you won't get it. The majority political sentiment in the country is going to insist on the equity aspect, which income relating and cost sharing try to deal with. Yes, it is a little more difficult, but we income-relate all the time, with tax credits for instance. We now have a medical deduction. It is just imperfect; it doesn't provide a ceiling on people. We have a whole set of deductions and tax credits that are income-related, such as joint versus separate filing. Why is it of greater difficulty for this particular tax credit than for all the other ones that we now have? There is always some gaming, but I don't see why that is a new problem.

Ehrlich

Larry, I want to say just one thing. It is not that I'm opposed to equity, but I can point out an alternative that you did not discuss: the Feldstein Plan.

Seidman

Oh, no, my proposal is just a version of the Feldstein Plan.

Ehrlich

The difference is that you propose an income, or a major last resort, type of insurance in addition to the Feldstein Plan. I also got the impression, though you didn't work any of the specifics out, that you wanted more graduation and more detail in connection with the subsidization. This would involve large administrative costs, and we want to take that into account because we are always interested in the balance of marginal costs versus marginal benefits.

Chapter 11 Notes

1. *Editor's note:* Jones's rebuttal is in connection with my oral comments on his paper presented in this session. I have later pursued the analysis of the accuracy of the cost estimates for the Kennedy Plan with Gordon Trapnell, the original author of these estimates. For my comments on Jones's paper and my findings concerning these cost estimates, see the second part of my paper appearing in this volume (chapter 9).

Section III

Some Lessons for the Future

Increasing the Role of Competition in the Market for Health Services

*Clark C. Havighurst**

The failure of the 1970s to yield a coherent national health policy has finally produced both (1) a new willingness on the part of some policymakers to reappraise government's role in the health services industry and (2) a new openness to the possibility that market forces could be primarily relied upon to guide the industry's evolution toward greater cost consciousness in the use of society's resources. My own thinking has long been that the potential of government regulation for dealing with the problem of health care costs has been greatly overestimated and that the market's capabilities have been correspondingly underestimated. It is naturally gratifying to see many policymakers gradually coming to share this perception.

Although it is reassuring to witness the beginning of a reconsideration of the roles to be assigned to regulation and competition in the future, I confess to an uneasy feeling: I fear that it will prove to have been much easier to open up the policy debate than it will be to identify and finally bring about all of the interrelated policy and behav-

*Professor of Law, Duke University. Work on this paper was supported in part by Grant No. HS 01539 from the National Center for Health Services Research, United States Department of Health and Human Services.

ioral changes that are needed to make the market alternative work satisfactorily. Just in the past year it has become incumbent on scholars of my persuasion to do more than simply hold out a lightly sketched alternative. We have to come up with a coherent and practical legislative program. Even though one may yearn to return to an earlier era, when it was sufficient simply to carp in academic terms about the unwisdom of the drift to regulation, it now seems necessary to offer a specific set of proposals that meets the tests of practicality and political feasibility.

These remarks are meant to outline my view of the things that need to be done. I have tried to address and overcome as many of the constraints as I can perceive, and I think the result is a viable approach. My list of proposals is far less definitive, however, than Alain Enthoven's Consumer-Choice Health Plan. For this reason, my approach, even though it includes elements that are very much like the innovations currently being sponsored by Congressmen Ullman, Gephardt, and Stockman and Senators Schweiker and Durenberger, lacks the programmatic character and identity that aid so much in giving ideas prominence in public debate. In fact, I have somewhat greater hope for a piecemeal approach, which addresses specific market defects and specific needs on an ad hoc basis, than for an all-embracing legislative solution. Consequently, this paper is not so much a blueprint for a national health plan as an agenda for governmental action (and occasional inaction in the nature of benign neglect) at several levels.

The 96th Congress's Rediscovery of a Role for Competition

At the outset, I would like to remark upon the extraordinary way in which the 96th Congress has taken the lead in commencing a re-examination of the assumptions that guided health policy development throughout most of the 1970s. Whereas the inevitability of heavy regulation in health services was nearly everyone's working hypothesis up until 1979, Congress has now begun to question that assumption and to consider whether it may not be possible, instead of trying to employ regulation to suppress the myriad symptoms of the market's malfunctioning, to address the root causes of market failure. It now seems at least possible that the 96th Congress's new emphasis on addressing health issues at this fundamental level will be viewed in time as a departure of historic significance.

Let me briefly list some of the ways in which Congress, in the space of little more than one calendar year, and with no help at all from the executive department with responsibility in the field, has opened the health policy debate to possibilities that only a few academics had previously had the independence of mind to entertain.

Procompetition language in the health planning amendments The most tangible endorsement to date of competition as a potentially useful force in health policy appears in the Health Planning and Resources Development Amendments of 1979 (Public Law 96-79), enacted in September 1979. That legislation and the accompanying committee reports reveal a dramatic reversal of the previously dominant premise that market forces cannot function in health care, and a new commitment to make them work wherever they can.[1] Although the reports do not go overboard for competition and do recognize that the demand side of the market (subsidized by poorly designed third-party insurance) currently requires supply-side regulation, the reports clearly acknowledge the potential for demand-side change. This legislation is the first to make health policy consistent with the new national awareness of the limitations of government regulation. Indeed, at the time of its enactment, the amended health planning act provided a clearer blueprint for deregulation—to the extent that the public interest would in fact be served thereby—than any other federal regulatory statute, with the possible exception of the Airline Deregulation Act.[2]

Exemption of HMOs from certificate-of-need requirements The health planning amendments also granted to health maintenance organizations (HMOs) a statutory exemption from certificate-of-need requirements,[3] thus embracing the fundamental principle that consumers' choices in a competitive market can be trusted to allocate resources appropriately. It is notable that the exemption extends to HMOs that are not regulated under the federal HMO Act, again expressing a judgment that consumers with incentives and opportunities to economize do not need federal regulators to prescribe the choices that they can make.

Development of the "multiple choice" concept The 96th Congress also gets nearly all of the credit for bringing the "multiple choice" idea into the public debate. Both in proposals to offer private employees a wider range of choice of health plans[4] and in proposals to allow Medicare beneficiaries to choose competing health plans on the basis of comparative efficiency,[5] Congress has begun to lay the groundwork for legislation that will restore market forces to useful functioning.

Serious attention to the distorting effects of tax subsidies Proposals to change the tax treatment of health insurance premiums[6] represent another breakthrough in the health policy debate. For years, the tax law's dilution of economizing incentives was acknowledged to be a significant cause of health care cost inflation, but it was widely said that regulation was politically inevitable because Congress would never bite that particular bullet. Developments in the 96th Congress have cast considerable doubt on those political prognostications.

Defeat of the hospital cost-containment bill The defeat of this 1977 bill (S 1391 HR 6575) is another achievement of which the 96th Congress can, in my view, be proud. While widely regarded as a victory for industry lobbyists, that action reflected more fundamentally a recognition by many legislators of the full implications of continuing down the road to arbitrary governmental controls. Congress's hard work at the task of devising alternative strategies addressed to fundamentals of the health care market—strategies which the Department of Health and Human Services (DHHS) has totally ignored—shows that its efforts, including its rejection of the Carter administration's bill, have been not only consistent but highly responsible. The Carter administration's criticisms notwithstanding, Congress takes the problem of health care costs seriously, but it has recognized, as the administration has yet to do, that the problem must be solved not by regulatory palliatives and placebos, but by stronger medicine that is intended to cure the disease.

Despite the Congress's major achievements on behalf of competition in the health services industry, its work is not yet done. Although the debate and many previously closed minds have been opened up, many issues and implications have yet to be fully recognized and understood, and many technical problems have yet to be resolved. Nevertheless, many of the essential ideas are already embodied in specific proposals,[7] and none of these seem so complex or so controversial that a bill cannot be enacted fairly soon. There is danger, however, that, if the 96th Congress fails to act in a definitive way on competition, Congress will lose the initiative on health legislation that it has so effectively seized and exercised. Following the presidential election—whatever the outcome—the executive branch will seek to resume its customary leadership on policy development, and it cannot be assumed that even a new administration of the other party will be any more capable of embracing the market strategy than previous administrations have been.

At the time this is written (March 1980), the 96th Congress has an opportunity to put the capstone on what could prove to be the most significant development in health policy since the enactment of Medicare and Medicaid. Without imposing a new federal program or massive federal spending, Congress can put the private health care market on a firmer footing—and on to the path toward privately initiated, competitively stimulated reform—simply by focusing on the incentives at work and on structural features of the market. That the political world and the media have not fully recognized the public significance of the changes being considered is no guide to their potential importance, but only a reflection of the fact that they will yield no programmatic monument to which congressional sponsors can point with pride. Indeed, because the political reward system and legislators' normal inclinations do not predispose Congress to address policy problems with primary attention to restoring the market's ability to function, we are witnessing a classic instance of the challenge that Charles L. Schultze posed in his landmark book, *The Public Use of Private Interest*.[8] Chairman Schultze observed how government has always been biased in favor of regulatory and bureaucratic solutions to policy problems, even when those problems might be more readily and effectively addressed by restructuring incentives and rectifying the causes of market failure. I must admit that I was one who scoffed out loud when Schultze expressed at the end of his book the hope that "a steady maturing of both the electorate and political leaders" might in time restore a more balanced approach to policy choices.[9] Although I still have grave doubts that Congress can in fact overcome the antimarket tendencies that political processes necessarily generate, at the moment I am full of admiration, as I have indicated, for the way in which the 96th Congress has begun to address health policy questions.

Of course, it remains to be seen whether Congress will in fact follow through in its procompetitive efforts. It is still not at all clear whether a majority of this Congress is promarket in a constructive sense or only irresponsibly antiregulation. For example, the recent vote in the Senate narrowly defeating a proposal to limit the Federal Trade Commission's (FTC) antitrust enforcement powers with respect to state-regulated professions, including organized medicine, indicates a discouraging level of understanding and a depressing receptivity to pressures from privileged interest groups.[10] Unfortunately, a failure by Congress to carry the competitive strategy forward could significantly strengthen the case for returning to the old and downward path toward regulatory strangulation of yet another critical industry.

The Problem to be Addressed:
Private Financing Without Cost Controls

A careful diagnosis of the health care sector's cost problem leads quickly to the conclusion that it results from Americans having too much of the wrong kind of financial protection against burdensome medical expenses. It is not third-party payment alone that is the problem, however, but rather the nature and breadth of the coverage provided and the absence in the various financing programs of any significant administrative checks on the price or utilization of services. Indeed, most of the allegedly unique characteristics of the health services industry that are usually cited to justify regulation are merely reflections of the dysfunctional financing mechanisms that have developed. For example, the central decision-making role of the physician, widely cited as making consumer choice irrelevant, is a significant problem only because, as health insurance expanded, no other accountability for the cost of care was substituted for the doctor's previous professional obligation to be concerned about his patient's financial well-being (along with his physical health). By the same token, the consumers' obvious ignorance in obtaining medical services looms large as a problem only because third parties, while removing most cost constraints, have not brought available expertise, selectivity, or bargaining power to bear on the consumers' behalf, thus leaving patients to the costly, though presumptively tender, mercies of the unconstrained physician. Finally, hospitals' ability to tolerate inefficiency both in operations and capital investments is a direct result of their decreasing need, under automatic third-party cost reimbursement, to keep the cost of care within patients' reach.

The deficiencies of third-party payment are frequently observed, of course, in explanations of the need for direct public intervention to control costs. Such analyses, however, nearly always stop conveniently short of tracing the precise reasons why financing mechanisms have taken their present form and of assessing the remediability of the underlying market failure. Public financing plans take their present form, of course, only because of a legislative choice to model them after the private financing mechanisms that were in place at the time of their enactment, particularly the Blue Cross and Blue Shield plans.[11] Thus, even though public plans are a major factor in the industry, their present characteristics can be viewed not as an inevitability but as a symptom of problems that arose initially in the private sector. Moreover, recent shifts in the health policy debate (for example, the redesign of Senator Kennedy's national insurance proposal) indicate that further expansion of direct public financing is unlikely and that the private market will continue to be heavily relied upon to provide financial protection against health care costs. Thus, even reformers dedicated to increased public subsidies for needy populations are redirecting their attention to the private sector's defects and potential strengths. The emphasis here is on the failures of the private market to generate financing mechanisms that respond adequately to the cost problem. If the private sector can be restored to economic health, the redesign of public programs to build on, rather than to undercut, the private sector's strengths should not be too difficult.

It seems to me that excessive growth in the private sector of the wrong kinds of financial protection against medical care costs can be traced to just two major causes, neither of which has until recently been widely recognized as the pernicious influence it is, and both of which are subject to remedy through measures that do not supplant private decision making with government control.

The first main cause of the market's failure is the tax law's treatment of health insurance premiums. The second is provider dictation of the type of financial protection available to consumers. The latter problem is currently being addressed by stepped-up antitrust enforcement, which is focusing in particular on the various ways in which organized providers exercise influence over private third-party payers and restrain both innovation in private insurance plans and the development of alternative delivery and financing systems, such as HMOs. Recent antitrust enforcement and new scholarship[12] have made it increasingly clear how effective organized provider-interests have been in suppressing the market's efforts to respond to consumers' problems, which flow from their ignorance and dependence on professional judgment as well as from the payment system's inducements to excessive spending of money in the common funds. Although eliminating the heritage of generations of minimal antitrust enforcement in this industry will take considerable time, energy, and persuasiveness, significant progress is being made by the FTC, the Justice Department, and some state attorneys general. Assuming that Congress's threats to interfere rashly with the FTC's jurisdiction in this area do not significantly depress prosecutorial zeal, the environment should become increasingly hospitable to privately initiated change. Although the antitrust enforcement effort is an essential item on the procompetition agenda, it will not be discussed further here. The focus of the discussion that follows is the legislative moves needed to implement the market alternative.

The Distortions Attributable to the Tax Treatment of Employer-Paid Health Insurance Premiums

Because antitrust enforcement is beginning to deal effectively with one of the two major causes of the health care market's failure to contain costs, efforts to remove the other major cause are of even greater importance. Let me try to capture in a nutshell the magnitude of the distortions created by the exclusion of employer-paid insurance premiums from employees' taxable income and wages.

Although the exact extent of the subsidy varies for individuals according to their tax bracket and whether incremental wages are subject to Federal Insurance Contribution Act (FICA) taxes, Martin

Feldstein and Bernard Friedman estimate that the tax law provides a discount (before administrative expenses) of roughly 35 percent for all health services purchased through an insurance plan.[13] (Because the FICA tax benefit accrues only to lower tax bracket employees, the discount is relatively uniform and in the 35 percent range for most workers.) The size of this discount means that people have a powerful incentive to pay as many bills as possible through insurance. Because bills can be paid with untaxed dollars only if paid from the common fund, coinsurance and deductibles are not favored, and people seek insurance coverage for services that could be readily paid for out-of-pocket. In other words, insurance is valued not simply as a means of obtaining essential financial protection but as a vehicle for obtaining federal help in paying routine bills. The subsidy is, of course, generally greater for upper tax bracket taxpayers and minimal for low-income persons having little tax liability.

The overinsurance that results from the tax subsidy has consequences that far exceed the dollar amount of the subsidy—which, at more than $13 billion in the recent Congressional Budget Office (CBO) estimate,[14] is itself a nonnegligible figure. By inducing the purchase of insurance that would not otherwise be purchased, the tax subsidy extends third-party payment's distorting effect on the demand for medical care to a much wider range of health care transactions than would otherwise be affected. Feldstein and Friedman describe the tax law as providing "a subsidy of a subsidy."[15] I call it piling one distortion of demand on top of another. The effect of this on health care spending, by removing cost considerations from provider and patient decision making, is probably incalculable, but certainly very large. The obvious solution to the problem (developed later in this paper) is to put some kind of limit on the exclusion, so that, while the purchase of basic financial protection is encouraged, the employee-consumer is made conscious, beyond a certain point, of the full value of the marginal dollar that is spent by his employer on health insurance rather than paid to him in wages.

Overinsurance induced by the tax law takes other forms as well. Excessive liberality on the part of insurers in the payment of claims, less than optimal use of dollar limitations on indemnity payments, and an undue preference for paid-in-full service benefits are other consequences of the tax law's penalization of out-of-pocket payments. By the same token, cost-containment efforts by third parties are not valued as highly as they should be, since any saving in premium that is achieved and paid out as increased wages becomes taxable income. Thus, because a dollar saved is not a dollar earned, insurers have been unduly passive in dealing with providers and in their attempts to curb the so-called moral hazard—the name that economists have given to the recognized propensity of the insured to spend an insurer's money without due regard to whether benefits exceed costs. Although much of the passivity of third-party payers results from restraints of trade imposed by providers, the tax law has greatly reduced the incentives of insurers and consumers to resist provider dictation.

This recitation of the ways in which the unlimited tax subsidy for private health insurance has distorted the industry's performance suggests why a change in the tax law would be in the public interest. My basic contention is simply that, with consumer incentives to economize appropriately strengthened and the market freed of professionally imposed restraints on innovation in the financing system, private initiatives can reasonably be expected to move us closer to efficient levels of spending on health care than we can hope to get by any other available means. Obviously, attainment of other social objectives may well require that public subsidies be redesigned and extended to some currently underserved groups, but these policy moves are not incompatible with the market's functioning; indeed, they will be facilitated if greater efficiency and competitiveness can free resources to meet, and reduce the cost of meeting, currently unmet needs.

The policy agenda set forth later in this paper is intended to satisfy the minimal conditions that must exist before the competitive market can be deemed to serve consumers well. Whether a tax law change is an essential precondition to primary reliance on competition and consumer choice is debatable; but, as Glenn Hackbarth and I have argued, continuation of

> the existing tax subsidies for the purchase of health insurance would not automatically justify government regulation, which may still be criticized as more self-aggrandizing than socially imperative. Tax subsidies are common in the overall economy and do not, in themselves, invalidate reliance on the marketplace to allocate resources. Moreover, if government lacks the will to change tax rules to improve private incentives, it is fair to ask that

it accept the consequences to that choice and not meddle further in the private market. Even with the tax laws as they are, the private market can be made to function usefully, although the equilibrium it seeks will obviously be affected by the tax subsidy. In short, heavy-handed regulation is not even a second-best strategy when compared with the market's ability to correct the defects in private insurance that are not tax induced.[16]

Be that as it may, it is still the case that no other single move could have a greater impact than a significant tax change in immediately stimulating needed change in the private sector. Indeed, the impetus that a tax change could supply may be essential to overcoming the atrophy that currently affects competition in this industry. While antitrust enforcement can remove the overt barriers, it may be that only a tax change strengthening consumer pressure for cost containment can break down the tacit conspiracies and other obstacles to competition that also exist. The ensuing discussion, assessing the market's ability to generate needed innovation, suggests reasons why a tax change may be a necessary condition to getting the competitive process started.

Assessing the Private Sector's Cost-Containment Capability

It is possible to doubt the premise that enhanced competition under appropriate incentives—that is, with the tax law revised to sharpen cost consciousness—can bring about changes in health care financing and delivery that will help materially in bringing costs under control. Some who challenge this expectation demand proof that the changes brought would all be desirable and that the level of spending achieved would satisfy their notion of what is right and proper. These observers are, of course, victims of a planning mentality that accords no prima facie legitimacy to the results of even smoothly functioning markets. Let me dispose first of this type of objection to reliance on the unpredictable marketplace before moving on to estimate the prospects for meaningful change.

To my mind, the process by which a particular configuration of financing and delivery and a particular level of spending are achieved is much more important than the results themselves, which we have no benchmark for judging. For this reason, I do not regard as decisive (even if accurate) the view—expressed, for example, by Mel Glasser of the United Auto Workers—that, even with changed incentives, employees would choose the same kinds of cost-escalating insurance they now have.[17] Even if this were true—and I am certain it is not—it would not affect the desirability of making employed people pay their way without the help of government subsidies beyond some minimum point. Only when people are spending their own rather than the government's money can we be sure that what we are seeing is what people in fact want. Thus, if auto workers chose to spend their own money to buy the most expensive kind of insurance, that would be their business. Even if they did so because their union gave them no meaningful option in a multiple choice situation, that would be a problem solely between them and their union's leadership, including Mr. Glasser, and would not be a problem to concern the government. The important thing for health policy is that the supply side of the market not be precluded from making a full range of choices available and that the demand side not reflect government-induced biases. If these conditions are reasonably well satisfied, then the market's verdict should be accepted as an expression of people's preferences.

Although under this rationale it is not necessary to have assurances that the market, once unleashed, will produce dramatic changes, I have considerable confidence that it will. The crucial insight (which has escaped most people, it seems to me) is that the way in which health services are currently paid for, though well established and familiar, is in no sense inevitable. Cost containment is a complex administrative and organizational problem that can be addressed in numerous ways, none of which is so clearly superior that other approaches should be legally discriminated against or foreclosed. Thus, although people are coming to an awareness that HMOs are a useful alternative to traditional payment and delivery mechanisms, there has been an unfortunate tendency to see HMOs as the only alternative. In fact, the range of alternatives that could serve the public well is probably much wider, and it is therefore essential that we stop equating the competitive strategy with HMO development. Health maintenance organizations are indeed important features in the competitive landscape, but there is a broad and largely unexplored spectrum between closed-panel HMOs on the one hand and traditional payment mechanisms on the other. Contrary to conventional wisdom, competition is entirely compatible with third-party payment for health services; it is incompatible only with the kinds of third-party payment that currently exist.

Evidence suggesting the potential for competitively stimulated cost-effectiveness in the private financing system can be gathered from many places and can only be outlined here. First, one can have reference to theory and to the powerful logic behind practical steps that might be taken but have not been attempted in medical care. In our recent article, Hackbarth and I attempted to conceptualize the ways in which health insurers, competing among themselves for the business of cost-conscious consumers, might go about the cost-containment task by redefining their benefits.[18] We identified two essential strategies that, although they are conceptually distinct, might often be mixed in creative ways in practice. One approach is to use carefully designed exclusions from coverage, or limitations on payments, to maintain cost awareness wherever the moral hazard problem was particularly acute; the theory here is simply the theory of insurance[19] applied to discrete health services, with the result that the appropriateness of buying particular coverage can be seen as a function of, among other things, the price elasticity of demand for the service in question.[20] The contrasting strategy, revealed in the HMO model in particular, is to limit the providers who are eligible to provide covered services. In a competitive world, I would expect, a priori, to find not only relatively pure models of both kinds—selective plans with large deductibles and copayments on the one hand and comprehensive group-practice HMOs on the other—but also a variety of hybrid plans offering a somewhat wider choice of provider than group-practice HMOs but using provider-participation agreements to impose administrative controls on utilization (that is, to effectuate exclusions from coverage) and to exclude high-cost providers from eligibility to treat plan subscribers on favorable terms.

A second source of my confidence in the market's ability to change is evidence that insurers in closely analogous fields—including limited areas of health insurance (particularly dental insurance)—have taken effective action to curb the natural propensity of consumers to spend the insurance fund on benefits not worth their costs. They have thus recognized the moral hazard phenomenon, characteristic of all insurance, as a problem that they must combat if they are to compete effectively. Among the techniques employed are insurance adjusters, multiple estimates, fixed cash benefits, and contracts with service providers (e.g., auto body shops). It cannot be emphasized too strongly that the immediate cause of the persistent rise in health care costs is the failure of health care providers and insurers to develop analogous cost-containment techniques or to develop altogether different forms of financing and delivery, such as HMOs. Although analogies to other types of insurance are far from perfect and the administrative costs of medical cost control would sometimes be prohibitive, the range of strategies neglected by medical care insurers still seems great enough to suggest that other inhibiting factors are at work. I have collected some specific examples of promising strategies in recent articles.[21]

An enlightening source of impressive anecdotal evidence that major change is possible is the antitrust enforcement effort, which is uncovering restraints by organized providers on specific moves attempted by individual insurers. In one case being pursued by the FTC, a state medical society organized an explicit boycott to force a Blue Shield plan to reconsider its cost-containment policies, which included aggressive use of provider participation agreements.[22] In another case, dental societies organized a conspiracy to withhold X rays from insurers seeking to implement a program for predetermination of benefits.[23] Organized providers' historical domination of third-party programs, such as Blue Shield plans, has been shown to curb insurer initiatives, and the FTC can be expected to take some measures to reduce or eliminate such domination.[24] In a recent decision, the FTC found the medical profession's restrictions on "contract practice" (a physician's sale of his services on a negotiated basis to lay-controlled third parties) to be an illegal restraint on competition.[25] In another set of antitrust cases, providers are hoping to persuade the courts that participation agreements and insurer selectivity in making providers eligible to provide covered services are anticompetitive;[26] these cases, which are not likely to be successful, reveal both increased use of such agreements to contain costs and the providers' distaste for the competition they stimulate.

Historical research on how the financing system reached its present condition also provides convincing evidence that private institutional arrangements could have evolved very differently and could be much

more responsive to consumers' concerns about costs. The record reveals that the medical profession itself has long realized that third-
party payment can be consistent with price competition in medical
markets. Indeed, in the early days, the profession resisted the growth of
private, voluntary health insurance precisely because it might lead to
what the profession considered "destructive" competition among physicians.[27] To a greater extent than today, the profession's leaders were
candid about their desire to suppress competition and third-party initiatives on behalf of patients. For example, when the prestigious Committee on the Costs of Medical Care issued its report in 1932, the
accompanying minority report, drafted in part by members of the medical establishment and endorsed by the American Medical Association,
was filled with criticism of lay-controlled insurers who were then seeking to secure medical services for their policyholders on advantageous
terms by contracting with individual physicians or organized physician
groups.[28] Rather than dealing only with the patient and reimbursing
him for whatever the provider charged (the almost universal practice
among commercial insurers today), these insurers dealt directly with
providers themselves and used their customers' combined financial resources to obtain care on favorable terms. These insurers certainly
were not the passive payers we know today but rather were aggressive,
cost-conscious buyers of medical care. The history of prepaid medical
care in Oregon, as gleaned by Goldberg and Greenberg from the record of an early antitrust case, demonstrates powerfully that the natural propensity of early third-party payers was to control physician
spending decisions and that it required strong concerted action by
organized medicine to make the early plans conform to the profession's
preferred model.[29]

Finally, promising signs of a revival of innovation in financing and
delivery are already beginning to appear, even though the tax law remains unchanged and even though antitrust enforcement is only beginning to reduce the effectiveness of professional resistance. Health
maintenance organization development has been steady and in some
markets has created competitive conditions that reveal the market's
promise.[30] Blue Cross and Blue Shield plans have taken some steps in
the right direction, even though they have not yet been pushed very
hard by competition. Experimentation with second-opinion programs
suggests that the innovative spirit is not wholly dead among commer-

cial health insurers. Even though this latter element of the industry apparently would prefer to have government assume prime responsibility for health care costs,[31] HMO development by some insurers (an innovative program created by the Safeco Insurance Company using a closed panel of primary care physicians[32]) and a few other scattered initiatives reveal that some capacity for independent action does still exist.

Even though there is good reason to believe that dramatic change in the private financing system is possible, it must be recognized that the private insurance industry is tightly wedded to its dysfunctional payment methods and, as a practical matter, will find it hard to change. Commercial insurers are, for the most part, neither oriented nor well enough organized to undertake the needed restructuring. The HMO movement has shown that health services must be organized and integrated with financing at the local community level, where traditional insurers are not accustomed or currently well equipped to function. For these reasons, insurers are anything but anxious to act competitively as cost-conscious purchasers of providers' services in negotiated transactions, and they will not look favorably on legislation, particularly changes in the tax law, that will strengthen the competitive pressures they feel in this regard. Indeed, the commercial insurers' recent pattern of collectively embracing all proposals for governmental cost-containment regulation is reminiscent of other industries' invocation of government's protection when faced with imminent competition. Blue Cross and Blue Shield plans are not very different in their attitudes toward government—though with their larger market shares, localized operations, and closer associations with providers, they have a reasonable hope of maintaining their position without new government support.

Breaking out of their current passivity in dealing with providers remains risky for insurers, even though antitrust law now inhibits the more overt forms of concerted provider retaliation. Such innovation would require incurring substantial costs in devising administrative controls, negotiating with providers on an individual basis, and selling new types of coverage. Moreover, as Mark Pauly has observed,[33] any success in changing providers' mode of practice may have spillover effects benefiting not only the innovator but also his competitors. Finally, successful innovation may, in many cases, be readily imitated, thus creating conditions in which perceptions of oligopolistic interdependence will deter significant initiatives. While it is difficult to assess the significance of these problems, it must be conceded that there are some remaining uncertainties surrounding the prospects for immediate change even if most of the artificial obstacles to it are removed.

In this connection, it may be helpful to observe some reasons why insurers may have emphasized HMO development over other kinds of innovation. Although in many cases the risks of provider retaliation and competitor imitation have been avoided by working closely with organized medicine in establishing individual practice associations (IPAs), other HMO initiatives have had a more competitive thrust and are indicative of a willingness to innovate in competitive ways. It seems plausible to conclude that these closed-panel ventures owe something to government's intervention in the market. First of all, government has legitimized the HMO model, carried some of the burden of public education, and subsidized developmental costs. Moreover, by giving the first federally qualified HMO in an area an inside track under the HMO Act's dual-choice provisions[34] and by the de facto limiting of subsidies to only one HMO per community, government has maintained substantial entry barriers to further HMO growth, thus reducing the risks associated with the first initiative. If obstacles to innovation by insurers are in fact as great as was suggested in the preceding paragraph, perhaps other governmental strategies similar to the HMO Act could be helpful—though obviously such strategies should be temporary measures designed only to get the process of innovation started. In thinking about these problems, I have lately been intrigued by the prospect of intervention in aid of innovative ventures in local markets by well run health systems agencies (HSAs). If they chose to do so, such agencies could greatly assist insurers in developing new cost-control techniques, in selling them to consumers, and in breaking down resistance to them on the part of providers. Perhaps, even with all their drawbacks, the 200-plus HSAs are potentially a better tool for fostering experimentation and change than an HMO program expanded to back other types of governmentally approved innovation.

Having laid many problems at the door of the health insurance industry, I must now observe that some, maybe even most, of these problems may lie ultimately with the customers. These customers often have not demanded—or even been willing to accept—cost containment, even to the extent that it would have been in the consumer's after-tax interest to do so. It is not contradictory to suggest that consumers do not want the health insurance they pay for. Most insurance is purchased not by the consumers themselves, but by employers and unions acting on behalf of employment groups, and these purchasers may not be good representatives of the individual consumer's interest. Thus, another important cause of the market's resistance to innovation—in addition to the tax subsidy and provider-imposed restraints—may be the incentives implicit in vicarious (employer) or collective (union) purchasing of health benefits. Even if employers become increasingly engaged in self-insurance or in the direct provision of care for their employees, their interests may differ enough from their employees' that their plans will not be ideal solutions to the cost problem. This is not to say that employers should not experiment with new techniques of financing and delivery as a way of stimulating competition among providers and encouraging change. It is, however, to suggest that ultimately employers and unions might do better to be less active as decisionmakers and to leave more to individual choice.

The incentives of employers and unions, affected in large measure by their paternalistic and/or quasi-political relationships with the rank and file, may indeed cause them to neglect legitimate economizing opportunities. Thus, the politics of employee benefits and the powerful symbolism surrounding medical care have combined to make comprehensive benefits and hassle-free administration the norm. On the other hand, individuals choosing for themselves might rationally prefer more selective but less costly coverage. This may result simply because, as a general rule, "politically" accountable decisionmakers, facing sensitive decisions, fear the repercussions of "Type I" errors (visible hardship due to economizing) more than "Type II" errors (excessive but well-spread and hidden costs). Also, costs and the trade-off with take-home pay are so effectively hidden from the workers that economizing usually appears only to enrich the employer or the insurer—at the expense of the individuals whose coverage is revealed to be inadequate in some respect. To complicate matters further, powerful ideologies frequently operate, and even when an employer or union becomes concerned about costs, past rhetoric and carefully nurtured expectations get in the way of change. Finally, all collective decision making carries with it the risk that some minority preferences will be neglected and that other minorities with a powerful incentive to exert their interests will be served at the majority's expense. In light of all these vagrant influences distorting the purchase of health insurance, one can reasonably suggest that the market failure we are witnessing may not be a problem of health policy at all, but may instead be a problem of labor and management relations and of a tax system that makes spending on health care a hostage to collective bargaining and other strange dynamics of the employment relationship.

Solutions to the problems presented by vicarious and collective decision making would appear to lie in somehow substituting individual for collective choice, thus better internalizing the costs and benefits of decisions. Because extending economizing opportunities to individuals is a strategy that employees and unions could adopt voluntarily, it is important to consider why it has not been employed. Although this intriguing issue cannot be explored here, it is useful to note as evidence of deep resistance to the idea of individual choice that employers concerned about health care costs have done very little in the way of cutting back on coverage and have instead pursued cost containment indirectly—behind the scenes, as it were—through collective attempts to influence health planning and provider behavior in general. The collective ethic would appear to be powerful indeed.

The remainder of this paper discusses ways in which public policy might, without giving up collective responsibility, seek to overcome obstacles that currently prevent placing increased reliance on individual choice. If competition is to operate effectively as the dominant allocational mechanism in health services, the overriding policy objective must be to assure that consumers have reasonable incentives to economize and that the market is free to offer them a reasonably complete range of choice.

An Overview of a Strategy for Promoting Competition

The foregoing perceptions have led me to the conviction that meaningful private-sector change, while perhaps harder to accomplish than is sometimes believed, is not only possible but is our best hope for getting serious and effective attention paid to health care costs. The scenario that I have in mind requires a series of interrelated policy moves.

The following paragraphs develop my proposed specifications for a legislative program to open up the private insurance and health plan market to more effective competition, particularly in obtaining needed inputs (providers' services) on competitive terms.

Multiple Choice Employers larger than a specified size should be required by law to offer their employees several health plan choices. The simplest and best requirement would be that at least three competing plans of any kind be offered; a purist approach, the case for which is developed more fully below, would call for eliminating the HMO Act requirements that currently empower federally qualified HMOs to displace other types in a multiple-choice situation.

One goal of the multiple-choice requirement is to get employers and unions out of the position of making the final choice of plans for their employees and members and to restore the ultimate choice of plan to the individuals concerned. For reasons already noted, it seems likely that the individual employee is better able to economize in selecting a health plan than his employer and/or union. On the other hand, employer or union screening of the choices to be offered should relieve concerns that would weigh in favor of close regulation of benefit packages and premiums in a totally free market based strictly on individual choice. Because it is difficult to predict whether employees and unions, given this new role, would permit a meaningful range of choice, the multiple-choice idea is not certain to achieve its entire objective. Nevertheless, employers who withhold desirable opportunities for economizing would be at some disadvantage in the labor market. Because consumer choice would operate at this level as well, the multiple-choice idea must be regarded as promising.

Despite the logic and desirability of expanded personal choice there are implementation problems that must be resolved. For example, actuarial risks increase as groups are split, and adverse selection (young versus old, well versus sick) could make some plans nonviable. The adverse selection problem can be overstated, however, since it is not inappropriate (up to a point) for people with similar risks to be grouped for insurance purposes. Nevertheless, price competition should also focus on efficiency and might not do so if risk selection were freely allowed. Systems for overcoming these problems for a single employment group, without raising costs unduly and without sacrificing competition, need to be considered; but, as noted under the next heading, employers can probably be left to decide for themselves just how serious the problem is and how best to cope with it. The need to allow experience rating—that is, price competition based on actual costs—in a competitive system should be clear, but some restrictions on it may be needed if the cost of individual enrollments is not to be prohibitive. There is also a question of how self-insuring employers should be treated. Small employers present another problem, which might be addressed by creating local clearinghouses, like "Project Health" in Oregon, to administer the choice mechanism for all but large employers. (This suggestion also goes quite far toward meeting Alain Enthoven's concerns about maintaining the employment-based insurance model.)[35]

Equal Contributions Employers must be required to make the same contribution on an employee's behalf, whichever plan he selects. The necessity to supplement that contribution or the opportunity to realize a cash saving provides the employee with the needed incentive to economize. Some technical limitations on this requirement may be necessary, however, to allow the employer to reduce the impact of adverse selection. Self-insurance again raises technical difficulties.

A possible solution to the adverse selection problem would be for the employer to require the health plans offered to quote premiums for a randomly selected sample of the employment group. These premiums would reflect only efficiency and benefits, not risk selection, and would be the basis on which employees' payments and tax treatment would be determined. By its contracts with the plans, however, the employer could adjust his actual payments from the premium pool on the basis of actuarial factors reflected in actual enrollments. Such a technique, which employers could adopt voluntarily as long as the law on equal contributions did not preclude it, would eliminate most of the adverse selection problem and cause plans to compete for enrollment of all employees within a group, not merely the best risks. The effect would be to foster experience rating (that is, price competition) for the group as a whole but not for self-selected subgroups. What is most noteworthy is that regulation is not only not needed to solve this seemingly complex problem but, unless carefully designed, could stand in the way of the most natural solutions.

Tax Considerations Among the proposals to change the tax law to reduce its demand-stimulating impact, the most common approach is to limit the amount of employer-paid premiums that may be excluded from income. Thus, Chairman Ullman's bill would include in taxable income for income tax purposes any contribution over $120 per month or $1440 per year. This approach, while beneficial, still fails to change incentives throughout the entire range in which economizing might be appropriate. Indeed, whereas the limit in the Ullman bill was chosen for the expressed purpose of subsidizing the purchase of comprehensive coverage, either through a federally qualified HMO or traditional insurance with modest cost sharing, my own conviction is that employees should not be discouraged by tax considerations from purchasing more selective plans; as noted earlier, one type of cost-saving innovation that should be given an equal chance to compete for consumers' and providers' favor involves strategic departures from comprehensiveness in benefit design. For this reason, it seems to me to be desirable to strengthen economizing incentives even further than under the Ullman bill by allowing employees to receive tax-free at least some of any additional savings that they might gain by choosing a low-cost plan. The following paragraphs discuss a proposal to change the tax laws to increase employees' economic incentive to be cost conscious when buying health insurance coverage. The proposal is not offered as a definitive solution to the incentive problem, since many questions, particularly concerning its revenue input, remain to be answered. Nevertheless, the idea has some possible advantages that at least merit further study.

While many variations are possible and many technical issues would need to be resolved, the specific proposal is, first, to impose a maximum limit of $1800 a year (the "maximum total exclusion") on the annual allowable exclusion from taxable income and wages for employer- or employee-paid health insurance premiums; this compares roughly with the $1440-per-year exclusion proposed in the Ullman bill, though the exclusion would not be limited to employer-paid premiums, and the limit would apply for FICA as well as income tax purposes. The unique new feature of the proposal is an additional exclusion from federal income and social security taxation for up to $800 of the unused maximum total exclusion—that is, the excess of $1800 per year over the employee's annual health plan premium; the effect of this tax exclusion for cash income is to make the employee see the last $800 spent on premiums below the $1800 level as whole dollars, thus encouraging economizing behavior in that range. Another aspect of the proposal is the suggestion that employee eligibility for the second (cash) exclusion should be conditioned on the employer's contributing at least $600 per year toward an appropriate catastrophic insurance plan. This latter condition would deny the favorable tax treatment for cash income not invested in health insurance to employers and employees who failed to obtain at least basic protection.

The chief advantage of this proposal over most other proposals is that it extends the employee's incentive to economize over a wider range. Under the Ullman bill, an undiluted economizing incentive exists only over the proposed maximum exclusion of $1440 per year. Under the proposed alternative, the incentive extends upward from $1000, as the employee trades off untaxed dollars and insurance coverage up to $1800 and spends after-tax dollars on insurance above that amount. Another advantage is the reduction of adverse tax effects on employees with costlier plans. Under the Ullman bill, employer contributions over $1440 would become taxable whether paid in cash or in premiums, and this would appear simply as a tax increase to beneficiaries of plans with premiums over $1440. The proposed alternative does not solve this problem entirely but is an improvement. Under it, the maximum exclusion is raised, but by sheltering any savings in premiums from taxes, the desired incentive effect is increased. While the dollar amounts may be varied, the operative principle seems sound, and the changed consequences for taxpayers seem likely to improve the political feasibility of a tax change. The revenue effects of the cash exclusion are obviously important as a constraint on how far the idea can be carried.

Although the cash exclusion feature may seem peculiar, it is in fact a quite logical extension of the perception that employees should be free to receive tax-free any saving achieved by selecting a low-cost rather than a high-cost option. Once it is perceived that taking this approach in the tax law would simply induce employers to offer new high options with premiums equal to the maximum exclusion (in order to shelter as much income as possible), it becomes obvious that the employees should enjoy the rewards of spending less than the maximum amount whether or not the employer offers the high-option plan in fact. Clearly there should be no artificial stimulus to the offering of a high-cost plan just so most employees can reject it. Also, the automatic cash exclusion approach greatly simplifies both the administration of the tax law and the paying of taxes.

In discussing the exclusion-limiting approach adopted in the Ullman bill and others, it is important not to lose sight of another, somewhat simpler way to improve cost consciousness with respect to the marginal dollar of insurance premium. In many ways, the fundamentally soundest approach would be to replace the present open-ended exclusion with a limited credit against the employee's taxes. All employer- and employee-paid premiums up to the limit of the credit would then be subtracted directly from the employee's tax bill, and all additional premiums would be paid with after-tax dollars. One of the advantages of this approach would be to end the disproportionately favorable tax subsidy for individuals in higher brackets. Moreover, a system of limited tax credits would make it possible to allow progressively larger credits for lower-income taxpayers, and could easily provide refundable credits for those persons who had income taxes insufficient to absorb the credit. The availability of a new tax credit would prompt the purchase of basic insurance protection by those persons who are not now covered adequately, yet the fixed limit on the credit would mean that people would be spending their own after-tax money for additional coverage beyond a certain point. A possible strategy might be to allow the maximum credit (say, $600 for a family) to be claimed for either (1) 100 percent of premiums paid for plans providing only approved catastrophic coverage or (2) 50 percent of premiums paid under a comprehensive plan also providing catastrophic protection. The maximum and the latter percentage could be adjusted upward for lower-income people for whom the credit might also be made refundable and payable in advance so as to solve their cash-flow problem and serve as a health voucher.

Mandatory Insurance Benefits Because the design of insurance benefit packages is, for the most part, best left to the market, the conventional idea that a minimum benefit package must be prescribed by law should be opposed. One reason is that, as argued earlier, exclusions from coverage may be a useful and appropriate cost-containment technique even when some desirable care is left uncovered.[36] Not all people need the same protection against out-of-pocket expenditures; indeed, only the very poor need truly comprehensive benefits. Moreover, the screening that employers and unions provide in multiple-choice situations would be entirely sufficient as a protection for consumers against glaring deficiencies in coverage. Finally, multiple choice and the tax change would make the consumer's cost savings palpable and should make well-conceived exclusions easier to accept (and to enforce). Thus, it is extremely important that a health insurer's most valuable cost-containment tool (that is, his ability to adjust coverage) not be taken away.

There are many marginally valuable services that should not be covered by health insurance, and competing plans must be allowed to find their own way of identifying them and implementing the exclusions. The prevalent idea that benefits should be made comprehensive and that everything not "medically necessary" can then be excluded is a trap. It is based on the idea that there is "one right way" to diagnose and treat disease, and any approach based on this mistaken premise leaves the medical profession to develop standards that reflect its own values, perceptions, and economic interests. This professional dominance, resulting in a kind of informally centralized decision making, is precisely what the health services industry must get away from before cost considerations can be given appropriate weight in medical decision making. Thus, some kind of decentralized decision making by competing health plans that are ultimately accountable to consumers is crucial if the difficult trade-offs are to be successfully addressed. Even though many observers find it difficult to conceive why it is dangerous to proceed on the assumption that there is some objectively identifiable standard of need and practice, this view must be overcome and supplanted by the conception that allowing a variety of approaches to coexist in a competitive environment is the best way to achieve efficient results.

Catastrophic Coverage Despite the good reasons for not specifying a minimum level of benefits in private insurance and other financing plans, there may be a justification (based on "free-rider" notions) for compelling all plans to provide adequate catastrophic coverage. The risk in compelling such coverage is that, in prescribing its form, a regulatory requirement may preclude ways of covering those risks more cost effectively. The tendency in nearly all current federal proposals is to insulate consumers from all costs after some initial outlay. Because the incremental costs of almost any significant hospitalization would be covered, cost constraints would disappear altogether. More work is needed to discover how catastrophic risks might best be covered in the face of the severe moral hazard, and out of such work might come some better ideas about how a requirement for mandatory coverage might best be framed. Although my article with two colleagues exploring these complex matters was somewhat inconclusive,[37] I have no doubt that current proposals would carry with them a powerful necessity to regulate system capacity to contain the costs and ration the availability of catastrophic care. Because such regulation is unlikely to be effective, for reasons we closely examined, alternative approaches are badly needed. Congress has so far been oblivious to the immense problems that current proposals, despite their political appeal, present.

Mandatory Offerings Under Multiple Choice Various pending proposals would require that certain specific options be made available in multiple-choice situations. The HMO Act already does this, of course, and several other proposals, including the Ullman bill, would require that one of the mandatory choices provide for substantial copayments. I do not find these specifications to be a sound idea. The HMO Act's dual-choice requirement should be repealed in enacting the multiple-choice requirement and not replaced by any other preference for HMOs. Any HMO definition is too confining and unduly limits the offering of other promising alternative delivery systems. On the other hand, the effect of proposals to require the offering of a plan featuring substantial copayments would not be to force a desirable change on the system. Because there is currently no obstacle to the offering of such plans, it must be that they are not deemed desirable by consumers. In the absence of some reason to think the market is artificially restrained in catering to consumer preferences, no mandatory offering can be justified.

If legislation was thought to be necessary to prod possibly recalcitrant insurers, employers, and union leaders into offering meaningful new options, I would simply require that one of the three mandatory choices be a "cost-sensitive health plan," defined roughly as a carrier, HMO, service-benefit plan, or other health services pre-payment plan that either (1) substantially limits its enrollees' choice of provider, or (2) to the extent that it permits free choice, establishes either its premiums or its benefits in such a way (as defined in regulations) that the incremental cost of choosing a high-priced provider is borne by the enrollee making such choice.

A plan such as an HMO or health care alliance that in effect shops for providers' services on behalf of its enrollees comes under clause 1. (Significantly, IPA–HMOs offering a choice of virtually any physician in the community would not qualify.) Clause 2 would allow a plan either to set premiums based on the insured person's advance choice of provider or to pay fixed cash indemnities, perhaps based on the cheapest available rates, leaving patients to make up the difference; a plan with ordinary cost-sharing provisions would not, it will be noted, be sufficient. An important point is that a free-choice plan under clause 2 could avoid the need for charging a patient for the very large cost differential in a high-cost tertiary care facility by imposing controls on referrals to such institutions, thereby limiting enrollees' choice in accordance with clause 2. All of the insured would thus have financial protection against the possible need for such high-cost treatment.

There should be no question that some limits on choice and/or increased responsibility for incremental costs are desirable, not undesirable, features of private health insurance. The absence of such restrictions in existing plans results not so much from free consumer choice as from employer and union policies and providers' preferences enforced on carriers by actions that would now be regarded as antitrust violations. It might be highly desirable for federal law, in this subtle way, to push carriers and providers into the kinds of arrangements that a truly competitive market would have yielded long ago. Because the ultimate choices would still be made by consumers, a regulatory mistake in defining one of the three options could do little harm and would be quickly apparent.

Insurer-Sponsored Choices A possibly desirable development would be the offering of more than one choice of plan by a single insurer. A choice between a high and a low option is less important, however, than a choice between an open panel and a closed panel of providers.

A way of encouraging development along these lines would be to count an insurer twice for multiple-choice purposes if it offers both open- and closed-panel options which are independently priced.

Encouraging Choices for Public Program Beneficiaries Congress should embrace the notion of choice for beneficiaries of Medicare and Medicaid, or of some future public program. Recent proposals to allow Medicare beneficiaries to enroll in HMOs are encouraging, although I understand that difficult technical problems, particularly in guarding against adverse selection, are being confronted. Medicaid programs should be encouraged to allow choice, perhaps using "Project Health" in Oregon as a model. Protection against "second-class" care can take the form of limiting public beneficiaries to some percentage of a plan's total enrollment. The "on–off" eligibility problem with Medicaid clients also needs attention. Most important, the door should be left open for non–HMO health plans to participate in the "voucher" program.

Antimonopoly and Market-Strengthening Strategies Protection of the competitive process can be provided through antitrust enforcement, but federal and state legislation should also be reviewed for obstacles to needed change. State premium tax and other tax exemptions and state mandatory benefit laws require particular attention. Information strategies should also be considered, and consumer protection legislation and regulation should be re-examined to see whether it helps or hinders the competitive process.

Chapter 12 Notes

1. For a discussion of the 1979 health planning amendments, see Clark Havighurst and Glenn Hackbarth, "Competition and Health Care: Planning for Deregulation," *Regulation*, 4 (May/June 1980):39–48.

2. See Pub.L.No. 95-504 (1978), *codified* at scattered sections of 49 U.S.C.

3. Pub.L.No. 96-79,§§117(a) and 117(b)(3), *amending* §§1527(b) and 1531 of the Public Health Service Act, respectively.

4. For example: U.S., Congress, House Report 5740, § 1485, and § 1590, 96th Cong., 1st sess. 1979.

5. For example: U.S., Congress, House Report 4000, § 1530, 96th Cong., 1st sess. 1979.

6. For example: U.S., Congress, House Report 3943 and House Report 5740, § 1485, § 1590, 96th Cong., 1st sess. 1979.

7. See notes 4, 5, and 6.

8. Charles Schultze, *The Public Use of the Private Interest* (Washington, D.C.: Brookings Institution, 1979).

9. Ibid., p. 90.

10. U.S., Congress, Senate, *Congressional Record*, Feb. 6, 1980, 126:1102–116.

11. For example, the cost reimbursement feature of Medicare Part A is modeled after Blue Cross reimbursement.

12. For example: U.S., Federal Trade Commission, *Staff Report on Medical Participation in Control of Blue Shield and Certain Other Open-Panel Medical Prepayment Plans* (Washington, D.C.: 1979); Lawrence Goldberg and Warren Greenberg, "The Effect of Physician-Controlled Health Insurance, U.S. v. Oregon State Medical Society," *Journal of Health Politics, Policy and Law* 2 (Spring 1977):48–78; Clark Havighurst, "Professional Restraints on Innovation in Health Care Financing," *Duke Law Journal* (May 1978), pp. 303–87; Clark Havighurst, "Antitrust Enforcement in the Medical Services Industry: What Does It All Mean?" *Milbank Memorial Fund Quarterly* 58 (Winter 1980):89–124; Clark Havighurst and Philip Kissam, "The Antitrust Implications of Relative Value Studies in Medicine," *Journal of Health Politics, Policy and Law* 4 (Spring 1979):48–86.

13. Martin Feldstein and Bernard Friedman, "Tax Subsidies, the Rational Demand for Insurance and the Health Care Crisis," *Journal of Public Economics* 7 (April 1977):156. Since 1977, when Feldstein and Friedman wrote the cited article, inflation has been pushing taxpayers into higher income tax brackets and Congress has legislated increases in the Social Security tax rate and wage base. Thus, effective marginal tax rates—and hence the value of the tax exclusion for employer-paid premiums—has been increasing.

14. U.S., Congressional Budget Office, *Tax Subsidies for Medical Care* (Washington, D.C., 1980), p. 5.

15. Feldstein and Friedman, "Tax Subsidies," p. 174.

16. Clark Havighurst and Glenn Hackbarth, "Private Cost Containment," *New England Journal of Medicine* 300 (June 7, 1979):1305.

17. For Mr. Glasser's view, see "Republican Cure Would Aggravate the Malady, Labor Leader Testifies," *National Health Insurance Report*, Feb. 22, 1980, p. 2.

18. Havighurst and Hackbarth, "Private Cost Containment." See also Clark Havighurst, "Private Cost Containment—Medical Practice Under

Competition," in Glen Misek, ed., *Socioeconomic Issues of Health, 1979* (Chicago: American Medical Association), pp. 41–65.

19. Cf. Martin Feldstein, "The Welfare Loss of Excess Health Insurance," *Journal of Political Economy* 81 (March/April 1973):251–80.

20. See Clark Havighurst, "The Role of Competition in Cost Containment," in Warren Greenberg, ed., *Competition in the Health Care Sector* (Germantown, Md.: Aspen Systems, 1978), pp. 287–89.

21. See Havighurst, "Professional Restraints on Innovation in Health Care Financing," pp. 321–26; Clark Havighurst, "Health Insurers and Health-Care Costs: Can the Problem Be Part of the Solution?" *Health Communications and Informatics* 5 (nos. 5 and 6, 1979):320–31.

22. Michigan State Medical Society, Docket No. 9129 (FTC, filed July 27, 1979).

23. Indiana Federation of Dentists, Docket No. 9118 (FTC, April 1, 1980) (initial decision).

24. See U.S., Federal Trade Commission 1979. *Staff Report on Medical Participation.*

25. American Medical Association, Docket No. 9064 (FTC, Oct. 12, 1979).

26. For example, Group Life & Health Insurance Co. v. Royal Drug Co., 440 U.S. 205 (1979); Manasen v. California Dental Service, Civil No. 75-0329 (N.D. Calif., May 16, 1980).

27. Note, "The American Medical Association: Power, Purpose, and Politics in Organized Medicine," *Yale Law Journal* 63 (May 1954): 976–97.

28. Committee on the Costs of Medical Care, *Medical Care for the American People* (Chicago: University of Chicago Press, 1932).

29. Goldberg and Greenberg, "Effect of Physician-Controlled Health Insurance." Supra note 12.

30. See for example, Jon Christianson and Walter McClure, "Competition in the Delivery of Medical Care," *New England Journal of Medicine* 301 (October 11, 1979): 812–18; John Iglehart, "HMOs Are Alive and Well in the Twin Cities Region," *National Journal* 10 (July 22, 1978):1160–165.

31. See for example, Robert Froehlke, "Promising Approaches to Cost Containment: The Health Insurance View," *Bulletin of the New York Academy of Medicine* 56 (January/February, 1980):152–56; see also Havighurst, "Professional Restraints on Innovation in Health Care Financing," pp. 339–42.

32. The Safeco plan is described and assessed in Stephen Moore, "Cost Containment through Risk-Sharing by Primary-Care Physicians," *New England Journal of Medicine* 300 (June 14, 1979): 1359–362.

33. Mark Pauly, *The Role of the Private Sector in National Health In-*

surance (Washington, D.C.: Health Insurance Association of America, 1979), pp. 37–38.

34. U.S., Congress, Public Health Service Act § 1310, codified at 42 U.S.C. § 300 e-9.

35. See Alain Enthoven, "Consumer-Centered v. Job-Centered Health Insurance," *Harvard Business Review* 57 (January/February, 1979): 141–52.

36. See notes 19 and 20 and accompanying text.

37. Clark Havighurst, James Blumstein, and Randall Bovbjerg, "Strategies in Underwriting the Costs of Catastrophic Disease," *Law and Contemporary Problems* 40 (Autumn 1976): 122–95.

Reimbursement Policies:
Lessons from Medicare

*Patricia Munch-Danzon**

Introduction

One purpose of any national health insurance (NHI) program is to stimulate the use of health care beyond the level that would be chosen privately, in the absence of government intervention. An increase in utilization of health care can be achieved by several alternative policies that differ in the degree of government involvement and in their effects on private markets for health insurance and health services.

The policy tool that minimizes government intervention in private markets for health insurance and health services is a subsidy to the private purchase of health insurance and/or health care. The current tax treatment of health-related expenditures provides such a subsidy.[1] As a further step, the government may mandate that private insurance policies cover some minimum level of services. This is a major feature of the Carter administration's 1979 NHI proposal. An important aspect of both these approaches is that the provision of insurance and of health services remain in the private sector.

Alternatively, the government may preempt the private insurance market and engage directly in the provision of insurance for at least

*Hoover Institution and the Rand Corporation

some subset of the population. This approach is embodied in the Medicare and Medicaid programs established in 1965 and is retained by several of the NHI proposals currently under consideration. A significant expansion of government provision of insurance, modeled basically on the Medicare precedent, is a cornerstone of the administration's proposal.

Government provision of health insurance to a large section of the population makes government the largest single purchaser of health services, albeit indirectly and without control over the quantity of services purchased. Consequently, government reimbursement policies (i.e., the criteria used to determine how much to pay providers of services to beneficiaries of the government programs) have important distributive and allocative effects. Most obviously, reimbursement policies affect the out-of-pocket costs to beneficiaries of public programs and hence their demand for health services. Reimbursement policies also affect revenue to providers, and hence their willingness to serve beneficiaries. Reimbursement policies of public programs may also have important effects on prices charged and availability of services to private patients.

When Medicare was introduced in 1965, Medicare reimbursement policies were modeled closely after practices in the private sector. Reimbursement for ambulatory care (physicians' services, out-patient lab tests, etc.) retained the fee-for-service systems. Limits on the amount Medicare would pay for specific procedures were tied to prices charged by physicians to private patients. For in-patient services, Medicare reimburses hospitals for the share of costs attributable to Medicare patients, where the Medicare share is determined by reference to charges to private patients.[2]

In all years (except 1972–74) since the introduction of Medicare, the medical care component of the consumer price index (CPI) has increased more rapidly than other items.[3] It is beyond the scope of this paper to determine the marginal contribution of various factors to the rapid increase in health care prices, but the introduction of Medicare and Medicaid in 1965 has probably played an important role, both directly and indirectly. First, the subsidy to program beneficiaries stimulated an increase in aggregate demand for health services which, with less than perfectly elastic supply, was bound to increase prices. Second, the Medicare reimbursement policies created incentives to providers to increase their charges to private patients above the level that would have prevailed for the same demand if Medicare reimbursement had been totally independent of charges to private patients. Third, the increase in the price of health services, induced by the stimulus to demand and exacerbated by the reimbursement policies of Medicare, has been one factor contributing to the increase in private demand for health insurance.[4] The vicious circle is well known: insurance increases demand for health services and decreases elasticity of this demand, which tends to increase prices, which further stimulates demand for insurance, and so on.[5] The current demand for national health insurance to protect people from the rising cost of health care is the next phase of the spiral.

The purpose of this paper is to examine the lessons for any future NHI policy that can be learned from experience with the reimbursement policies adopted under Medicare. Both the distributive effects (charges and availability of services to different patient groups) and the allocative effects (the mix of services used to produce health care) are discussed. To set the following discussions in the context of the current policy debate, the first section of the paper outlines the major features of the Carter administration's NHI proposal. The second section analyzes Medicare reimbursement for ambulatory services, first under the original system (which tied Medicare reimbursement to charges to private patients) and then under the system with exogenous fee controls that has been in effect for most of the 1970s. Problems of reimbursement for ancillary services such as lab tests are explicitly considered in the third section. Section four briefly discusses hospital services. Section five provides conclusions and relates them to the administration's proposal.

The Carter Administration's National Health Plan (NHP)[6]

The stated goals of NHP are five:

1. Assure all Americans of comprehensive coverage, including protection against the costs of major illnesses
2. Eliminate those aspects of the current health system that often cause the poor to receive substandard care

3. Reduce inflation in the health care industry
4. Be financed through multiple sources
5. Include a significant role for the private insurance industry

There are two major institutional features of the Phase 1 bill: (1) an expanded federal insurance program (Healthcare) and (2) the mandated employer coverage.

Healthcare

Covered population The federal insurance program, Healthcare, consolidates existing Medicare and Medicaid programs, which currently cover 24 million and 15.7 million persons, respectively. Coverage is extended to an additional 10.5 million poor persons and an estimated 11 million "near poor" persons, who "spend-down" to the eligibility level (55 percent of the official poverty level) on account of large medical expenses. An additional nine million unemployed or part-time workers, who would not automatically be insured under Healthcare or through mandated employer coverage, would be able to purchase Healthcare coverage at a national, community-rated premium.

Cost sharing For the aged and disabled, there is an annual deductible of $160 on in-patient care and a $60 deductible plus 20 percent coinsurance on nonhospital services.[7] Out-of-pocket costs are limited to $1,250 per individual. Persons eligible because they are entitled to cash assistance (Medicaid) and those additional 10.5 million persons who meet the low-income standard face no cost sharing. Those who spend-down face no cost sharing after they spend-down below the low-income standard. Individuals or employer groups who buy into Healthcare face a limit on out-of-pocket expense of $2,500 per family per year. Prenatal care, delivery care, and infant care in the first year of life are exempt from all cost sharing.

Benefits The Healthcare benefit package is more comprehensive than Medicare and more comprehensive than the current Medicaid program in roughly half the states. It includes:

1. Inpatient hospital services (unlimited)

2. Physician and other ambulatory services (unlimited), including lab but excluding dental and psychiatric care
3. Skilled nursing services (100 days per year)
4. Home health visits (100 visits per year)
5. Mental health (20 days of inpatient hospital care and $1,000 of ambulatory service)
6. Preventive care (complete prenatal, delivery, and infant care and a schedule of preventive services for all children up to age 18)

Reimbursement Reimbursement for physician and other ambulatory services provided to Healthcare patients is on the basis of a fee schedule. Initially, the fee schedule will be based on average Medicare payment levels. Subsequent alterations will be determined through negotiation between Healthcare and physician representatives. Physicians are required to accept the Healthcare fee as payment in full (i.e., patients cannot be billed for any additional amount).

The original proposal was to limit reimbursement for hospital services for both Healthcare and private patients by ceilings on the rate of increase of hospital expenditure. The hospital cost-containment proposal is not addressed in this paper.

Mandated Employer Coverage

Covered population All employers are required to provide full-time workers (persons who have worked at least 25 hours per week for ten consecutive weeks) and their families with a health insurance plan that meets federal standards. Coverage may be purchased from private insurance companies or be provided by self-insurance. Coverage must continue at least 90 days after termination of employment. Coverage cannot be limited due to preexisting conditions. Employees and/or their dependents must be given the right to continue to buy a comparable individual plan from the insurance company after termination of employment, regardless of their health risk.

Cost sharing Plans may include any configuration of deductible and coinsurance, subject to a limit on out-of-pocket liability of $2,500 per family per year. Prenatal, delivery, and infant care are exempt from all cost sharing.

Benefits Certified plans must provide at least the Healthcare benefit package, but they may be more comprehensive.

Financing Employers must pay at least 75 percent of the premium cost. No employer is required to spend more than 5 percent of payroll on a mandated plan. Subsidies for costs in excess of 5 percent are available either by purchasing coverage from Healthcare at a premium rate equal to 5 percent of payroll, or by applying for an equivalent subsidy to purchase coverage from private insurance firms. It is estimated that firms employing approximately seven million workers (out of a workforce of 73 million full-time workers) might take advantage of one of the two subsidy options.

Reimbursement Reimbursement of physician services by private plans is not regulated. Instead, NHP attempts to stimulate competition among providers by requiring that plans furnish enrollees with lists of physicians who agree to accept the plan's reimbursement as payment in full and by providing incentives to expand prepaid practice systems.

Summary

This proposal is likely to stimulate the demand for health services from several sources. The number of persons with fully subsidized coverage is more than doubled. Covered services are expanded and cost sharing reduced for Medicare beneficiaries and for the majority of persons with private coverage, since the current private benefit package is typically less comprehensive, both in terms of services covered and depth of coverage, than the mandated minimum. Moreover, NHP increases the federal subsidy to the private purchase of insurance.

In view of the certain increase in demand and the reduced patient sensitivity to price, equilibrium price levels must rise unless there is an offsetting increase in supply. This is not part of NHP. On the contrary, it is proposed to "revise federal health manpower policy to prevent a potentially costly physician surplus" and to limit capital expenditure by hospitals. Thus reimbursement policies will play a crucial role in rationing excess demand among competing users and in controlling the increase in health costs. The Medicare experience with similar reimbursement policies is examined in the discussion that follows.

Medicare Reimbursement for Physician Services

The Basic Medicare Formula

Medicare reimbursement policies for physician and other ambulatory services were grafted onto existing practices in the private sector. Basically, the physician bills patients on a fee-for-service basis and sets his own fees or charges. However, the amount Medicare will pay for any procedure is limited by a series of "fee screens" which are based on charges to private patients by the billing physician and other physicians in the locality. Specifically, the physician's "reasonable," or maximum, allowed charge is the lesser of (1) his actual charge, (2) his customary charge, defined as his median charge to all patients during the calendar year preceding the current fiscal year, and (3) the prevailing charge, defined as the 75th percentile of the customary charges, weighted by the number of services, of all physicians in his specialty in his geographic area. Thus the allowed charge is physician-specific, but applies uniformly to all Medicare patients served by the physician. Since Medicare has a 20 percent coinsurance rate for ambulatory services, the program pays 80 percent of the physician's allowed charge (after a deductible of $60 per calendar year).

The physician retains some flexibility to set different prices to different Medicare patients through use of the "assignment" option. If the physician chooses to assign a claim, he bills Medicare directly and accepts the Medicare-allowed charge as payment in full (except for the patient's 20 percent coinsurance, which is billed directly to the patient). Alternatively, if he chooses not to assign the claim, he bills the patient directly without constraint on amount. However, the patient's reimbursement from Medicare is limited to 80 percent of the physician's allowed charge. Thus the Medicare allowed charge is a ceiling on the physician's reimbursement on assigned claims. On unassigned claims, the allowed charge is a ceiling on reimbursement to the patient. Since the patient bears 100 percent of any increment, demand is expected to be much more elastic in the range above the allowed charge.[8] This limits the physician's profit-maximizing fee on unassigned claims. As a first approximation, the allowed charge therefore sets a ceiling on a physician's reimbursement from all Medicare patients. This ceiling on Medicare reimbursement is determined by charges to private patients, because the customary and prevailing fees screens are defined in terms of the median of the distribution of charges to all patients.[9]

Effects on Private Patients

Standard economic theory implies that tying Medicare fee ceilings onto charges to private patients will raise charges to private patients under certain plausible assumptions. The situation is analogous to constraining a monopolist to charge a uniform price to all customers, with an additional time dimension. To illustrate the potential inflationary effect of the Medicare reimbursement formula on charges to private patients, consider a physician who provides a single, uniform service to two homogeneous groups of patients, private (N) and public (M). The service is provided at constant cost per unit, w. If the prices charged to each market are totally independent, the standard theory of price discrimination applies. Charges to public patients will be greater (less) than charges to private patients if demand of public patients is less (more) elastic than demand of private patients:

$$\hat{P}_m \gtreqless \hat{P}_n \text{ as } |\varepsilon_m| \lesseqgtr |\varepsilon_n|$$

where $\hat{P}$ = profit maximizing price and ε = elasticity of quantity demanded with respect to price.

In fact, the Medicare reimbursement formula links the two markets by the requirement that allowed charges to public patients cannot exceed charges to private patients, in some prior period. If the constraint is not binding (i.e., $\hat{P}_n > \hat{P}_m$) the linkage has no effect. In the more likely case (where $\hat{P}_m > \hat{P}_n$) the linkage raises charges to private patients.[10] For simplicity, assume that only private patients are served in the first period, at a cost of w_1, and only public patients are served in the second period, at a cost of w_2 per unit. The physician's net revenue function can be written:

$$\Pi = P_{n+m}(M+N) - w_1N - w_2M \tag{1}$$

where P_{n+m} is the charge to both M and N, now constrained to be equal.[11]

$$\frac{\partial \Pi}{\partial P_{n+m}} = M + N + P_{n+m}\left(\frac{\partial N}{\partial P} + \frac{\partial M}{\partial P}\right)$$

$$- w_1 \frac{\partial N}{\partial P} - w_2 \frac{\partial M}{\partial P} = 0 \qquad (2)$$

or

$$\hat{P}_{n+m} = \frac{w_1 \varepsilon_{n+m} + (w_2 - w_1)\varepsilon_m s_m}{\varepsilon_{n+m} + 1} \qquad (2)'$$

where $s_m = \dfrac{M}{M + N}$

$\varepsilon_{n+m} = \varepsilon_n s_n + \varepsilon_m s_m.$

With independent markets, the charge to private patients is

$$\hat{P}_N = \frac{w_1 \varepsilon_n}{\varepsilon_n + 1}$$

which is less than

$$\hat{P}_{N+M} \text{ if } |\varepsilon_N| > |\varepsilon_M| \text{ and } w_1 < w_2.$$

Thus the Medicare reimbursement formula tends to raise private charges. The upward pressure is greater:

1. The more inelastic is public demand relative to private demand
2. The greater the expected rate of inflation of costs
3. The larger the fraction of services provided to the public market, s_M (as long as $s_M < .5$)

There are several important modifications to this general conclusion that tying Medicare reimbursement to charges to private patients has contributed to the inflation of the latter. First, since Medicare allowable charges are constrained to the median of actual charges, private charges are unaffected if over 50 percent of a physician's services are to Medicare patients. Second, even where over 50 percent of charges are to private patients, in principal only the median charge is affected. However, if the physician cannot predict with certainty the distribution of demand for his services during the year, then there is an incentive to increase all charges in the lower half of the distribution of unconstrained optimum charges. In other words, the inflationary impact falls most heavily on those private patients who would otherwise be charged relatively low charges. These are patients whose demand is relatively elastic, presumably because of little insurance coverage or low income. Thus the average rate of increase of physician fees induced by Medicare probably understates the actual increase that has been experienced by those least able to afford it.[12]

A further regressive aspect of the Medicare formula is that the inflationary effect is confined to physicians who expect their customary charge to be below the 75th percentile of customaries in the locality (the prevailing charge). For physicians in the upper quartile of the distribution, the binding constraint on their reimbursement from Medicare is the prevailing charge, not their own customary charge, so they have no incentive to raise charges to their private patients.[13]

Assignment: Exploitation or "Progressive" Price Discrimination?

The assignment option gives the physician some freedom to price-discriminate among patients. If the physician assigns a claim, he bills Medicare directly and accepts the allowed charge as payment in full. The patient pays 20 percent of the allowed charge. If the physician does not assign the claim, he can bill the patient without constraint. The patient pays 20 percent of the allowed charge plus 100 percent of any excess of the actual over the allowed charges. The patient then bills Medicare and is reimbursed 80 percent of the physician's allowed charge. The profit-maximizing physician will accept assignment only if the increment in fee (over the allowed charge) that can be obtained from the patient exceeds the incremental cost of billing the patient rather than Medicare:[14]

$$\hat{P}^i_m - \bar{P} - (k^i - \bar{k}) \geq 0.$$

where $\hat{P}^i_m$ = optimum charge to the ith patient, discounted for the risk of noncollection;

$\bar{P}_m$ = Medicare allowed charge;

k^i = cost of collecting from the patient; and

$\bar{k}$ = cost of collecting from Medicare.

Assignment is therefore more likely:

1. The more elastic the individual patient's demand
2. The higher the Medicare-allowed charge relative to the optimum charge to that patient
3. The lower the cost of collecting from Medicare, relative to billing the patient

Several studies have confirmed this theoretical prediction that charges on unassigned claims exceed charges on assigned claims.[15] It is erroneous, however, to attribute the lower charges on assigned claims to the assignment process per se. In the absence of assignment, profit-maximizing charges to these patients would be lower than charges to patients the physician opts not to assign: that is precisely why the physician selects assignment for some patients but not for others.

The advantage of the assignment option is the advantage of price discrimination in general: prices are higher to those patients most able (willing) to pay, and therefore prices are lower to those least able (willing) to pay. The above analysis of the distributive effects of constraining reimbursement for Medicare patients (who have relatively inelastic demand) to charges to private patients (who have relatively elastic demand) applies equally among public patients if assignment is made mandatory, as in the administration's proposal.

In conclusion, if reimbursement for beneficiaries of a publicly funded insurance program is uniform across patients and is determined by reference to physicians' charges to private patients, charges to private patients will be higher than they would be in the absence of the link with the public program.[16] Among both public and private patients, the incidence will be regressive; i.e., inflation of charges will be greatest for those who would face the lowest charges if physicians were free to discriminate through separate charges to private patients, public assigned patients, and public nonassigned patients.

The Medicare Formula with Exogenous Fee Controls

In 1971 the formula for determining Medicare-allowed charges (lesser of actual, customary, or prevailing) was modified by exogenous controls on the annual rate of increase of allowed charges. As part of the Economic Stabilization Plan (ESP) introduced in August 1971, the increase in allowed charges was limited to 2.5 percent per year. This placed binding constraints on physician fees from July 1972 through 1974.[17] Controls were lifted in 1975. Since 1976, increases in Medicare-prevailing charges have been limited to increases in an index of expenses and wages, the Economic Index.

An absolute ceiling on the rate of increase of Medicare-allowed charges breaks the link between Medicare and private charges, once profit-maximizing charges to private patients exceed the Medicare charge ceiling. Over time, private charges will rise increasingly above Medicare-allowed charges but will nevertheless be lower than they would have been under the basic Medicare formula, without an exogenous constraint on Medicare charges.[18]

Exogenous fee controls also affect assignment rates, charges, out-of-pocket costs to patients, and utilization by Medicare patients. Three groups of Medicare patients must be distinguished. To isolate effects, first consider each group separately, assuming a perfectly elastic supply of physician services.

The first group of patients is those whose claims are assigned (before and after the imposition of controls) and who face lower charges and lower out-of-pocket costs, since their out-of-pocket cost is limited to at most 20 percent of the (lower) allowed charge. Their demand for services is expected to be higher than it would have been in the absence of controls. This is illustrated in figure 13.1.[19] The solid demand schedule is drawn on the assumption of 20 percent coinsurance of all charges and no ceiling on the allowed charge. If the allowed charge is constrained to some price, $\bar{P}_1$, and the physician accepts assignment, the effective marginal revenue curve is horizontal at this ceiling price until it joins the demand curve, at which point it drops down to the original MR curve. If the ceiling price is lowered to $\bar{P}_2$, the out-of-pocket cost to assigned patients falls and utilization of services increases to Q_2.

The second group of patients is those who are unassigned, before and after the controls. The effect of controls on charges and utiliza-

FIGURE 13.1

Assigned claims

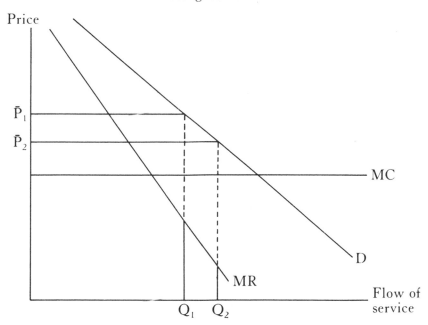

tion in this market is illustrated in figure 13.2. The solid demand schedule is drawn on the assumption of a constant 20 percent coinsurance rate and no ceiling on allowed charges. If Medicare reimbursement is limited to $\bar{P}_1$, the demand schedule becomes kinked at this point (the dashed line) because the patient's marginal coinsurance rate is 100 percent for all higher charges.[20] The profit-maximizing charge, $\hat{P}_1$, is slightly above the allowed charge. A decrease in the allowed charge lowers the kink, lowers the entire demand schedule at all prices above the kink, and shifts the intersection of the marginal revenue and marginal cost schedules to the left. Thus a reduction in allowed charge levels, as enforced under ESP, is expected to reduce utilization in the nonassigned market below the level that would have prevailed in the absence of controls.[21] This implies that out-of-pocket cost per unit of service must increase. In other words, the larger patient share of a lower actual charge results in a larger out-of-pocket cost to the patient.[22]

The third group of patients is those who were assigned but for

FIGURE 13.2
Nonassigned claims

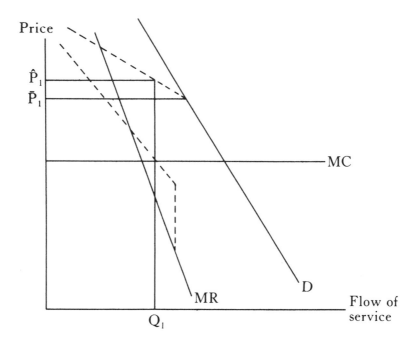

whom nonassignment becomes the more profitable option as a result of the decrease in allowed charges. Out-of-pocket costs must increase and utilization decrease for this group, relative to the situation with a higher allowed charge.

Thus a reduction in Medicare-allowed charges is expected to reduce out-of-pocket costs to assigned patients and increase their utilization, but increase out-of-pocket costs to unassigned patients and decrease their utilization. There will be some decrease in the fraction of patients assigned. The net effect on utilization by the Medicare population as a whole depends on whether the increase by those on assignment outweighs the decrease for the (increased) fraction of patients who are unassigned.

These conclusions depend critically on the assumption of a perfectly elastic supply of services for each subgroup of patients. More realistically, each physician's marginal cost schedule is upward sloping. His aggregate marginal revenue is the summation of the marginal revenue from the different subgroups: private, Medicare unassigned, Medicare assigned, and Medicaid. Medicare fee controls have been shown to reduce marginal revenue from the Medicare assigned and non-assigned markets. This may result in the curtailment of supply to the least profitable markets. This is illustrated in figure 13.3.

For simplicity consider one private market with demand D_n and one public market with an absolute fee ceiling, such as the Medicare assigned market or Medicaid. Demand from this market is assumed to be infinitely elastic in the relevant range. The aggregate marginal revenue schedule is therefore MR_n at prices above the Medicare fee ceiling and becomes horizontal at the fee ceiling. When the Medicare-allowed charge is set at $\bar{P}_1$, Q_1^n services are supplied to the private market and

FIGURE 13.3
Allocation of supply between public and private markets

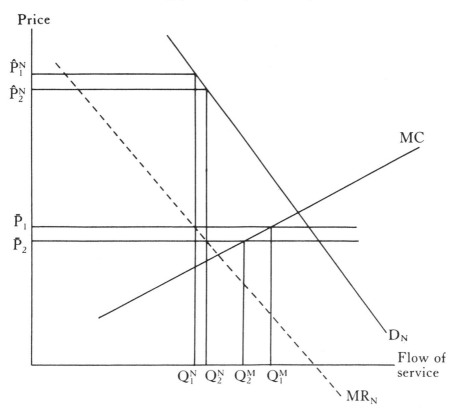

$Q_1^m - Q_1^n$ to the Medicare assigned market. When the Medicare-allowed charge is reduced to $\bar{P}_2$, output to the private market increases to Q_2^n but output to the Medicare market is curtailed to $Q_2^m - Q_2^n$. Since demand from in-Medicare market is expected to have increased (due to a reduction in out-of-pocket cost) some increase in nonprice rationing is necessary. This may take the form of physician refusal to take Medicare patients, longer waiting times for appointments, etc.

This theoretical analysis of the effects of exogenous controls on Medicare reimbursement levels (relative to the basic formula limiting Medicare reimbursement to private charge levels) concludes that utilization of services by private patients will increase and utilization by Medicare patients may increase or decrease. An increase in Medicare utilization is more likely, as the fraction of patients on assignment becomes larger and as the supply of physician services becomes more elastic.

This conclusion, that price controls may increase utilization, differs from that of Phelps (1976), Leffler and Lindsay (1976), and others, due to different assumptions about competition in the market for physician services. Imposition of fee controls in a competitive market unambiguously decreases the quantity of services supplied. A necessary condition for controls to induce an increase in supply is that the individual physician face a downward sloping demand.[23] If each physician is not a pure price taker, an increase in services under fee controls is entirely consistent with standard economic theory, with exogenously determined demand. It does not presuppose, as some have argued, that physicians are able to and do shift demand in order to maintain some target income.

Unfortunately, data necessary to test these predictions on the effect of Medicare fee controls are not available. Limited evidence on the effect of the ESP fee ceilings on charges and services to Medicare patients is presented in table 13.1, based on data reported in Holahan and Scanlon (1979). The data base consists of all claims paid by Medicare to a cohort of 1,261 northern California solo practitioners over a three-month period (April to June) for each of the years 1972 to 1975.[24] Controls on allowed charges became binding in July 1972, were in effect through 1974, and were removed by 1975. For each claim, the data include the actual charge, the allowed charge, and the procedure codes, (from the California Relative Value Scale [RVS]).[25] In computing average price changes in table 1, the unit of output is an

Table 13.1

Increases in physician prices and output under the economic stabilization program: California Medicare program[a]

	General Practice			General Surgery			Internal Medicine		
	1973	1974	1975	1973	1974	1975	1973	1974	1975
Allowed charge per RVS unit	1.1	0.9	7.3	0.7	1.7	5.3	1.4	2.3	6.0
Actual charge per RVS unit	2.6	6.0	11.3	3.0	5.9	10.6	0.8	8.2	9.8
RVS units per service	3.0	1.0	5.1	5.1	0.4	3.9	−0.3	3.2	2.4
Number of procedures	9.4	8.4	−7.8	10.9	9.5	1.3	8.7	14.6	2.5
Gross revenue[b]	11.9	12.4	3.6	10.1	15.6	9.1	12.9	19.3	12.3

a. Computed from data reported in Holahan and Scanlon (1979). Entries are percentage changes over the previous year, for all procedures.

b. These estimates are based on allowed charges and therefore understate actual revenue.

RVS unit, which provides a convenient basis for aggregating heterogeneous medical procedures.

The effects of price controls cannot be measured accurately without knowledge of what would have happened without controls, which is unobservable. However, the data in table 1 strongly suggest that controls slowed the rate of increase of charges temporarily. The rate of increase of allowed charges fell well within the ESP target of 2.5 percent per year during the control years but accelerated when controls were removed in 1975. Actual charges rose 3 percent or less during 1973 but accelerated to at least 6 percent in 1974.[26] The number of RVS units per service increased erratically over the period, but at least as much in the decontrolled year as under the controls. Thus there is no basis for concluding that the increased intensity was a response induced by the controls.[27]

The fourth row in table 13.1 shows that there was an increase in the total number of procedures provided to Medicare patients of between 8 percent and 11 percent in each year of the controls, with a strong reversal of that trend when controls were removed. For general practitioners, the number of procedures actually fell in 1975 and the largest increase was 2.5 percent for internists.[28] Thus fee controls appear to have increased the number of procedures per enrollee, on average. As a result, physician revenues and total program costs increased at least 10 percent per year, although allowed charges were held within the target range of 2.5 percent.[29]

Although we cannot prove that demand inducement did not occur, it is not necessarily implied by the increase in the number of services under price controls, as inferred by Holahon and Scanlon. As noted earlier, an increase in services is theoretically consistent with a movement along a well-defined demand schedule, as patients respond to lower prices. Unfortunately, we cannot test whether the observed increase is consistent with a reasonable elasticity of demand without information on prices actually faced by patients. The average out-of-pocket cost to patients is not known.[30]

Input Distortions: The Physician
as a Multiproduct Firm

The analysis so far has considered the effect of reimbursement policies on different patient groups, assuming that the physician produces a single service of a fixed quality. The only dimension of choice was price (or quantity) of service to different types of patients. In fact, the physician produces health care by combining a mix of inputs or services. These inputs include lab tests and X rays and a range of procedures involving different amounts of physician time. With the fee-for-service reimbursement system, the physician bills and is reimbursed for each individual procedure.[31] There is a maximum Medicare-allowed charge for each of these procedures. If allowed charges result in different levels of profit for different procedures, the physician's choice of inputs may be distorted. Thus the amount of physician time and other inputs per visit are dimensions of service the physician may adjust in response to fee controls.

In order to include these other dimensions in the analysis of physician response to fee controls, consider a simple model in which the demand for physicians' services depends explicitly on two inputs, time per visit and tests per visit, as well as on prices charged for both time and tests. Patients' basic demand is for health care, K, which is produced with inputs of physician time and tests. The total amount of care consumed by the ith patient is the product of the number of visits, n_i, and the average amount of care per visit, S, which is a positive function of hours per visit, H, and tests per visit, T:

$$K_i = n_i S(H,T)$$
$$S_h, S_t > 0; S_{hh}, S_{tt} < 0.$$

For convenience, we refer to the average amount of care per visit, S, as the quality of a visit. Strictly, S is the expected average quality of a visit as perceived by the patient, which may diverge from true quality due to imperfect information.[32]

The physician faces a demand for visits which is a function of the price and quality of the visit.[33] The composite price of a visit, p^n, has two components: the fee for physician time or office visit fee, P^v, and the fee for tests, $P^t T$. One purpose of this model is to determine the effects of a fee-for-service system in which reimbursement for physician time is not strictly proportional to the amount of time spent, whereas reimbursement for tests is strictly proportional to the number ordered.[34] To determine qualitative effects we make the extreme simplifying assumption that the charge and reimbursement for an office visit, P^v, is independent of the amount of time spent. Thus:

$$P^n = P^v + P^tT$$

We make the further simplifying assumption that demand depends only on the composite price, P^n, and is insensitive to the division of the total price between the office visit and lab test components. Thus the physician's demand function for visits, N, may be written as follows:

$$N = N(S, P^v, P^tT) = N(H, T, P^v, P^t)$$
$$N_{p^v}, N_{p^t} < 0; N_S \gtrless 0$$
$$N_h = N_S S_h = N_h^S \gtrless 0$$
$$N_t = N_S S_t + N_{pn} P^t = N_t^S + N_{pn} P^t \lessgtr 0$$

Demand is negatively related to price. The derivation of quantity of visits demanded with respect to quality per visit, N_S, is uncertain a priori. An increase in quality, holding price per visit constant, is equivalent to a reduction in the price per unit of care. Total quantity of care, and hence the number of visits demanded by existing patients, will only increase if the demand for care is elastic. However, even if demand of existing patients is inelastic, the demand facing the physician may be elastic ($N_S > Q$) due to the attraction of new patients to the practice.

The physician produces visits with two inputs (physician time and tests), which are supplied at constant cost, w and c, respectively.[35] Thus the composite cost of a visit, C^n, includes the physician time and test costs:

$$C^n = wH + cT \tag{1}$$

Given these demand and input supply conditions, the physician is assumed to maximize profit with respect to hours per visit, tests per visit, price per visit, and price per test:

$$\text{Max } \Pi = NP^n - NC^n$$
$$H,T,P^vP^t$$
$$= N[P^v + P^tT] - N[wH + cT] \tag{2}$$

Maximization of equation (2) subject to equation (1) yields the first order conditions:

$$\frac{\partial \Pi}{\partial H} = (P^n - C^n)N_h - Nw = 0 \tag{3}$$

$$\frac{\partial \Pi}{\partial T} = (P^n - C^n)N_t - N(P^t - c) = 0 \tag{4}$$

$$\frac{\partial \Pi}{\partial P^v} = N + (P^n - C^n)N_{pn} = 0 \tag{5}$$

$$\frac{\partial \Pi}{\partial P^t} = NT + (P^n - C^n)N_{Pn}T = 0. \tag{6}$$

Equation (3) implies that the marginal cost of increasing time per visit, Nw, is equated to the marginal revenue derived from an increase in quantity of visits demanded, due to the increase in quality. If $(P^n - C^n) > 0$, this implies that $N_h > 0$ and hence that $N_S > 0$. Equation (4), which is the analogous condition for tests, reveals two important differences between time and tests. First, in contrast to time, where an increase in time per visit does not directly increase revenue per visit, the direct net revenue effect in the case of tests is positive, as long as $(P^t - c) > 0$. Tests will therefore be increased until this direct positive effect on revenue is offset by a negative indirect effect as the increase in tests per visit raises the price of a visit and hence reduces quantity of visits demanded. Rewriting equation (4):

$$(P^n - C^n)(N_S S_t + N_{Pn}P^t) = N(c - P^t) \tag{4$'$}$$

Assuming $(P^n - C^n) > 0$ and $(P^t - c) > 0$, equilibrium requires $N^t < 0$. This requires that the positive demand shift effect, $N_S S_t$, be offset by the negative price effect, $N_{pn}P^t$. Thus if tests have a large positive demand shift effect (because they reveal problems hitherto undetected or permit treatment of conditions which might otherwise have gone untreated because undiagnosed) and if demand is inelastic with respect to price, the optimum frequency of tests may be very high. This is obviously one reason why screening tests are not covered by many private insurance plans.

Rearranging equations (3) and (4) illustrates the distortion in input mix induced by the payment mechanism which reimburses for tests in proportion to number of tests but reimburses for visits without regard to the amount of time per visit.

$$\frac{w}{c - P^t} = \frac{N_h}{N_t} = \frac{N_S S_h}{N_S S_t + N_{pn} P^t} \tag{7}$$

The efficient first order conditions would equate marginal input costs to marginal products in terms of quality of care:

$$\frac{w}{c} = \frac{S_h}{S_t}$$

Relative to this efficient input mix, equation (7) implies an excessive substitution of tests for time.[36]

Equations (5) and (6) both reduce to the equality of marginal cost and marginal revenue:

$$C^n = P^n(1 + \varepsilon^{-1}_{NPn}) \tag{(5)' = (6)'}$$

Thus if the patient is concerned only with the total price of the visit, there is a single decision as to the optimum composite price, P^n; maximization with respect to one component, say P^v, implies an optimum value of P^t, given T.[37]

Consider now the effect of fee ceilings. For simplicity assume that the insurer's ceiling on allowed charges is an absolute ceiling and that the physician cannot bill the patient for any additional amount.[38] If a constraint is imposed on fees for both office visits and tests, the composite price of a visit falls and the number of visits demanded increases (assuming no change in the number of tests per visit). This conclusion follows from the assumption that each physician faces a negatively sloped demand for his services, as discussed above. Thus the total number of procedures performed is expected to increase.

Fee ceilings may also change the amount of time and tests per visit, but the effects are uncertain a priori.[39] The ambiguity arises because the increase in number of visits induced by the lower composite price per visit increases the total consumption of tests and time, and hence reduces the demand-stimulating effect of time and tests per visit. It can be shown, however, that a ceiling on office visit fees is likely to reduce physician's time and increase tests per visit. This is more likely, the more price-elastic the demand for visits is and the less rapidly the marginal value of tests diminishes. If fixed patient-time costs per visit and a rising marginal cost of physician time are also introduced into the model, the likelihood increases that ceilings on allowed charges will induce increased frequency of tests per visit, rather than increased number of visits. Thus the increase in "intensity" (RVS units per claim) observed in the California Medicare data (table 13.1), is a theoretically plausible response to price controls (in the context of a reasonable model of the physician as a multiproduct firm facing an exogenously determined demand for its services). It does not imply induced demand or fraudulent billing.[40]

Inpatient Hospital Services

Inpatient hospital services are covered under Part A of Medicare. Providers are reimbursed for Medicare's share of "reasonable" costs. Medicare's share of costs is calculated by computing the ratio of hypothetical charges to Medicare patients to total charges, and applying this ratio to total cost for each revenue-producing department.[41] "Charges" are prices charged to private patients.[42] This formula is referred to as the ratio-of-charges-applied-to-costs (RCCAC). Costs of the non-revenue-producing departments are allocated to the revenue-producing departments. Thus total costs of each revenue-producing department include its direct costs (labor, supplies, depreciation) plus some fraction of the overhead costs of the non-revenue-producing departments.[43]

Thus Medicare's share of costs for the jth department is:

$$\text{Medicare Reimbursement} = \frac{\sum_{i \in j} p_i q_i^m}{\sum_{i \in j} p_i Q_i} \times \left(\sum_{i \in j} c_i Q_i + \alpha_j Z \right)$$

where P_i = charge for the ith service in department j

q_i^m = amount of ith service due to Medicare patients

Q_i = total amount of ith service

c_i = average direct cost of ith service

Z = total hospital overhead cost (non-revenue producing departments)

α_j = fraction of overhead allocated to department j.

If the department only produces a single service, Medicare's share is simply the fraction of that service provided to Medicare patients. If the department produces many services, Medicare's share is a weighted average of all services, where services are weighted by their respective charges.[44]

There are three potential limits on costs reimbursable by Medicare. First, certain costs are disallowed. These include bad debts to non–Medicare patients, luxury accommodations, gift shop, etc.; depreciation is calculated as straight-line depreciation at historic cost. Second, there is a ceiling on the per diem cost for day services, gross of the 8½ percent nursing cost differential but excluding the cost of intensive care units. Third, since 1974, Medicare pays the lesser of costs and charges (i.e., total reimbursable costs, aggregated over all departments, cannot exceed the charges that would be attributable to Medicare, if Medicare paid charges). This charge limit is computed by multiplying all services provided to Medicare patients by their respective charges to obtain a hypothetical charge bill to Medicare. This total is then multiplied by the fraction of charges to charge-paying patients that is actually collected. The hospital is then reimbursed the lesser of (1) this fraction of hypothetical charges and (2) Medicare's share of costs, obtained by the RCCAC method summed over all departments and subject to the per diem limit on day service.

Elsewhere (Danzon 1980b), I have developed a theoretical and empirical analysis of the effect of this system of cost-based reimbursement on the level of costs and charges. The basic thesis is that accounting "costs" reported for reimbursement purposes should not be interpreted as economic costs but rather as the price charged to cost-paying patients. A hospital that serves both cost- and charge-paying patients is effectively able to utilize two price schedules. If "costs" are viewed as simply the prices charged to cost-paying patients, an accounting profit ratio (ratio of total charges to total costs) is not a measure of economic profit but of the relative prices charged to these two groups of patients.

It can be shown that if the hospital's objective is to maximize net revenue, the basic Medicare cost reimbursement formula, ceilings on per diem costs, and the constraint that Medicare pays the lesser of costs or charges all imply that profit maximizing charges to charge-paying patients will be higher than the simple profit-maximizing level.

The logic is simply that in raising charges, there is some increase in revenue from Medicare that offsets the loss in revenue from private patients. Furthermore, since Medicare reimbursement is limited by the charges to private patients actually collected, the Medicare formula increases the cost to hospitals of providing charity care. This result is analogous to that found in the ambulatory sector: tying Medicare reimbursement to charges to private patients creates incentives for providers to raise charges to private patients.

Conclusions

The Carter administration's National Health Plan or any national health insurance program which extends coverage and reduces patient copayment will increase demand for health services and reduce patient sensitivity to price. Equilibrium price levels must rise unless there is an offsetting increase in supply. This is not part of NHP. On the contrary, it is proposed to "revise federal health manpower policy to prevent a potentially costly physician surplus" and to limit capital expenditures by hospitals. Thus reimbursement policies will play a crucial role in rationing excess demand and in controlling the increase in health costs. What are the likely effects of the proposed reimbursement policies?

For physician and other ambulatory services, reimbursement for Healthcare patients will be on the basis of a fee schedule, set initially at average Medicare levels, but revised thereafter by negotiation between Healthcare and physician representatives. Tying the initial Healthcare fee schedule to Medicare charge levels creates incentives for physicians to raise Medicare charges in anticipation.[45] The crucial issue in subsequent revisions of the fee schedule will be the extent to which it is linked to charges to private patients. Upward pressure on private charges is expected because of the increase in private insurance coverage. If Healthcare fees are linked to private charges, this will create additional upward pressure on private charges, as in the case of the Medicare customary and prevailing formula described above. If Healthcare fees are not linked to private charges, there will be increasing divergence between the reimbursement physicians can receive from private patients and from Healthcare patients. The greater the divergence, the greater the fraction of services that will be allocated to private patients and the greater the problems of lack of availability and non-price rationing of services for Healthcare patients.[46] Thus a repeat of the Medicaid experience is to be anticipated.[47] One of the stated goals of NHP is to eliminate those aspects of the current health system that often cause the poor to receive substandard care. Attainment of this goal is unlikely to be compatible with use of a fee schedule for Healthcare patients that constrains reimbursement for public patients below fees from private patients.

Mandatory assignment of claims for public program beneficiaries, as proposed by NHP, will exacerbate the problem of access. The fact that assignment of Medicare claims was not mandatory effectively gave Medicare patients the option of supplementing the Medicare-allowed charge and hence obtaining the services of physicians who would be unwilling to treat them at the allowed charge. The administration estimates that mandating assignments will save Medicare patients $1 billion out-of-pocket costs. Against any saving due to mandatory assignment must be counted the reduced availability, and presumably lower quality, of care that Healthcare patients will be constrained to buy because they cannot supplement the Healthcare allowance.[48] Thus the first general conclusion is that given the implied increase in aggregate demand without a commensurable increase in supply, a reimbursement policy that uses a mandatory fee schedule for public patients but no controls on charges to private patients cannot simultaneously achieve the two stated goals of equal access and reduced inflation of costs.

Growing pressure to extend controls to private charges seems inevitable. Fee controls may have at least two adverse effects. First, their effect on the supply of services is uncertain. If physicians have some degree of monopoly power, then constraints on fees will increase the supply of services, in the short run, relative to the unconstrained situation.[49] In the long run, however, the supply of physicians may contract if controls reduce incomes to the medical professions. If prices are not used to ration excess demand for services, more costly forms of rationing will have to be used.

Second, it has been shown that fee controls in the context of a fee-for-service system tend to distort the mix of services used to produce health care. An increase in the ratio of other inputs to physician time is expected, assuming the supply of physician time is less elastic than the supply of lab tests and other ancillary services.[50] If utilization is controlled directly, it is likely to be even less cost-effective for tests than for other services because the value of most tests is low relative to monitoring costs.

One proposal for constraining the use of tests, which has been implemented in a few states, is to require that the lab performing the test bill the patient directly, rather than bill the physician, who in turn bills the patient.[51] Direct billing would eliminate the profit to physicians from tests and hence reduce the incentive to order tests. However, against any savings from reduced use of tests must be counted two additional sources of waste. First, collection costs are almost doubled, since the patient must be billed twice, once for the physician's services and once by the lab.[52] For many routine tests, billing costs are a substantial fraction of the total cost. Second, direct billing laws create an incentive for the physician to perform tests in-house, in order to save the additional billing cost and to retain the potential profit from tests, even if the production cost of doing tests in-house is higher than the production costs of tests sent out, because of diseconomies of small scale. It is quite possible that direct billing would decrease the total number of tests performed but increase the total expenditures of resources on performing and billing for tests. Thus the second general conclusion is that fee controls will increase inefficiency in the production of health care by distorting the mix of inputs.

These results are derived from standard analysis of the behavior of markets. There is ambivalence underlying the NHP as to whether market forces operate in the health sector. On the one hand, NHP includes specific measures to stimulate competition and relies on competition to regulate physician prices to private patients. On the other hand, the subsidy to private purchase of insurance is not reduced and is increased for those whose premium cost exceeds 5 percent of payroll.[53] Thus the incentive for private patients to be concerned about health care prices is not increased. Also, the proposal to reduce the supply of physicians is premised on the assumption that physicians can and do shift demand for their services. It has been argued that the increase in services provided under the Economic Stabilization Program does not necessarily imply physician ability to induce demand or that health markets are intrinsically different from other markets.

Assuming that health care markets function like other markets, the above analysis suggests that if the government operates a large insurance program, with little incentive for its beneficiaries to be concerned about price, reimbursement policies face a basic dilemma. If allowed fees for public patients are tied with charges to private patients, private charges will be pushed up; and this effect is greater, the larger the public sector and the more inelastic private demand are, because of the tax subsidy to private insurance. If allowed fees for public patients are constrained to increase less rapidly than private charges, the rate of price inflation will be less; but the problem of "two-tier medicine," lack of access for public patients, nonprice rationing, and distorted input mix will emerge. There are many ways of subsidizing health care other than through a government-operated insurance program. I conclude that, on the basis of the Medicare experience, this is one of the less attractive options.

Chapter 13 Notes

1. The value of this subsidy has been estimated at $9 billion in 1975. (Phelps 1976.)

2. This is described in detail in a later section of this paper.

3. For the period of 1965–1977, the medical care component increased 126 percent while other items increased 90 percent. (Social Security Bulletin 41:71, December 1978.) From 1972–1974, price controls were in effect under the Economic Stabilization Program. The role of Medicare and Medicaid should not be exaggerated, however. Over the fifteen year period prior to 1965, the medical care component increased more than twice as fast as the total CPI (66.7 percent versus 31.1 percent).

4. Rising incomes and the tax subsidy to health insurance have also stimulated the growth in private insurance coverage.

5. Phelps (1973) shows that, as a theoretical proposition, an increase in the price of medical care need not induce an increase in the demand for health insurance. However, the empirical evidence suggests a positive relation.

6. This section is based on the Detailed Fact Sheet, dated June 12, 1979, entitled "President Carter's National Health Plan Legislation."

7. Currently (1979) Medicare has a $160 hospital deductible per spell of illness and a flat $40 daily charge after 60 days in the hospital. For nonhospital services, there is a $60 deductible plus 20 percent coinsurance.

8. Out-of-pocket costs to Medicare patients may be covered by Medicaid or by private purchase of supplemental insurance.

9. Reimbursement under Medicaid varies by state. In California, Medi-Cal has used a formula similar to that used by Medicare, but with less frequent updating of allowable charges. For example, 1968 charge ceilings remained in effect throughout 1975, except for a 2.5 percent increase in 1972. All claims are assigned under Medicaid since patient cost sharing is typically zero.

10. Since Medicare copayment is only 20 percent, and this may be partially covered by Medicaid or supplemental private insurance, Medicare demand is expected to be less elastic than private demand.

11. Discounting is ignored.

12. The impact may be mitigated if the physician does not enforce collection of all charges from patients with low income and shallow coverage. But, in the long run, physicians are unlikely to continue to serve patients from whom they do not collect.

13. Precisely the same analysis applies to private insurance plans which limit reimbursement to the lesser of the physician's "usual, customary, and reasonable" (UCR) charge, where "usual" is the physician's median charge (Medicare's "customary") and "customary" is analogous to Medicare's "prevailing," but set at the 95th percentile of median charges in the area. During the 1960s, UCR plans increased in market share, at the expense of indemnity plans, in which the insurance contract specifies an absolute fee schedule for specific procedures. Because the patient pays 100 percent of any charge above the schedule allowance, indemnity plans preserve the patient's sensitivity to price and hence reduce moral hazard and waste in utilization of health services. Because of their greater inefficiency, the growth of UCR plans is puzzling. One explanation may be that they impose an externality on insurers and consumers using indemnity plans, because of the incentive to physicians created by UCR to raise charges at the lower end of the (unconstrained) charge distribution which are likely to be charges to persons on indemnity plans. Labor and trade unions, which have above average coverage and hence are expected to be charged above average fees if physicians are free to price-discriminate without constraint, have favored UCR plans. One reason for union support of UCR plans may be that the UCR formula tends to limit price discrimination against those with relatively complete insurance coverage.

14. Strictly, in the analysis in the previous discussion ("Effects on private patients") each patient's individual demand function incorporated in the physician's aggregate demand function from Medicare patients is the maximum over the assignment and nonassignment options for that patient. The assignment decision is determined simultaneously with the selection of optimum charges.

15. For example, Danzon 1980a.

16. This assumes that the demand of public patients is less elastic than private patients because of more complete coverage.

17. Holahan and Scanlon 1979.

18. Utilization by private patients is therefore greater than it would be without the constraint.

19. The analysis is in terms of the imposition of a fee ceiling on a previously uncontrolled market, rather than a limit on the rate of change. It ignores deductibles.

20. The marginal revenue schedule is discontinuous below the kink.

21. The reduction in the fee ceiling is not shown in figure 13.2 to avoid cluttering, but the reader can readily satisfy himself that the results are as described.

22. This conclusion differs from that of Hadley and Lee (1978), who argue that the net effect of a decrease in the Medicare-allowable charge on unassigned patient out-of-pocket cost is ambiguous a priori. Inconsistently, they argue that output in the nonassigned market will increase. Their analysis differs in at least three important respects. (1) They ignore the fact that movements along an exogenously determined demand curve must be induced by change in price to the patient, i.e., in out-of-pocket cost per unit of service. (2) They assume that fees charged to private and unassigned Medicare patients must be equal. Although regulation prohibits charging Medicare patients more than private patients, the converse is not prohibited. Thus the assumption of equal charges is unnecessarily strong. (3) They ignore the kink in the Medicare demand curve at the allowable charge, the downward shift in the kink, and the upper portion of the demand curve with lower charge ceilings.

23. This seems plausible, given the weak incentives of patients to search for lower prices, because of the high level of insurance coverage. The fact that many physicians serve different patients at different prices is consistent with the hypothesis that physicians are not price takers. However, some price differences may reflect differences in "quality" of service.

24. Data are also available for MediCal but are not reported here. The effects of MediCal fee controls cannot be distinguished from the introduction of limited coinsurance and utilization controls which occurred simultaneously.

25. The RVS assigns all medical procedures a unit value roughly proportional to input cost. It was designed to establish the relative values of different procedures for reimbursement purposes.

26. One can speculate that this was in anticipation that allowed charges after removal of controls would be based on actual charges during the last control year. In fact, in the case of Medicare assignment (and Medicaid),

billing an actual charge in excess of the allowed charge can have no purpose other than to influence future fee ceilings.

27. It will be argued later in this paper that increased intensity is a theoretically possible response to fee controls, given certain demand assumptions, even absent physician ability to shift demand or bill for more complex procedures than they in fact perform.

28. Since the number of Medicare enrollees only increased by 2.5 percent each year over the period covered, it cannot account for the observed increase in the total number of procedures.

29. This understates the actual increase because the gross revenue figures are computed using allowed charges, hence omit any revenue from billings in excess of allowed charges on unassigned claims.

30. It is some fraction of a weighted average of the reported actual and allowed charge, with weights depending on the proportion of patients assigned.

31. Lab tests may be performed in the physician's own office or be sent out to an independent lab. Even if tests are sent out, the lab typically bills the physician, who then bills the patient, so charges for tests remain at the discretion of the physician. This discretion is constrained by direct billing and truth in billing laws.

32. The expected marginal product of a test, S, must be positive, although for some minority of tests the actual marginal product may be negative, due to false positive or false negative results.

33. We abstract from patient time costs and health insurance. Thus the charge billed by the physician is the full cost to the patient and is assumed paid in full.

34. There has been increasing flexibility in reimbursement for office visits, depending on the amount of time spent. The number of different categories of office visits recognized by the California Relative Value System increased from 2 in 1956 to 28 in 1974. By 1979, Medicare recognized 10 different categories of office visit. To the extent reimbursement for time is still less flexible than an hourly rate, the analysis applies.

35. The constant cost assumption for physician time is appropriate if he can purchase time of other physicians or auxilliary personnel at the same cost in terms of efficiency units. The constant input cost assumptions simplify without qualitatively affecting the results of analysis.

36. If physician time is reimbursed on an hourly rate, P^h, equation (7) becomes:

$$\frac{w - P^h}{c - P^t} = \frac{N_h}{N_t} \tag{7}'$$

The use of tests relative to time is excessive or suboptimal as:

$$(P^t - c) \gtreqless (P^h - w)$$

37. If the patient is insured for visits but not for tests, then more of the total charge will be loaded onto the visit fee and the distorting incentive to use too many tests relative to physician time may be reversed.

38. This corresponds to the proposal for assignment of all health care patients in the administration's National Health Insurance plan.

39. The results summarized here are proved in Danzon (1980a).

40. While the model developed here shows that demand inducement is not a necessary inference from the observed response to price controls, it cannot prove that demand inducement does not occur. I would like to thank Uwe Reinhardt for emphasizing this point. For an analysis of the problems of measuring demand inducement, see Sloan and Feldman (1978) and Reinhardt (1978).

41. Prior to 1975, hospitals with less than 100 beds had the option of using the combination rather than the departmental method described here. Under the combination method, all ancillary departments are combined and a single ratio of Medicare charges to total charges is applied to total costs, summed over all ancillary departments; under the departmental method there is aggregation over services within a department, but Medicare's share of each department's costs is computed separately.

42. Commercial insurers pay charges. Some Blue Cross plans pay charges, other Blue Cross plans pay their share of costs.

43. For example, administration costs are allocated in proportion to the direct costs of the revenue-producing departments, cafeteria is allocated in proportion to meals served, etc. There are certain guidelines for the allocation of overhead across departments, but some flexibility remains.

44. In the case of day services, Medicare's share is the number of Medicare days multiplied by the average cost per day. This is equivalent to the RCCAC formula used for the ancillary departments for the case of a department producing a single service. The average cost per day for Medicare patients includes an 8½ percent markup on the nursing component on the grounds that aged patients require more nursing attention than the average patient.

45. This tendency may be constrained by existing controls on allowed charges through the Economic Index.

46. The previous analysis relating to figure 13.3 is relevant here.

47. Burney et al. (1978) report that, nationally, Medicaid specialist fees are 77 percent of Medicare specialist fees.

48. Eliminating the physician's ability to price-discriminate among Healthcare patients tends to raise charges to those who would have been offered the lowest charges if price discrimination were permitted. Whether this last effect is operative depends on how Healthcare-allowed charges are determined.

49. Whereas an increase in output in a monopolized market is usually assumed to increase social welfare, that presumption does not hold in the health care market because of distortions due to subsidies, insurance, and barriers to entry.

50. The use of tests will also be stimulated by the extension of insurance coverage for tests embodied in the Healthcare benefits package.

51. Bailey (1979) strongly advocates direct billing.

52. If the lab bills the physician, then a single bill for tests performed for all patients can be sent.

53. Since health expenditures exceeded 9 percent of GNP in 1979, if the distribution of expenditures were uniform across the population, everyone would be entitled to the subsidy. Since coverage is increased by the mandatory minimum benefit package, the 1979 figures underestimate the potential population qualifying for a subsidy.

Chapter 13 References

Bailey, Richard M. 1979. *Clinical Laboratories and the Practice of Medicine.* Berkeley: McCutchan.

Burney, Ira L.; Schieber, George J.; Blaxall, Martha; Gabel, Jon R. 1978. "Geographic Variation in Physician Fees." *JAMA* (September 22, 1978).

Danzon, Patricia Munch. 1980a. "Economic Factors in the Use of Laboratory Tests by Office-Based Physicians." R-2525 HCFA. Santa Monica: Rand Corporation.

Danzon, Patricia Munch. 1980b. "Profits in Hospital Laboratories: The Effects of Reimbursement Policies on Hospital Costs and Charges." R-2582 HCFA. Santa Monica: Rand Corporation.

Frech, H. E. III, and Ginsberg, Paul. 1978. *Public Insurance in Private Markets.* Washington, D.C.: American Enterprise Institute.

Hadley, Jack, and Lee, Robert. 1978. "Physicians' Price and Output Decisions: Theory and Evidence." Working paper 998-8, Washington, D.C.: Urban Institute (March 1978).

Holahan, John, and Scanlon, William. 1979. *Physician Pricing in California:*

Price Controls, Physician Fees and Physician Incomes from Medicare and Medicaid, Washington, D.C.: Urban Institute.

Leffler, Keith B., and Lindsay, Cotton M. 1976. "The Long Run Effects of National Health Insurance on Medical Care Prices and Output." In *New Directions in Public Health Care*. San Francisco: Institute for Contemporary Studies.

Mitchell, Bridger, and Phelps, Charles E. 1976. "National Health Insurance: Some Costs and Effects of Mandated Coverage." *Journal of Political Economy* (June 1976).

Phelps, Charles E. 1976. "Public Sector Medicine: History and Analysis." In *New Directions in Public Health Care*. San Francisco: Institute for Contemporary Studies.

Phelps, Charles E., 1973. "The Demand for Health Insurance: A Theoretical and Empirical Investigation." R-1054-OEO. Santa Monica: Rand Corporation.

Reinhardt, Uwe. 1978. "Comment." In *Competition in the Health Care Sector*, ed. Warren Greenberg. Maryland: Aspen Systems.

Sloan, Frank A., and Feldman, Roger. 1978. "Competition Among Physicians." In *Competition in Health Care Sectors*, ed. Warren Greenberg. Maryland: Aspen Systems.

Health Policy: A Payer's Perspective

*Willis B. Goldbeck**

Introduction

Four assumptions lie at the heart of this paper: (1) it is both desirable and possible to change the U.S. medical system into a true health system; (2) improvements in health status and control of waste are not incompatible with maintenance of quality; (3) the only alternative to more government is a cooperative effort among the private sector factions and between the private and public sectors; and (4) none of the above will be possible without the participation of the major private payers—business and industry.

Historically, employers have been passive purchasers of medical insurance. The health component of compensation was not designed to have a positive or negative impact on national health policy or medical care costs. Not unlike the rest of our medical system, the benefit package was not designed to be cost effective, to improve health, or to change the economic incentives of providers. On the contrary, employee benefits were designed to support unquestionably the status quo as it was defined by the providers.

With few exceptions, it has been only in the past five years that employers have begun to re-examine the way they do business with the medical industry. The reasons are clear: in the post-economic-stabili-

*Washington Business Group on Health, Washington, D.C.

zation period, medical benefit costs rose at a rate considerably out of proportion to increases in either persons covered or benefits provided.

Ford Motor Company provides the most compelling single example with its premium rise of $100,000,000 in a single year despite no benefit expansion and no changes in the covered population. Dramatic numbers such as this, along with the growing concern that a national health insurance plan might become law, prompted industry in 1974–75 to begin applying a new level of scrutiny to its insurance purchases.

Alternatives to Government

Despite decades of antigovernment rhetoric by business representatives, I would suggest that the only way we will ever make major, effective changes in our health system is through a private–public partnership.

There is no indication that the private sector is prepared to run those programs now under the government's control. There will be isolated examples of private firms taking over the management of public hospitals, of increasing use of service-provider contracts by local government, but no massive assumption by the private sector of public programs or of the responsibility for the poor—a responsibility which most people in the industry feel should reside within the public sector.

Unfortunately, there is also little indication that the government is prepared to run those programs very effectively. If the Indian Health Service, the migrant health programs, Veterans Administration, Renal Disease Program, Medicare, and Medicaid are the examples of government at work, then one can easily understand the very real fear many have of the same government agencies trying to run a full-scale national system. If the Veterans Administration is able to build more unneeded hospitals, how can the government's efforts to close unneeded private sector hospitals be taken seriously? If the Southwest Texas migrant health problem, which concerns only a few hundred thousand people, cannot be promptly resolved by the Public Health Service and the state of Texas, how can the private sector expect national health insurance (NHI) to help all 220 million of us? If we have a major physician distribution problem, and simultaneously, an oversupply of physicians (with resulting cost escalation), why do we see the government spending millions on new medical schools, while failing to exercise control over the work locations of those whose education is publicly supported? If the Medicaid program, more than a decade after its inception, remains unimplemented in one entire state, is bankrupt in others, and is frequently crippled by fraud and abuse, how can the private sector have confidence in government management? If the Health and Human Services (HHS) and Housing and Urban Development (HUD) in 1980 cannot solve the lead-based paint poisoning problem that was solved in West Germany before 1900, and which, according to Government Accounting Office (GAO), is the second largest generator of nontreatment Medicaid hospitalization days, what faith should the public place in promised interagency cooperation?

Why is the entire federal and state system seemingly unable to agree upon a process to resolve the medical liability mess that causes billions of dollars in wasted procedures annually? How much more must we waste while we study the problem?

Lastly, if Medicare cannot adequately serve today's elderly, what can we expect in ten years when the demographics so clearly predict a dramatic increase in the size of our elderly population? My point is not to castigate government, but to suggest that only by working together can we resolve these difficult problems, which, by all existing measures, do not lend themselves to regulatory solutions or to changes in economic incentives unless all payers play by the same rules.

Forces for Change

There are those who believe that the only way to improve our health system is to essentially start over, to establish a new system based upon federal budget controls, or conversely, upon new market forces. Anything less is generally designated as mere tinkering and at best is referred to as a short-term approach. I reject this attitude because the history of social and economic policy development in the United States is, and will continue to be, evolutionary rather than revolutionary. Certainly, this is appropriate in the health care sector when the vast majority already feel well served.

Change has to be a blend of short- and long-term goals and tasks, because inherent in such change are significant shifts in public values and private choices, which, in aggregate, become our public expression of will—the genesis of public policy.

Industry—the payers—reflects values in the design of the benefit package. Normally, design follows value as expressed through negotiations, tradition, the demands of providers, and the personal attitudes of executives. Today, we are asking, through design, to lead and to take an active, aggregate role in the evolution of our sickness system into one which is more health oriented, more publicly accountable, less wasteful, and more affordable. These multiple objectives can only be achieved through a strategy that predicates long-term systems reform upon a wide range of short-term actions.

Basic to this approach is the belief that the forces which have been, and are, influencing our system today will be more receptive to a multi-faceted strategy rather than a single-purpose bludgeon of massive reform. The medical system does exactly what we have designed it to do, thus rendering our public gnashing of teeth over cost escalation to be little more than a somewhat naive substitution of self-flagellation for real action that could be far more effective in both cost efficiency and improved health outcomes.

As we enter a new decade and contemplate major changes in our health system, it would be irresponsible if we did not recognize that such changes may last for a very long time and must be adaptable to a future that will be quite different from our present condition. To the extent that NHI is conceived largely as a financing mechanism, it is but one element of an all too frequently ignored larger issue: the need for a national health strategy.

I realize that the call for a health policy is not new; however, the call remains unanswered. Let me suggest that one of the reasons the business community is reluctant to endorse any specific NHI approach is because the preferred alternatives are based largely on the population, economic, medical, and health conditions as they have been, rather than on what they are becoming. A health policy, or at least a health strategy, reflecting and leading public values is equally needed, regardless of whether the system as we know it becomes more or less regulated by the federal government. Few look ahead and do not realize that the major determinants of health policy in the 1980s will be exogenous to the health or medical industries. Aging, balance of trade, environment, communications technology, inflation and unemployment, the value of the dollar, dwindling food supplies in the face of massive worldwide impoverished population growth, defense spending, and energy—these are the factors that will determine what we are able to do about domestic health issues. The unfortunate truth is that not one of these factors, when measured by even the most conservative standards, bodes well for our capacity to make vast new investments in medical care. Congress is left with the dilemma of trying to improve services, increase access (which means increased utilization), and decrease costs while facing an extended era of limited economic resources.

We feel strongly that any new health policy that is unmindful of this full range of forces will have inherent design flaws of a major magnitude. As payers, we see the current forces for change as including:

1. Fear of financial catastrophe
2. Patient ignorance
3. Public and private acquiescence to the myth of provider omniscience
4. Absence of economic incentives for providers
5. Absence of incentives for patients to be effective consumers
6. Misuse and misunderstanding of medical technology (i.e., technology assessment clashing with ethics, and the history of innovation, which makes a strong case for letting use determine ultimate cost effectiveness)
7. Court actions on issues such as malpractice, affirmative action, and actions regarding the physically or mentally handicapped
8. The rapid explosion in population
9. Deinstitutionalization—humane and cost effective, but acceptable only in "your neighborhood rather than mine"
10. The unserved and the underserved—the gaps that must be filled but which, due to the relatively smaller number of people concerned (12–20 million), cannot be the primary reason to change the medical system for the other 200 million who are rather well served.

To these, one might add maldistribution of providers: rapidly growing oversupply of providers with neither the economic forces nor regulation to direct them to the needed locations or specialties; and consistent failure of existing government programs to meet management, economic, or service delivery expectations.

Competition: Pros and Cons

From the moment the incentive reform, or market force, or consumer choice approach to NHI was renamed "competition," people expected business to join the bandwagon of support. Not only was that expectation incorrect, so too is the name: competition is not the antithesis of regulation; it is the shifting of regulation from provider to payer, a shifting of emphasis from access to price. There is no question that we are encouraged by this new direction, which represents the recognition that a fully federalized, comprehensive health system is no longer to be seriously considered. We have felt for a long time that not only was such an approach undesirable for economic and philosophical reasons but that it was also unneeded.

The incentive reform approach can address the priority objectives that we feel represent the hierarchy of health policy needs: (1) correcting the economic incentives now in the system which, if left unaltered, guarantee a continuing increase in medical care costs; (2) increasing the nation's commitment to health rather than continuing the unsupportable overemphasis upon medical treatment; (3) addressing the specific, identifiable gaps in protection in the current system; and (4) removing the problem of financial catastrophe deriving from illness and/or accidents. If one were to set priorities from the standpoint of political pressures, one would start from the bottom of the list. If one sets these goals from the standpoint of major improvements in the medical system, one would start at the top. Herein lies the dilemma we face when working with these issues.

While finding the concept of competition attractive and having the long-range potential to address the incentive reform objective, we caution against premature reliance upon markets that historically have dumped the poor into second-class government programs and upon alternative delivery systems that do not yet exist. We are also concerned about systems that have a natural incentive to either keep out or underserve the medically indigent and the elderly precisely because of the extensive services they require. Even though we are strong supporters of alternative delivery system developments, we must recognize the problems as well as the potential of these systems.

There are several major questions about the legislative proposals designed to create new market forces. Whom does this approach actually reach? Whom does it serve? It is difficult at this point to get a firm sense of how many employers would, in fact, be activated by the $120 trigger proposed by Congressman Ullman. The average family insurance premium for major employers in 1979 was $804. This suggests that there is a rather large gap between that and $120 a month. The all-too-common inference that the prices paid for insurance in the auto industry are in fact the national norm, needs to be corrected. Of course, if the legislation were not to pass until the early or mid 1980s, that $120 may be a realistic target.

As a business group vitally concerned not only with the health issues, but also with broader issues of economic policy, we at Washington Business Group on Health applaud the new directions in NHI proposals. To be successful, the competition approach must bring with it certain changes not attainable by mandating the shape of employee benefits only.

1. Physicians and all other providers must be allowed to advertise, including price information.
2. Schools must no longer be allowed to ignore health education, as the vast majority do now. Consumer choice will never be really meaningful without an educated public. Today, we consciously guarantee that each generation of new adults will be ignorant of health, of their own bodies, and of the medical system. And these are the consumers we wish to have making intelligent choices. We pay an awful price for this ignorance, a price compounded by the more than one million teenagers who annually become pregnant—thanks, in part, to a society that says 700,000 babies and more than 300,000 abortions for teenage mothers is acceptable, but that sex education in our schools is not.
3. Medical schools receiving any public financing or tax support must teach health economics and educate providers to know how to value the products they order as well as the services they provide.
4. Quality and performance standards for hospitals and other medical facilities must be established, and each institution's periodic evaluation must be made known to the public. To provide consumer

choice without addressing some of the underlying value questions that make consumers today choose as they do, fails to recognize the motivations of the consumers we are seeking to serve.

We are also concerned about legislation that would make the level at which additional benefits become taxable so close to the current premium levels that new, innovative benefits designed to slow cost increases would be counted as employee income. This is especially onerous for benefits such as mental health and health promotion, which are the very essence of the kind of new directions we are all trying to set in the health care delivery system. The advent of a competition system would open the door to creative benefit design based on tax incentives that favor prevention and wellness programs.

Employee Rebate

The employers have mixed feelings about the employee rebate proposals because many negotiate benefits, not dollars, and thus feel any financial savings that do not come from a reduction in offered benefits rightfully belong to the company. However, many employers also see the long-term advantage of encouraging employees to be wiser buyers and users of their benefits. As with any other advantage, there must also be a price. Therefore, we would recommend that any legislation which addresses this subject simply require that the savings be shared by the employer and employees. This will meet the objective of providing a cost-consciousness incentive for employees and maintain the employer's incentive to push for cost containment through benefit redesign, claims management, participation in the local health planning system, etc. The individual consumer cannot be expected to change the economic incentive of the delivery system—a system with which most are satisfied—as fast as can the major corporate purchasers.

I would also note that there is certainly no reason to assume that employees would behave any differently than other consumers with their rebate. There is nothing to suggest this money would go towards healthy products or healthy behavior. As a nation, we are not nearly as concerned with the amount we spend on smoking and drinking as we are about the amount we spend on health. The few early tests of employee preferences (done by Citicorp and American Can, for example) show that rebates or low-option plans hold little attraction.

Multiple Choice

The multiple-choice requirement seems to come from a basically sound concept. Many employers do offer the health maintenance organization (HMO) option, and certainly most could not claim that offering a low option addition would be administratively too onerous to handle. However, there are several issues which call into question the ultimate value to be gained by this offering.

The one major example which currently exists is the Federal Employee Health Benefit program. In this program, the employees have shown that they can indeed make sound economic choices (for example, choose low options except when they want to schedule a baby or elective surgery). The resulting adverse selection does not save the health system needed resources even though it may be good for certain individual consumers. Standard Oil of California had the same experience. A two-year enrollment period may be a partial solution.

If there is to be a mandated low-option plan, we would recommend that its price be set at a regional level and be determined by a process which considers hospital cost, provider availability, consumer demographics, and health planning, as well as HMO costs.

Capital Investment

This is one issue which might be favorably addressed through the market force approach. Any national health plan and any financing mechanism that ignores the needs of the medical complex to maintain its infrastructure ignores the needs of the future by hiding today's costs in the overutilization of capital resources for operating funds. This view is a short-term perspective that drives the hospital into a borrowing circumstance that only increases the interest rates that must in turn be passed on. Ultimately, the private hospital is driven out of that borrowing market and into the public sector market at a time when neither the administration nor the Congress has expressed an interest in increasing the federal budget.

Accountability

Many providers take great umbrage at the idea that they should be held accountable to the public for their professional tasks, let alone for the cost of their performance. These attitudes have a long history predicated on the traditionally elitist design of our postgraduate education system, the very real public ignorance about medical matters, and the acquiescent attitude of payers and patients. A heritage of well-financed political clout aided these attitudes. The 1960s saw a boom of consumerism and even the inroads of some principles of socialism in medical care financing and new attention to patients' rights.

While not as openly activist as the 1960s, the late 1970s and early 1980s appear to be legitimate heirs to their accountability-oriented parents of the 1960s. Increasingly, industry is matching or exceeding the individual as concerned consumers. Industry will stop unquestioning acceptance of the wide variations in physician fees for the same service in the same town, the absence of comparative mortality and infection rate information about hospitals, the Friday admission for Monday treatment, the rate escalations for the hotel aspects of a hospital stay, and the cost shifting that results from unfair reimbursement by publicly funded programs. The list goes on, but the point is clear: just as industry has been and is a supporter of local hospitals, so too does it owe a human, moral, and fiduciary responsibility to its employees and shareholders to become a knowledgeable and prudent purchaser of care. The payers will get what they pay for. Physicians can get around any regulatory system. Therefore, it is incumbent upon the payers to aggregate their efforts to establish methods of data collection and analysis, and to be of clear voice in demanding accountability from all three key parties: providers, patients, and insurance carriers. An attitude of accountability will do more for the system than will any legislated cost-containment program. Accountability can result from public–private cooperative efforts using professional standards review organizations (PSROs).

Specific Company Examples

Four points should precede the following examples: (1) employer experience with utilization review (UR) and PSRO is very recent, and thus long-term statistics are not available; (2) many companies do not keep records of the UR activities of their local plants or divisions; (3) physician and administrator behavior changes, resulting from the review process, may be more significant in the long run than any short-term dollar savings; and (4) all UR programs should be very careful not to oversell the dollar savings. Quality enhancement is the greater virtue of good programs.

Sundstrand In Rockford, Illinois, they have contracted with the PSRO for the past two and a half years. They do not have an exact "before and after" data, but feel confident that the PSRO has been a positive experience because the length of stay for their hospitalized employees is very favorable compared to the area and national averages. The company can find no reason for this other than their PSRO involvement.

National average	7.1 days per thousand population
Area average	6.4 days per thousand population
Sundstrand average	5.9 days per thousand population

A second Sundstrand program, using a hospital's own UR committee, has resulted in a 15 percent reduction in per employee health care costs in that area.

Caterpillar Working with PSRO in the Peoria area, the Caterpillar employee's average length of hospital stay in 1979 was down 10 percent from 1977; the employee patient-days-per-thousand were down 19 percent; and their employee hospital admission rate was down 10 percent. These reductions resulted in a cost–benefit ratio of $4.00 saved for each $1.00 Caterpillar expended in the PSRO program.

Goodyear The Goodyear company calculated a savings of $30,000 on a basis of only 600 hospital admissions in Springfield, Illinois. Length of stay dropped one day and has remained at that level. The company makes the point that the same scrutiny applied to different hospitals will lead to different results depending on the quality of management present in the hospital prior to the initiation of a review system.

Bethlehem Steel The Bethlehem steel company contracted with the Baltimore City (MD) PSRO and has experienced an immediate decrease in length of stay. Final first-year accounting is not yet complete, so the degree of savings is not yet known.

In Tidewater, Virginia, the Blues' Focused Review Program saved Ford's 2,256 employees over $80,000 in health care costs through a 13.8 percent reduction in absenteeism, a 12.8 percent reduction in hospital length of stay, and a 23.5 percent reduction in hospital days per 1,000 persons.

Other examples abound, but they are not necessary in making the point demonstrated by the examples presented here: i.e., everyone will benefit from an increasingly accountable system, including the truly excellent physician.

Wellness: The Healthy Alternative

While it would be misleading to suggest that all of industry has accepted the concept of health promotion, it is important to note the progress made in just the past three years.

Several reasons for industry's increased interest in health promotion are: (1) increased understanding that employees' lifestyles are a (some would say *the*) major determinant of medical benefit utilization, absenteeism, and diminished productivity; (2) increased evidence of the effectivenesss of wellness programs; (3) increased acceptance of these programs by the medical and scientific communities; and (4) increased government attention to wellness as a method of reducing costs and improving quality of life.

Each of these reasons warrant a word of explanation. Studies show that upwards of 80 percent of industrial accidents are due to personal problems, not the equipment or the work setting itself. Similarly, HEW and the Department of Labor (DOL) note an annual productivity loss of more than $20 billion due to alcoholism; combined with medical costs, alcoholism costs this country over $44 billion—an amount that exceeds the total Gross National Product (GNP) of all but 14 nations! And the President's Mental Health Commission estimated that 15 to 20 percent of the work force have serious emotional problems. One company, Weirton Steel, found that 61 percent of its absenteeism was due to psychiatric problems.

Washington Business Group on Health (WBGH) conferences, seminars and surveys all demonstrate a growing attention to personal behavior through a spectrum of wellness programs and insured benefits, and insurance carrier and employee programs are increasing the number of participants. Employee values are increasingly calling employer attention to the desirability of providing wellness programs, especially for physical fitness. Kimberly-Clark, for example, frankly notes the recruiting advantages resulting from its fitness program, and Canadian National Life Assurance credits its wellness program with a dramatic reduction in turnover.

Health Research Institute did a cost-containment survey in late 1979. They found that among responding firms, the per employee health insurance cost in 1978 was $827.00 for those without a major prevention/promotion effect, while those with such a program averaged only $564 per employee. In addition, a collection of 22 evaluations shows a mean reduction in hospital/medical/surgical utilization of 24 percent by participants in mental health programs and 45 percent by participants in alcoholism programs. These numbers are supported by the California Psychological Health Plan (24 percent reduction); Blues, which show a better than 50 percent drop after outpatient psychotherapy was made available; and Kennecott, with a 74.6 percent reduction in indemnity costs for the users of its Insight program. Allis Chalmers found a 200 percent reduction in absenteeism due to its alcoholism program, and Equitable reports a 3–1 return in productivity in its small stress management program.

The following facts illustrate the growing acceptance of the healthy alternatives: the August 1979 editorial in *Science* magazine was entitled, "Self-Care: A Nation's Best Health Insurance"; the visibility of the American College of Preventive Medicine has significantly increased (its current president was just named the new medical director of IBM, explicitly due to the company's desire to emphasize health promotion); the Council on Wage and Price Stability, at the request of the Washington Business Group on Health and HEW's Office of Health Information and Promotion, exempted wellness programs in industry from the 1979 wage guidelines; the Surgeon General's report, *Healthy People*, positions the federal establishment in concurrence with the view that future health improvements are dependent more on lifestyle than medicine; employers are mandated to provide employee prevention benefits by state laws that have more extensive mandates than some of the NHI bills now before Congress; and there is an in-

creasing number of HEW studies and conferences aimed at document-
ing and encouraging health promotion programs in the workplace.

Despite these and many other positive examples, the prevention end
of the health spectrum remains the least financially or politically supported. Many employers have had bad experiences with overpromoted,
poorly designed, and undermanaged prevention programs. The federal
government still spends far more on every other aspect of the health
system than it does on prevention. Physicians still often note that they
are trained to cure, not prevent. Hospitals rarely offer wellness programs, and most of those that do are primarily interested in protecting
their share of the acute-care market. Unions have a wariness that wellness is often enhanced by management as a method of evading or de-
laying their workplace safety responsibilities. Finally, we as individuals are far more willing to invest in self-destructive behavior than
healthier, but less exciting, lifestyles. Clearly, many obstacles to prevention programs remain.

We would like to see Congress assist the health promotion movement by assisting employers to do even more than that which is already under way. For example, currently the cost of in-house promotion programs is exempt from the Council on Wage and Price Stability's guidelines. However, reimbursement for the same services provided outside the company on an individual basis are counted as wages
and taxed, thus decreasing the employee's incentive to use these services.

Those who would like to see the movement toward health promotion delayed are quick to point out the paucity of scientific evidence,
which would prove the effectiveness, in either health or cost–benefit
terms, of specific promotion programs. Others counter that there is at
least as much evidence of the effectiveness of promotion as there is of
many medical procedures for which we now pay vast sums; that evidence is growing in both quality and quantity; that if everyone waits
to begin a program until "proof" is in hand, such proof will never be
available, since there will have been no programs to generate measur-
able data.

Between these two poles lies the real world of promotion. As the
trends indicate, promotion programs in industry are relatively new,
and most were started because someone felt it was the right thing to
do. Most programs are neither comprehensive nor subject to serious
evaluation. In fact, were evaluation, which is expensive and time con-

suming, a requirement, many companies would simply not bother to establish the program in the first place.

There have been no studies of industry programs that are both long-term and comprehensive (ten years or more and of a multifaceted program). But the evidence of effectiveness that does exist is encouraging and would tend to support those who took the first leap of faith to start promotion programs.

Effectiveness, according to the 1978–79 surveys by the Washington Business Group on Health (WBGH), is often measured by such soft criteria as "improved morale." In an attempt to bring order to the evaluation issue, WBGH members are working with HEW in two ad hoc groups. We view wellness as a viable alternative to the status quo and to more money being thrown at health problems for which solutions simply cannot be purchased. The promotion of wellness programs is not the final answer to the health dilemma; it is part of the changing values which will allow our medical system to evolve into a true health system. Without acceptance by the payers, wellness will never be more than an appendage to the medical system. The growth of effectiveness evidence, combined with increased frustration at cost increases seemingly unrelated to health, is causing the payers to be increasingly inclined to forego the promotion/prevention system that will ultimately determine whether or not this nation will have a true commitment to health.

Industry and Planning: A Legitimate Alliance?

It should come as a surprise to no one that many employers in industry feel uncomfortable participating in an effort which is both governmental in its origin and regulatory in its purpose and design. Equally concerned are many planners whose gut reaction to industry is largely negative and whose view is clouded by the environmental and occupational health hazards associated with industry. The production and massive advertising of unhealthful products is another reason for skepticism about the sincerity of industry's commitment to an improved health delivery system.

All these concerns are serious and, like most stereotypes, have some basis in fact. No health system association (HSA) or industry contemplating a cooperative relationship should be unaware of these problems. However, we respectfully but adamantly reject any of these problems as sufficient excuse for either industry to ignore planning or for planners to reject industry participation.

For health planning to be successful, it must take a long-range perspective as well as meet mandated short-term goals. Industry has many health-related roles which are often in conflict: it is a payer of benefits; a provider of direct and referred care; a consumer of health and medical care resources; a producer of medical technology (which must be sold); a producer of products known to be unhealthy, and products specifically designed to improve health; a "host" to work settings of great danger and others of remarkable safety; a hospital trustee and financial supporter; a spoiler, cleaner, exploiter, and rejuvenator of the environment; a regulator, through control of reimbursement, as well as by participation, in such systems as HSA and PSRO. The list could be longer, but the point is clear: industry cannot be seen as all good or all bad, and increasingly, a single company has components which fit all the categories listed above.

Based on real experiences, the following are a few of the ways industry can contribute to the HSAs. It can provide shared facilities, electronic data processing expertise and time, meeting space, audio-visual equipment and facilities, and medical/health promotion programs and facilities. (The HSAs are also employers whose business is too small to warrant or afford independent programs and facilities.) It can give technical assistance such as banking and investment analysis, architectural review, bulk processing, information systems design, and technology assessment. In addition, it can provide human resources such as actuaries, financial managers, and long-range planners.

Simply put, health planners cannot ignore the payer, provider, and consumer roles and the resources that industry represents. In time, the more the planning system becomes an integrated private–public effort working independently at the local level, the better the planning system will be.

Similarly, industry cannot let its traditional antipathy to the regulatory process blind the companies to basic facts for the following reasons: (1) if the local HSAs fail or are eliminated by budget restrictions, the next step will not be less regulation, but rather, more federal controls and shifting of regulation onto the employers; (2) the future directions of the health/medical system will be set by a combination of competitive and regulatory forces, by which neither side wins at the expense of the other; (3) participation is both an opportunity and an obligation—an obligation to the employees, dependents, stockholders, and others for whom an unplanned, wasteful health system is a direct and unnecessary drain on needed economic resources; and (4) planning will continue with or without industry. Most companies and most planners, we believe, will see the wisdom and mutual benefit to be gained from a cooperative relationship.

Coalitions

A basic tenet of the employer's perspective is to keep health systems controls, whether public or private, at the local level. Even granting the obvious problems this can cause the multistate employer, most prefer administrative complexity to increasingly centralized government controls. The Business Roundtable Task Force on Health and the Washington Business Group on Health are two responses to this concern. However, both of these are Washington-based and thus deal primarily with federal actions. To supplement this narrow force, employers in many communities are forming coalitions—local business groups on health. The latest is a regional effort, The Midwest Business Group on Health, which was started through the efforts of the WBGH and Jim Mortimer, who left a vice-presidency at Continental Bank to become the group's first director.

In several cases, most notably in Cincinnati, there is compelling evidence that a local coalition can, over time, work with both the providers and the public sector regulatory efforts, such as health planning, to bring about lasting cost savings without reduced quality of, or access to, needed care. Following are examples of this type of coalition.

Minneapolis-St. Paul Citizens League: a large nonpartisan citizen study group with heavy business involvement. The league is working on tough issues such as bed reduction and hospital closings. An industry group was also responsible for the surge of HMO development in Minneapolis. Observers of local health care efforts consider Minneapolis to be the best example of planning and competition working together for cost containment with increased quality of care. Industry is credited with being the stimulator of this effort. In addition, a statewide coalition is being formed as an outgrowth of the Minnesota Cost Containment Commission.

Cleveland (1) Associated Industries Health Care Committee and (2) Greater Cleveland Coalition on Health Care Cost Containment.

Fairfield-Westchester IBM has joined with some two dozen other major employers to form a local business group on health.

Philadelphia (1) Philadelphia Area Committee on Health Care Costs and (2) Chamber Joint Cost Containment Program.

Dayton Dayton Health Care Coalition.

San Diego Employers Health Care Cost Committee of San Diego Industry (Rohr, General Dynamics, etc.) and public employers working together.

Cincinnati The coalition does not have a separate organization. The business community, Blue Cross, and hospitals work closely with CORVA, the local Health Systems Agency. Proctor and Gamble, for example, has not had an increase in their insurance rates for three years.

Nashville An ad hoc business and labor committee that works to broaden the perspective and capacity of the Middle Tennessee HSA.

Rochester, NY Rochester Coalition on HMOs (Kodak, Xerox, Blue Shield and Blue Cross, labor, and providers). Two of the three HMOs started are now doing very well. Interestingly, the one that failed was the one run by the medical society.

State examples Maryland Health Care Coalition: Instigated by Health Insurance Association of America with employer involvement initiated by the Washington Business Group on Health, the coalition is now an ongoing effort which works with the state's Health Services Cost Review Commission. A significant aspect of the employer involvement has been the evolution from participation by the companies' local division/plant personnel in Maryland.

Michigan Coalition on Bed Reduction: A coordinated effort involving the auto companies, UAW, Blue Shield and Blue Cross, the state

Health Department, and state legislators, the project has resulted in new state legislation on bed reduction and has been closely involved with the new HMO development at Henry Ford Hospital in Detroit.

In at least two other states (Florida and Oklahoma), the governor has initiated a new coalition effort.

Regional example The Southeastern Association of Health Systems Agencies, with consultation by the Washington Business Group on Health, HEW, and others, has formed a regional industry advisory committee.

Trends and lessons There are two basic trends to report: (1) the issues of cost containment are providing new stimulus to the older coalitions, many of which were started more for resource development and (2) the HSAs are the focal point of many of the new coalitions but serve as a catalyst for implementation with the coalition typically becoming independent.

Lessons from these coalitions are many and in a constant state of change, but are nonetheless informative for those who would consider starting such an effort.

1. There is no single format for success at the local level.
2. These efforts are complex, difficult, fraught with conflict, and expensive (costs, if accurately accounted for, must include time contributed).
3. The coalitions will be successful only if there is business participation.
4. Labor participation is often very hard to get, but is essential.
5. Success should not be measured by short-term cost savings only.
6. While some traditional organizations such as chambers of commerce have successfully internalized a coalition, the greatest chance of success seems to come when the coalition is independent.

Despite the examples listed and a steady growth in these coalitions, the fact remains that most communities have neither coalitions nor evidence of strong business concern for health care costs. This, however, at least among the large companies, is rapidly changing.

Employer Actions

Current employer actions to become a more active influence in health policy can be viewed in several categories. (Examples of each follow with some of the participating companies identified.) On the international level we have seen: employer involvement with development of President Carter's 1978 International Health Policy (Westinghouse, American Medical International); increased awareness of U.S. multinational corporations' roles in public health as well as employee health and medical insurance, especially in developing countries (IBM, GE, GM); sponsorship of the International Health Resource Consortium (Metropolitan Life, Pfizer); and increasing attention to issues of environment and product dumping abroad.

Examples on the national level are: the Business Roundtable Task Force on Health; the creation and growth of Washington Business Group on Health (from one member, Ford Motor Company, to 175 WBGH members currently); U.S. Chamber Health/Action Strategy; Boston University Center for Industry and Health Care; Voluntary Effort (VE); National Steering Committee; Labor Management Group Health Policy Project; and appointed memberships of employers on the Carter NHI Advisory Committee and other national-level advisory organizations, both public and private.

On the state and local level, more than half the HSAs now have industry participation and support. There is participation in state health legislation, training for personnel who serve on hospital boards (IBM, Midwest Business Group on Health, Deere, Chrysler), VE Committees, and employers working with school boards for health and sex education programs. There is a growth of "Industry and Health" coalitions (Cleveland, San Diego, Chicago, Philadelphia, Fairfield and Westchester County, Miami, Cincinnati, etc.). And the WBGH feels this will be the "hot" development of the early 1980s.

On the corporate level, we see control of philanthropic contribution and investments for health facilities based on real need, not traditional affiliations or standard measures of return on investment (e.g., Continental Bank, IBM, Citicorp); tying reimbursement to HSA-approved facilities (e.g., Boeing); self funding (e.g., Goodyear); and cooperative cost-containment projects with labor (auto–UAW 1976 contract).

In the area of care delivery and employee safety, we see employers helping establish and support alternative delivery systems, HMOs, IPAs, etc. (Ford, Deere, R. J. Reynolds, Burlington Industries); contracting for utilization review such as PSRO and Foundations for Medical Care (Caterpillar, Motorola); expanding corporate medical departments to full primary care service (Gillette); providing off-job safety (ARMCO Steel); employee environmental health screening (IBM); preretirement counseling (Sun); and encouraging health promotion (wellness) through incentives (Hospital Corporation of America), fitness (Kimberly-Clark, Xerox, Exxon, and others), community resources for dependents (IBM), stress management (Equitable), hypertension prevention (Campbell Soup), smoking cessation (AT&T, Metropolitan Life), mental wellness (Kennecott, General Foods), alcoholism treatment (Ford, Allis Chalmers, and most others), and a variety of other programs.

In the area of benefit design, employers help reduce the economic incentives for unnecessary inpatient care by providing reimbursement for home health care, ambulatory care, surgi-centers, mental health residency programs, hospices, use of nonphysician providers (such as psychiatric social workers, nurse practitioners, physician extenders, and paramedics), second and third surgical opinion, preadmission testing, disability review, innovative mental health insurance (California Psychological Health Plan), managed care delivery (SAFECO), and cost sharing (deductibles and/or coinsurance).

Conclusion

Business, a payer, has more potential clout than it has ever elected to use to alter the medical delivery system. The reasons it has not used this clout are many, but trends suggest a new attitude of business—one that is more concerned, aggressive, and demanding. Dollars saved through reduced waste can be applied to categories of real need.

Employers cannot shirk responsibility for their unhealthy products, job designs, work settings, environmental pollution, etc.; but none of these major issues should be used as an excuse by management or labor to avoid doing what is needed to improve the incentives emanating from the benefit package. The trends are toward more mental health coverage, more health promotion, greater accountability, better data management, and more direct health policy involvement.

Industry, even with its purchasing power, cannot solve all our health needs. The private sector payers must work with their public sector counterparts. This country does not need a new medical care delivery system. We do need a new approach to health with all payers, providers, and consumers participating. As a populace, we cannot look only to the payers or to government for guidance. We must articulate the values that make a commitment to health politically and economically compelling.

Discussants' Comments on Section III

Richard Egdahl

Diana Dutton

Richard Egdahl

I guess it helps to know where people are coming from. I'm still a practicing endocrine surgeon and university and medical center administrator who is very interested in these issues; and I have read these papers, heard their discussions, and have a few comments on each of the topics. Clark Havighurst and I have had these discussions before. Basically, I feel that he often doesn't place the physicians in as friendly an equation as he might. That is unfortunate because it is going to be necessary to achieve a partnership with the physicians to accomplish some of the things he feels are needed.

First, I do not think it is realistic to expect that we will be able to require three plans for consumers to choose from. I wish we could, but those of us who work with HMO development know how hard it is to restructure the delivery system. Frequently, I discuss with industry groups the possibility of a closed- or an open-panel plan or a very vigorous utilization control program; but these don't arise easily for a variety of reasons. I think it is academic to require three competing plans, when many groups are working very hard to start one alternative delivery system. You can mandate it, but it isn't going to happen in the near future in most places.

Clark talks about restoring the ultimate choice to the individual, and I agree very much with what Willis Goldbeck has said, that there is information out there that is available, which, when used, may have amazing effects. The Evanston Hospital in Evanston, Illinois, for example, as well as other hospitals around the country, are putting together information about the credentials and practice patterns of doctors in the area—where they went to school, how long they've practiced, whether they take Medicaid patients, how long a waiting time they have in their office, and what fees they charge. This information is made widely available. Maybe the consumer can't choose wisely or easily, but he can find out if a physician has his specialty boards or if he doesn't see people without a half-hour wait. This information gives a feel for many factors that are going to be increasingly important. There can be no choice if the information is not made available.

I do worry about the fate of self-insured plans under Clark's competition model. Many large corporations are self-insured, and this gives them access to data so that they can understand what is happening to their employees. This provides the basis for instituting utilization-control programs that are based upon the ready availability of the right kind of data. Goldbeck talked about nosocomial infections. There are some very interesting data, for example, concerning the 200-bed Kaiser Hospital in San Diego, which does almost as much surgery as hospitals with twice as much bed capacity. They admit almost everybody on the same day of their surgery, and there is good evidence that the rate of nosocomial infections is less than in hospitals where the patients are admitted a few days before surgery. It takes very good preoperating arrangements to do this. But it is true that there are changes that will contain increasing health care costs, but also will move in the direction of better patient care.

One of the problems with Havighurst's statement that there is not just one right way to diagnose and/or treat, is that we are just in the infancy of setting safety standards. For example, only a few years ago we didn't have the data that demonstrate that if a hospital doesn't carry out at least two open-heart operations a week in a unit, the mortality rate is excessive. If a hospital carries out only one open-heart procedure a month, we now know that it is just not right, because of a probable high mortality. There are papers coming through now indicating the same kind of phenomenon for other complicated surgical procedures as well—a critical mass of cases is necessary for optimal results. (Years ago it was suggested that one way to test the confidence of the surgeon in radical mastectomy would be to let him do whatever operation he thinks is best, but to pay him at the simple mastectomy rates. That would quickly settle the issue and remove any possible economic motive for doing a more radical procedure.) As the years go by, I think we will find society demanding that specialized centers do the things that are associated with a very high morbidity and mortality when not performed frequently.

There is another problem with Havighurst's concepts and paper about antitrust and doctor coalitions. In Wausau, all 105 doctors joined the fee-for-service HMO set up by the Employers Insurance of Wausau. Despite the fact that all local physicians belonged to the HMO, radical changes occurred in their practice patterns. I don't think the reason that the Individual Practice Association (IPA) "works" is because of financial risk, but rather because of peer review information and physicians not hospitalizing patients more than is absolutely necessary.

When you don't have an IPA in an area, you still can have a utilization-control program by appropriate informational campaigns. In hospitals where the doctor bills the patient and truly sees the very high costs of everything, real changes in physician ordering practices occur. Just discussing the subject at patient rounds can result in major changes in physician practices. The key is information and physician leadership.

Now, Pat Munch-Danzon's paper on fees focuses on a tremendous dilemma. There are increases if you tie Medicare and Medicaid fees to private fees, and a possible lack of availability of doctors who opt out if you don't. I have no answer to that, except to say that there is a creative dialogue beginning now on fees that has never really existed before. Under the freedom of information act, it is now possible to get information about Medicare fees in regional areas, and this has been done in Washington, D.C., and other places. The findings are quite startling. You find surgeons that take out from one to thirty gall bladders a year on Medicare patients, and their fee range is between $400 and $900, with no apparent rationale. The same thing is true for hysterectomies. Now, the credentials of these people and the years they have been practicing often have little relationship to the fees they charge. My graduating chief residents often receive higher fees their first year out than I do because of the profile I established when I first came to Boston, using Richmond fee levels. The point is that there is little rationale when it comes to fees.

In 1930, doctors, lawyers, and dentists all had about $4,500 as their net income. In the late 1970s, physicians netted around $60,000, and the others netted a little over half of that. I'm not saying this is wrong, but is certainly wasn't planned rationally. In Ontario, Canada, where they have negotiated fee schedules, it was decided years ago that the specialist/generalist ratio of income should be about 1 to 0.7. Previously it was about 2 to 1. For the last several years, they have kept the rate of increase for specialists at a few percentage points and have had increases of over 10 percent for generalists. That has led to a modest exodus of specialists, but it is not certain that they will end up with too few specialists. Within the closed doors of HMO physician fee committees, the specialists and generalists (who have to give comprehensive services to a defined patient group with a fixed pot of dollars) must work out their differences. There is also the problem of inadequate work loads. Group practices do not have to take in more specialists than they need, and in the future neither will the IPAs. But what of unstructured fee-for-service practices in areas that are attractive to live in?

Goldbeck mentioned in his paper that there is no provision by the private sector for giving care to the poor. This is a critical issue. The question is whether tax money should be used to permit the poor to receive health services in the private system or whether we should establish a separate public system, also paid for with tax dollars. There are arguments for both approaches, but I prefer that the public buy into the private system, with a minimum benefit package to which everyone is entitled. Then, if you want the frills for which there is no proof of efficacy, these may be purchased with discretionary income, if you have any.

The issue of quality is critical. I work at a city hospital, a Veterans Administration (VA) hospital, and a university hospital, and everybody in our city knows that if you are badly hurt in a car accident, you are as well off at the city hospital as any other, and you certainly don't want to go to a slick private hospital that is not specifically geared for a major trauma. For some other things, the city hospital is better too; although they may not have some of the amenities in the wards, there is usually a top-flight house staff, and that is often not true at community hospitals. So the quality argument is much more complex than we sometimes hear.

My final point has to do with the industry coalitions. I feel that coalitions often become discussion groups that don't move on specific targets. If the industry coalition doesn't involve the doctor who writes the orders, there isn't much chance for success. I spent several days, recently, talking with top AMA officials about how doctor–industry partnerships can work to contain costs. We are all worried about more and more governmental regulation, and although the doctor has been knocked a good bit in the press recently, most doctors want to give very good care to their patients. They put in many years to get very complex training. The private practice of medicine is on the line, and whether it will survive as we now know it depends upon whether we can exercise enough restraint, and at the same time keep up the kind and quality of health services that the public appears to want. An industry partnership with physicians could result in major breakthroughs.

Our Center for Industry and Health Care recently received a grant from the Hartford Foundation that lets us work in industries and, using claims forms data that are now used exclusively for paying purposes, lets us accumulate a data base that can be used to spot outlying hospitals and doctors. We will then work with the doctors in the area, presenting data to them for a utilization-control program. I have great faith in the private sector and the potential of industry–physician partnerships to contain costs without increasing regulation.

Diana Dutton

Like Dr. Egdahl, I too will begin with the warning that I am not an economist—as will probably become clear—nor am I a lawyer or a doctor, but rather a health sociologist. Consequently, I have a rather different point of view on some of the matters we have been discussing.

In reading the papers for this panel, particularly those by Munch-Danzon and Havighurst, I had two basic questions: (1) how valid are the economic models employed? and (2) would more competition really produce the benefits assumed? I will not try to answer these questions, but perhaps I can suggest why these papers also do not provide satisfactory answers.

First, how valid is the economic model? By validity, I mean how accurately does it reflect the forces which actually motivate people's behavior. Patricia Munch-Danzon's paper presents a very sophisticated mathematical analysis of a theoretical model, but the model includes only two variables: time and money. I do not see how such a model can be valid, for it vastly oversimplifies the nature of medical care transactions. Surely physicians, while certainly not devoid of venal instincts, allocate their time according to many factors in addition to personal financial gain. (Indeed, many physicians are deeply offended by the suggestion that financial considerations play *any* role in clinical decisions.) Considerable research indicates, in fact, that patterns of care reflect a complex set of factors including (in addition to economic incentives), professional, ethical, organizational, and personal considerations (Mechanic 1975; Dutton 1979; Eisenberg 1979).

For patients as well, many things are often more important than money in choosing a doctor or deciding to undergo a medical procedure. In fact, lacking any better evidence, patients may actually use price as an indicator of quality—the higher the price, the better the quality. If patients do react to medical prices in this way, either ignoring them or actually preferring higher prices, such behavior throws all the gears of the conventional economic model into reverse. Thus, not only does the scope of Munch-Danzon's analysis seem unduly narrow, but it may not even adequately represent the economic issues which it includes.

Munch-Danzon's model also involves a number of "simplifying" assumptions, some of which tax the imagination. For example, she assumes that "the charge and reimbursement for an office visit ... is independent of the amount of time spent"; that "demand depends only on the composite price ... and is insensitive to the division of the total price between the office visit and lab test components"; and "that the insurer's ceiling on allowed charges is an absolute ceiling and that the physician cannot bill the patient for any additional amount." Such assumptions are clearly at odds with the realities of medical practice, and one can only guess at how they affect the results.

In short, Munch-Danzon's portrayal of the physician as a "multiproduct firm facing an exogenously determined demand for its services" seems to be a serious distortion of the nature of health care transactions. If this theoretical model does not, in fact, adequately reflect the various peculiarities of patients' and physicians' behavior with respect to either economic or noneconomic factors, it does not provide a convincing basis for drawing policy conclusions.

That this model may yield plausible conclusions does not, per se, provide support for the model. Munch-Danzon's two general conclusions are very reasonable: (1) future health care reforms probably won't solve the dual problems of access and cost inflation; and (2) the use of lab tests and other technological procedures will increase at a higher rate than will total physician time. But these conclusions are hardly new and do not require special theoretical or mathematical analysis. Simple extrapolation from past experience would lead to the prediction that future reforms will fail to solve the problems of access and cost inflation. Most explanations of the continuing failure of such efforts point to a variety of political, social, cultural, and professional (as well as economic) forces.

The second prediction, that the use of lab tests will accelerate, could also be derived quite independently of the analyses Munch-Danzon presents. Noneconomic factors (such as the increasing emphasis on high technology practice in academic medical training, the psychological reassurance such tests give to both patients and doctors, and the prestige of high-technology medicine) play an important role, which can be distinguished from that of economic motives. Moreover, even the economic forces would seem to be more complex than indicated in Munch-Danzon's model, which deals primarily with physician behavior at the individual level. The focus on individuals ignores important forces which are more evident at the aggregate level, such as the aggressive promotional efforts of the drug industry (see, for example, Silverman 1976). Such efforts, which exceed mere response to demand (patients' or physicians'), play an important role in shaping attitudes toward desirable modes of practice.

At a more detailed level, I think the validity of some of Munch-Danzon's concepts is also open to question. One example is her use of the term "quality" to refer to a variable which she defines as the amount of physician time spent per patient visit multiplied by the number of laboratory tests ordered. This definition implies that the more tests ordered, the higher the quality. This implication is particularly unfortunate in light of the point made yesterday concerning the subtle but powerful ways in which terminology can shape our perceptions of issues. Equating more tests with higher quality runs directly counter to current policy efforts to promote greater concern for cost effectiveness. More seriously, it is probably also incorrect in many situations. Increasingly, evidence suggests that higher quality medicine sometimes involves fewer lab tests and procedures (Korvin et al. 1975; Spitzer and Brown 1975; Bergman 1977; Barkin et al. 1977).

Another example of terminology that I consider misleading (and its use extends far beyond Munch-Danzon's paper) is the concept of "consumer demand" in health care. To me, this term implies that patients rather than doctors control the bulk of decisions about health care utilization. Patients do control the initial decision to seek care during an episode of illness. After that, however, they rely heavily on doctors to tell them how soon and how often to return and what procedures to undergo. While patient compliance with doctors' orders is not perfect, achieving better compliance is a widely accepted goal among health policymakers. The concept of "demand" gives little recognition to the crucial role of physicians in influencing patients' behavior, a role which seriously undercuts the usual assumption of consumer sovereignty in the economic model.

Moreover, by focusing attention on patients rather than on physicians, this conceptualization diverts attention away from the factors that influence health care providers. The demand for health care is usually operationalized as the annual number of physician visits per person, combining patient-controlled and physician-controlled visits. Only when patient- and physician-controlled visits are distinguished is it possible to analyze the factors that increase or inhibit either. Empirical evidence indicates that these factors differ. For example, fee-for-service payment often creates a cost barrier which discourages patients from seeking care initially, while also creating a financial incentive for physicians to increase the volume of follow-up visits (Dutton 1979). Organizational and social factors also affect patients and physicians in different ways. The typical measure of demand—annual per capita visits—thus makes it difficult to identify the role of factors which have a differential impact on patients and physicians.

Let me now turn to my second question concerning these papers: would more competition produce the benefits assumed? As Clark Havighurst notes, "It is possible to doubt the premise that enhanced competition . . . can bring about changes in health care financing and delivery that . . . will all be desirable." Of course, Havighurst labels people who raise such doubts as "victims of a planning mentality." I think it is important to note that, Havighurst's intent notwithstanding, "a planning mentality" is not considered a mark of disrepute in many academic and policy circles. Indeed, planning is an essential step in designing appropriate social policy, and should include careful and critical examination of the expected consequences of many different policy options. Some situations will call for market solutions; others will require regulatory approaches, and still others may call for yet-untried alternatives. It would be irresponsible not to question the benefits of different options in trying to find the policy which best fits the particular circumstances and seems most likely to yield the desired results.

The way that Havighurst disposes of doubts about the benefits of competition is also somewhat cavalier. He begins by arguing that there are no benchmarks for judging the outcomes of health care delivery, and so only the process involved can be judged; in fact, really only one aspect of the process—whether or not "people are spending their own rather than the government's money." Thus he contends that only when people pay for the care themselves can we be sure that they are getting what they want. The catch is that this system only works if certain market conditions are, as he notes, reasonably well satisfied. These conditions are simply the standard requirements of the competitive model of economic theory: "that the supply side of the market not be precluded from making a full range of choices available and that the demand side not reflect biases artificially induced by government." (He does not mention other sources of bias besides the government, such as deceptive marketing practices, inadequate information, discrimination by providers, the convergence of low income and severe illness, and so on.) But restating the theory does not make it any more relevant to reality, and ample evidence has been presented at this conference and elsewhere to indicate that the realities of health care often diverge sharply from the ideal conditions of economic theory. Many of the doubts about the benefits of competition hinge on the perceived failure of these conditions in the real world. Thus, restating the theoretical conditions without addressing how they will be fulfilled in practice can hardly be said to dispose of such doubts. Once again, the economic theory seems to float untrammelled over the awkward realities of health care.

Turning now from theory to data, let us examine Havighurst's contention that when people spend their own money, they get what they want. Table 15.1 and figure 15.1 bear on this point. Table 15.1 lists

TABLE 15.1

Average annual out-of-pocket health expenses for persons with such expense, and proportion with expenses, by type of expense and family income (United States, 1975)

| Family income | Average expense in dollars | | All types of expense (including insurance premium) | Average annual expenses (all types), as percent of family income | Percent of income group with health expense during year |
	Hospital	Doctor			
All persons	264	107	285	2.1	86
Less than $3,000	714	156	345	17.3	65
$3,000–$4,999	457	141	355	8.9	72
$5,000–$6,999	333	120	303	5.6	76
$7,000–$9,999	262	117	282	3.3	85
$10,000–$14,999	239	96	263	2.1	91
$15,000 or more	179	98	275	1.5	93

Source: Adapted from NCHS 10:122, 1978, pp. 27 and 31.

the average annual out-of-pocket health expenses for persons with expenses by family income, and as a proportion of income; it also shows the proportion of families at each income level with expenses. These data indicate that, despite Medicaid and other public programs, out-of-pocket expenses for people with expenses are much higher among the poor than among the more affluent (consuming 17.3 percent versus 1.5 percent of family income, respectively). Moreover, a sizeable proportion (65 percent) of the poor had some health expenses, meaning that the majority of the poor had to bear this disproportionate burden of

FIGURE 15.1

Percent more dissatisfied than the median person in the national population with aspects of medical care by family income level (CHAS national sample, 1976)

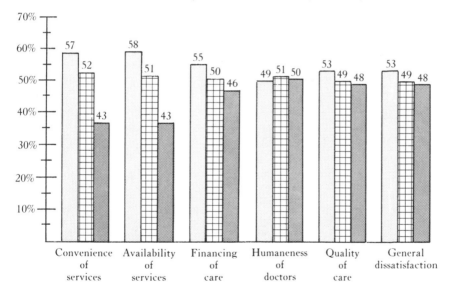

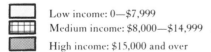

Low income: 0—$7,999
Medium income: $8,000—$14,999
High income: $15,000 and over

Source: Aday, L.A., Andersen, R., and Fleming, G.: *Health Care in the U.S.: Equitable for Whom?* Table 4.2, p. 150. Copyright 1980 Sage Publications, Beverly Hills, CA, with permission of the publisher.

health costs. Figure 15.1 compares various measures of satisfaction with medical care reported by persons of different income levels; it shows that on almost every measure, the poor were more dissatisfied than the more affluent. For the poor, therefore, it is clear that spending their own money for health care is no guarantee of getting the kind of care they want.

An important reason for the greater dissatisfaction among the poor is probably that they tend to use different sources of care. As seen in table 15.2, the poor are far more likely than others to be seen in hospital clinics than in doctors' offices. These patterns often reflect practical necessities, and not personal preferences; private doctors are less likely to locate in low-income areas, and many are unwilling to treat patients on Medicaid. Table 15.2 also shows that telephone contacts

TABLE 15.2

Physician visits of children under age 18 in the United States
(average annual 1975-76)[a]

Family income and race	Visits per 1,000 children under age 18	Percent of visits occurring		
		In doctor's office[b]	In hospital outpatient clinics[c]	By telephone
All children[d]	4,204	64.0	13.1	17.8
Family income				
Less than $5,000	4,324	55.8	23.0	11.1
$5,000–$9,999	3,702	57.4	20.7	13.3
$10,000–$14,999	4,096	65.1	12.5	18.3
$15,000 or more	4,449	67.1	9.3	20.0
Race				
White	4,289	65.3	11.9	18.2
Nonwhite	3,254	50.9	29.1	8.5

a.   Data are based on household interviews of a sample of the civilian noninstitutionalized population.

b.   Includes private doctor's office, doctor's clinic, and group practice.

c.   Includes hospital outpatient departments and emergency rooms.

d.   Based on children under age 15 in 1976.

Source: DHEW, *Health: United States*, 1978, p. 270.

(the least expensive and most convenient form of medical care) are much more common among the affluent than among the poor. Even though the poor, with higher levels of disability and lower levels of health knowledge, could probably benefit most from the advantages of telephone advice, they are currently the least likely to receive it.

In addition, the use of hospital clinics as a source of primary care is growing at the fastest rate among children, the poor, and minorities. These are the very groups who most need access to preventive, comprehensive, and continuous primary care, which many hospital clinics are poorly suited to provide. More competition seems unlikely to solve such basic structural problems of geographic access and fragmentation. Indeed, increased cost sharing might even make matters worse for the poor by adding further strain to their already limited financial resources and doing nothing to counteract physicians' disinclination to practice in rural or inner-city poverty areas.

But perhaps there is another way to look at the problem. Even if there are presently many individuals who are spending their own money on health care and not getting what they want, perhaps society gets what it wants—perhaps the resulting patterns of care represent a kind of societal optimum. One way to explore this possibility is to examine how charges and other kinds of barriers affect use rates, particularly those of the poor. (Surprisingly, there appears to have been very little empirical research in the economics literature testing the seemingly plausible hypothesis that the poor have a different—more negative—price elasticity of demand than the nonpoor.)

Table 15.3 presents some empirical evidence on this point based on regression analyses of survey data from Washington, D.C. (For further detail, see Dutton 1979.) These results indicate how particular financial and organizational barriers as well as the use of different ambulatory care settings affect the frequency of children's preventive examinations. The model also tests whether or not each of four barriers (price, distance, office waiting time, and appointment lead time) has a differential effect on poor children. I focus here on children's preventive care because regular physical examinations are widely agreed to be an essential part of good primary care for all children, but especially for low-income children who are at special risk for nutritional deficiencies and developmental disorders.

The results in table 15.3 suggest that among this sample of children,

TABLE 15.3

Estimated effects of various financial and organizational barriers and type of regular provider on frequency of children's preventive checkups (Washington, D.C., 1971 sample)

Independent variables	**Dependent variable** (Frequency with which children are taken for preventive health examinations) Standardized regression coefficient	(F value)
Barriers		
Relative charge index (based on average of charges for pediatric exam, treatment of ear infection, urinalysis, hemoglobin, and throat culture)	.224[a]	(16.43)
Relative charge index (poverty children difference)	−.129[a]	(9.09)
Distance to provider (miles)	−.006	(0.03)
Distance to provider (poverty children difference)	−.058[b]	(2.22)
Office waiting time (minutes)	−.114[a]	(8.68)
Office waiting time (poverty children difference)	.091[b]	(3.78)
Lead time to get appointment (days)	.048	(1.38)
Lead time to get appointment (poverty children difference)	.025	(0.34)
Mixed income practice (0=low income only, 1=mixed income)	.123[a]	(17.09)

Type of regular provider setting

Solo fee-for-service practice (omitted variable)		
Group fee-for-service practice	−.004	(0.01)
Prepaid group practice	.172[a]	(23.46)
Public clinics	.123[a]	(6.18)
Hospital outpatient departments	−.045	(1.86)
Hospital emergency rooms	−.114[a]	(17.95)

$R^2 = .247$

$N = 1409$

a. p<.01
b. p<.10

Note: The department variable was coded: 1=never, 2=when needed, 3=every year, 4=every 6 months. The OLS regression model also contained variables representing child's age, sex, first-or-subsequent child, race, age and sex of head of house, family size, income, education of mother, blue- or while-collar occupational status of head of house, length of residence in Washington D.C., welfare coverage, and private health insurance.

the single most important cause of infrequent preventive exams was the use of hospital emergency rooms as a regular source of care. These results control for patient group differences as well as particular financial and organizational barriers. At the opposite extreme were children using the prepaid group practices, who were significantly more likely to have preventive exams than children using any other setting.

Another very important determinant was the economic level of the patient clientele (regardless of practice setting); children in predominately low-income practices had significantly lower rates of preventive care than those where patient clienteles were mixed.

Of the specific barriers, the charge index had the greatest differential effect on poor children (although overall higher charges were associated with higher rates of preventive care for both poor and nonpoor children). There was also weak evidence that both distance and office waiting time affected poor children's rates of preventive care differentially; distance had a stronger negative impact on poor than nonpoor children, while office waiting time had a less strong negative impact on poor children.

These results illustrate a situation which is well known and widely documented: despite Medicaid and other public programs, the poor and minorities bear the brunt of current deficiencies in health care organization and financing. For the poor, such deficiencies make access to adequate care difficult to impossible. The irony of the situation is that it is precisely these disadvantaged groups who, with higher levels of illness and unmet medical needs, would most benefit from greater access. The current distribution of access barriers (both cost-sharing and organizational factors) thus produce a distribution of services that varies inversely with medical need. This is a far cry from what most people would consider to be a societal optimum.

But this situation is not only inequitable, it is also socially inefficient. True efficiency—defined as achieving maximum health benefits from the available medical resources—would require that care be allocated according to potential medical benefit (or, roughly speaking, medical need). The present mismatch between the distribution of care according to need and its actual potential for cure results in large part from a highly skewed distribution of access barriers and other structural problems. But it also reflects a fundamental flaw in the operation of the "market model" in health care; namely, that consumer preferences provide an unreliable measure of true clinical need (or potential for therapeutic benefit). As extensive sociological research has shown, perceptions of symptoms and attitudes toward the use of medical care are conditioned by various social and cultural factors and are often quite unrelated to (objectively defined) therapeutic need (Zola 1966; Linn et al. 1980). Therefore, distributing services according to consumer preferences—the only legitimate currency of the market model—may not result in a very good match between care and cure. Cost sharing, if it bears most heavily on the poor, as is likely, will only make matters worse.

The likely consequences of the competitive market model in health care are well summarized in the following quote from Paul Ellwood in the HMO Act of 1972: "The emergence of a free market economy could stimulate a course of change in the health industry that would have some of the classical aspects of the industrial revolution—conversion to larger units of production, technological innovation, division of labor, substitution of capital for labor, vigorous competition, and profitability as the mandatory condition for survival" (Roy 1972, p. 250). But are these the conditions society wants to promote in health care? Massive hospital complexes and large group practices are already frequently criticized for being excessively bureaucratic, rigid, and alienating. Technological innovation and other forms of substitution of capital for labor, while the source of many medical marvels, have also been the bane of cost control and have contributed to deteriorating doctor–patient relationships. Division of labor and the resulting professional specialization have further compounded problems of communication and fragmentation, threatening the survival of comprehensive, family-oriented care. Vigorous competition, with profitability as the condition for survival, is indeed likely to foster care that is profitable (for doctors); but without strict controls, such competition is likely to expand services in areas where consumer perceptions of needs are vulnerable to influence, such as cosmetic surgery and other elective luxury procedures. And, based on evidence to date, there is little reason to expect competition to meet the needs of the poor. Indeed, in assessing the relative success of various public programs for the poor, Foltz (1980) concludes that "one factor which seems to help public programs to function is the *absence* of competition from the private sector" (p. 54, emphasis added). In short, existing evidence about how each of the "classical aspects of the industrial revolution" has affected health care appears to be, at best, mixed. It is important for those who advocate stimulating competition and further development of industrialization in health care to address the negative as well as the positive aspects of the experiences to date and to propose creative ways to minimize the negative consequences in the future.

Chapter 15 References

Aday, L. A.; Andersen, R.; and Fleming, G. 1980. *Health Care in the U.S.: Equitable for Whom?* Beverly Hills: Sage.

Barkin, J.; Vining, D.; Miale, A., Jr.; Gottlieb, S.; Redhammer, D. E.; and Kaiser, M. H. 1977. "Computerized tomography, diagnostic ultrasound and radionuclide scanning. Comparison of efficacy in diagnosis of pancreatic carcinoma." *JAMA* 238:2040.

Bergman, A. B. 1977. "The menace of mass screening." *American Journal of Public Health* 67:601.

Bloomgarden, Z., and Sidel, V. W. 1980. "Evaluation of utilization of laboratory tests in a hospital emergency room." *American Journal of Public Health* 70(5):525.

Dutton, D. B. 1979. "Patterns of ambulatory health care in five different delivery systems." *Medical Care* 17(3):221.

Eisenberg, John. 1979. "Sociologic Influences on Decisionmaking by Clinicians." *Annals of Internal Medicine* 90:957–64.

Foltz, A-M. 1980. "The organization and financing of child health services." Paper prepared for the Select Panel for the Promotion of Child Health, U.S. Department of Health, Education, and Welfare (March 1980).

Holman, H. R.; Hopkins, J.; and Ewy, J. 1980. "Seeking effective, efficient and equitable health care." Paper presented at Health Services Research Seminar, Stanford University (March 31, 1980).

Korvin, C. C.; Pearce, R. H.; and Stanley, J. 1975. "Admissions screening: clinical benefits." *Annals of Internal Medicine* 83:197.

Linn, M. W.; Hunter, K. I.; Linn, B. S. 1980. "Self-assessed health, impairment and disability in Anglo, Black and Cuban elderly." *Medical Care* 18(3):282.

Roy, W. R. 1972. *The Proposed Health Maintenance Organization Act of 1972.* Sourcebook Series Vol. 2. (Washington, D.C.: The Science and Health Communications Group.) p. 250, appendix XI.

Silverman, M. 1976. *The Drugging of the Americas*. Berkeley: University of California Press.

Spitzer, W. O., and Brown B. P. 1975. "Unanswered questions about the periodic health examination." *Annals of Internal Medicine* 83:257.

Zola, I. K. 1966. "Culture and symptoms—an analysis of patients' presenting complaints." *American Sociological Review* 31:615.

General Discussion of Section III

Clark Havighurst's Paper

Havighurst

First of all, the multiple-choice idea doesn't require that we have closed-panel plans already available. The requirement would be that three options of any kind be offered. The hope is that such a requirement would stimulate the creation of new plans, but I agree that it is a lot 'to hope that there will be such plans in every community any time soon. I am not as interested in promoting the traditional kinds of closed panels, such as HMOs, as I am in encouraging other kinds of innovation in the insurance system. It seems to me that if we could increase the competitive pressures on insurers to provide somewhat different products, such innovations would happen.

As to the question of whether individual choice will really result in significantly less comprehensive coverage, I agree there is evidence that some people sometimes seem irrational. It is usually a better policy, however, to allow people to be irrational than to maintain a system that is irrational and that subsidizes irrational behavior. In line with what Diana said, my argument was that if you get the incentives right and still perceive that people are making foolish decisions and buying more insurance than you think they should, that perception provides no clear basis for intervention to require them to take less or to devalue what they have purchased by back-door regulation of the supply side. It seems to me that it would be hard to make a case for intervention if people were spending their own money in ways that suit them, particularly if they were getting more care than we would regard as appropriate for them. People spending their own money have an incentive to learn of economizing opportunities, and we should probably regard decisions to overinsure (as we perceive it) as expressions of individuals' preferences. The public's role should be confined to assuring a full range of choice and accurate information.

Dick Egdahl's comments raise one very large and important question. He points out that the medical profession is working hard at providing information and leadership in an effort to change physician practices at the local level. The Voluntary Effort was cited, and there are other reasons to conclude that the medical profession is indeed trying harder than ever before. But let us ask why. Why does organized medicine let progressive doctors like Dick Egdahl work to improve efficiency and lower costs? It must be that they feel threatened politically and feel that there is a need to present a better image to the world than they have done in the past. But it doesn't seem realistic to expect a medical organization allied with organized medicine to behave as a totally benign monopoly. To my mind, this "partnership-with-physicians" notion is just asking us to trust the doctors.

The Wausau HMO has probably done fine things. But why do all the doctors in Wausau have to be in the same health plan? Why can't we have a number of such plans? I agree that doctors have to be organized better than they are, but not all in one plan. It seems to me that competing plans could provide all the benefits of integration without the costs that are associated with monopoly and could provide a much greater assurance that changes beneficial to consumers will be stimulated.

One should not, of course, be too cynical about the medical profession's efforts. Many individuals working in the Voluntary Effort and the Individual Practice Association (IPA) movement are doing so for impeccable reasons. Moreover, the medical profession's efforts to improve the quality of information and to emphasize cost considerations are worthwhile and deserving of respect. But the notion that somehow this information will eventually trickle down to practice and that doctors will bring their behavior into line with consumers' interests is not satisfying and is certainly no substitute for competition. For this reason, I strongly support using the antitrust laws to limit collective professional efforts affecting price and utilization. Aside from efforts to improve the quality of information, I see real dangers in profession-sponsored reforms. They perpetuate the traditional view that there is "one right way," which we look to the profession to define. I have every confidence that it would be a better world if people were given the chance to opt out of the system designed by the medical profession, and if professionals and others could offer new alternatives. That is what we are talking about when we stress the need for competing systems that offer the consumers opportunities to gratify their different preferences. Diana Dutton's remarks attach no importance to the idea that preferences differ, but I think it is an important fact. People ought to be allowed to register their preferences but should pay the differences if their preference involves a higher cost.

Finally, what I said had really nothing to do with the problems of the poor, which Diana addressed. This society probably wants to do somewhat more for the poor than has been done, but the problem is to define what the appropriate minimum of medical care is. There is no question that we must face the choice between defining an appropriate minimum and embracing what Uwe Reinhardt calls the solidarity principle, which would put us all in the same boat. Only the former is compatible with maintaining a competitive system; but there should be no doubt that adopting competition as a strategy leaves plenty of room for the government to subsidize care for the poor better than it does now, thus assuring reasonable access for those who cannot pay their own way. Certainly more comprehensive benefits and less cost sharing are appropriate for low-income people. Ideally, I have yet to see any reason why a workable voucher system could not be designed to meet the needs of public beneficiaries.

Perlman

I think one point that has come from this morning's discussion is that there is no essential contradiction between Egdahl's and Havighurst's positions, unless you assume that the discussions between parties are discussions between bilateral monopolies and are secret. If these discussions are open (and that, after all, is what Egdahl is talking about), you have a kind of situation that is not the conventional bilateral monopoly picture. I think this is one point that Egdahl is making very strongly, and his position is not in contradiction to Havighurst's; it just builds on the assumption that there will be publicity given to the discussion.

The argument about the Wausau HMO is that the discussion is insufficiently open. If it were sufficiently open, who cares whether they are all members of one IPA or not? You have given an opportunity for counter-organization.

Havighurst

I still think there is a difference between Egdahl and myself that is probably irreconcilable. I would prefer not to rely on keeping political pressure—even stronger political pressure—on the medical profession as the main vehicle for promoting change. The competitive process provides a stronger force for change because we don't have to persuade them to go along. While I think we need both forms of pressure, I don't think we can put enough political pressure on to do the job consistently and effectively over time.

Egdahl

My key point on Wausau is that the insurance industry, not the doctors, set up a plan for their own employees (the Employers Insurance of Wausau), and then they extended it to everybody else. This is a voluntary plan, and I think it is better than more regulation. The Employers Insurance of Wausau had every doctor look at every other doctor's admitting practice—all 105—and ancillary use patterns, and this changed things radically. It wasn't just a change in the IPA work of the doctors, but a very radical change in terms of the other types of master medical work they did.

Havighurst

My problem is still that the insurance companies who set up the Wausau arrangement had no alternatives. The medical profession wouldn't have tolerated a system that split the doctors into competing groups, and that is why the insurers chose the method they did. That is just the way you do business with the medical profession. You treat it as a monopoly, you address it as such, and try to persuade it to do things more the way you want them done. But, if you can't persuade them, you have no alternative. Competition allows you to deal with providers individually and in groups—not as a monopoly—and that is the only way for the consumer to get all the changes he is entitled to.

Patricia Munch-Danzon's Paper

Munch-Danzon

First, I'd like to respond to the suggestion that I was implying that physicians only respond to money. I certainly didn't mean to imply that. It is one factor among others. It is an empirical question how important money is relative to other things.

I have done an empirical analysis of the use of lab tests by physicians and the prices they charge. I find that both the frequency of tests and the prices charged for these tests are responsive to economic factors, such as the insurance coverage of the patient, the cost of tests to the physician, and the cost of malpractice insurance premiums. I also find that the frequency of tests is affected and constrained by medical factors too. There are substantial differences across specialties, which would not exist if physicians had the ability to prescribe as many tests as they wanted to; so one does find empirically that physicians respond to both medical and economic factors.

Second, on the question of whether using more tests means higher quality. In the paper, I explicitly define quality as the expected quality as perceived by the patient. I admit this type of quality may differ from some objective quality, that in some cases the marginal value of some tests may be negative because of false results. I disagree, though, that on average the expected value should be negative, unless there is substantial consumer ignorance. If there is consumer ignorance, the ignorance applies to all forms of health care and is not confined to lab tests.

I do agree that we probably have reached the point where, relative to physician time, we have too much testing—that we have become too test-intensive in the production of health care. I would argue that this has been induced by the reimbursement system, and we would be better off with somewhat more time in contact with the physician and fewer tests. If Diana agrees that we have too many tests but says physicians are not responding to economic factors but rather to medical factors, then how does she explain their excessive use of tests?

Finally, on whether models are necessary or useful in predicting things that are obvious (for example, that in the past we didn't get control of inflation or equal access, and therefore in the future we won't get them either): the point of the model is to try to isolate those factors in past institutional arrangements that led to the results that we didn't like, in order to prevent the recurrence of those results in the future. It is only by systematic thinking about what occurred in the past that we can hope to improve the future.

Ricardo-Campbell

As chairman, I want to comment briefly about the demand for medical care and consumers' influence on that demand.

The demand for medical care is largely a demand for chronic disease care. It is not demand for emergency care, where the physician has full control over utilization because the patient may be unconscious or because the patient is so upset by the emergency that he cannot influence his own demand. Eighty percent of medical care is for chronic disease. Here the patient does have some control over utilization of medical care. In the surplus physician areas of the United States—Palo Alto is one of them and Boston is another—some physicians recycle patients with chronic disease too frequently. They rationalize this mode of practice with the knowledge that, eventually, persons with a chronic disease will need a return visit and, as physicians, they know best the preferred timing. However, lengths of remissions vary. By timing return visits more frequently than the patients would set them on their own, physicians create their own demand. However, some patients go back only when they feel that they should go back. Those patients do have an influence on demand, and this has been documented.

Moreover, if you look at the drug sector, compliance in filling prescriptions or renewing prescriptions is entirely within the patients' control. Eight to ten percent of the health care dollar in the United States is spent on drugs. Drugs can be substitutes for medical treatment, hospital days, and surgery and are often complementary to other forms of medical care. Patients probably have more influence on demand than was suggested by Diana.

Dutton

I have three brief responses to the points which were just made. First, whether the average expected value of tests would on average be positive or negative is, I think, an open question. But some actual experiences in health care settings suggest that the value of tests is generally less than believed and may actually be negative in some cases. For example, the Division of Immunology here at Stanford began to cut back over the last decade on the amount of testing done and in the use of medications. They found that their patient mortality and morbidity rates improved, and their costs decreased. Another encouraging experience along the same lines is a local health plan (Mid-Peninsula Health Service), which is experimenting with ways to cut down on testing and institutional health care. Only preliminary results are available so far, but they are consistent with the claim that it is possible to reduce the use of tests and other forms of medical intervention, and at the same time to improve health levels and reduce costs (Holman, et al. 1980). A recent study of the use of lab tests in a teaching hospital emergency room concluded that "the number of tests per visit showed a strong negative correlation with the necessity and with the quality of care" (Bloomgarden and Sidel, *AJPH*, 1980, p. 525).

The second point is by way of clarification: I certainly didn't intend to suggest that economic factors don't affect both patients and physicians; they do. But it is still important to keep the role of such factors in perspective. My view is that a model of either patient or physician behavior which deals solely with economic factors will often be inadequate, and that a more comprehensive model is more likely to produce reliable conclusions because such a model can more accurately represent the complexity of reality.

Third, in response to Rita's point, I also didn't mean to suggest that patients don't have any control over utilization decisions, even in the follow-up visit stage. Again, I think it is a question of degree. It is true that the bulk of patient visits now are for chronic disease, but I think that even in chronic care, the balance of control between patients and providers remains quite unequal. Patients are still heavily dependent on their physicians for the initial determination of the course of treatment, and, later on, for guidance in handling new stages of the disease as it evolves as well as for unforeseen circumstances that inevitably arise. In other words, the physician plays a more important part in determining patients' patterns of utilization, even in the care of chronic disease, than the passive role implied in the economic theory of consumer demand.

Ingbar

I just wanted to pursue some of the problems that our discussion on laboratory tests illustrates. Some very broad questions go back to the point that we now have a different market structure in the health services sector. We have inserted an insurer between our consumer and our producer. We have created a different kind of big buyer and big producer structure, and we have individual consumers. What do we really want our reimbursement structure to do? Should insurance like Blue Cross, Medicare, or Medicaid go into the business of monitoring the numbers of tests?

Munch-Danzon

I would argue that this is prohibitively costly. The average test costs maybe $5.00, and monitoring tests would cost as much as it would to prevent them.

Ingbar

We are looking at a bill-paying system left over from a time when individuals paid the bills. We are not asking how equitable is the reimbursement structure, which we should. If we want solidarity, that's one thing. If we want Medicare to pay in proportion to resources used by Medicare participants, that's another. But our billing structure is one in which the bill is allegedly somehow proportional to the resources used by an individual person, when in fact I think you can question this. Even without that, you can ask, what services are we really buying? Are we buying lab tests, days of care, an episode of illness, or are we maybe buying time requisitions? We really have got to stop looking at a fee schedule that was constructed when the individual patient paid the bill. We should ask what the price is for.

Of course, once we begin to ask what the equity of the reimbursement is from the payer's point of view or what is the best device to use in defining a service, we also must ask, what is the best way to pay providers? We may decide that we want to pay them on the basis of some revamped service, say on the basis of time.

Pat's paper mentions a point that to me is probably the most disastrous aspect of the original Medicare–Medicaid legislation: the Part A–Part B distinctions, which, under the guise of trying to ensure equity for everyone, called for a private physician for everyone. It sounds great, but in fact the whole notion of delegation of authority and responsibility that had been going on beautifully in the teaching hospitals was eliminated. It transformed a teaching hospital from a salary deal into a fee-for-care system. This fee-for-care system doesn't show up because people are officially paid a salary, but they have to earn their salary through group practices.

Goldbeck

I just want to make a comment on whether or not it is worthwhile to supply some form of review process and scrutiny to the testing side of the agenda. From the payer's standpoint, I completely disagree with what Munch-Danzon has said for several reasons. One, if we put up the signal that we're not going to apply any scrutiny in the entire spectrum of provider care, then that is where most of the fraud, abuse, and overutilization will take place, because these are very clearly what human behavior leads to. Second, we are not just talking about saving the cost of one test. We generate a change in the behavior of providers once the attitude of scrutiny has been applied. We see this in systems where some scrutiny already exists. There is a big spillover effect, and it is very beneficial.

I think that you have to look at a larger set of costs than just the price of that individual test. There is a negative side: a cost to the people who are made ill from unnecessary testing, the people who die from unnecessary testing, and the people who have to spend an extra day in the hospital for unnecessary testing. There is the $25 test that necessitates hospitalization the night before. The scrutiny is not just to save the $25—it is to save the $310 lodging/hotel charge. We need to apply scrutiny to every element of the system.

Munch-Danzon

I agree that you might initially get some reduction in tests if you let it be known that you are going to monitor them, but that bluff is only going to work in the short run. You have to go ahead and consistently monitor the medical system for this benefit to persist. Then you have the costs of actually determining how many tests are being done for each episode of illness and whether or not that number is appropriate. Monitoring the tests may be worthwhile. I haven't done any cost-benefit analysis. But it looks certainly more worthwhile for procedures that are relatively costly, simply because there is a fixed cost in monitoring anything, and the larger the cost of the procedure relative to the fixed monitoring cost, the more worthwhile the monitoring.

I agree that there are other costs associated with the excess tests. Whether there are more such costs resulting from tests than from other forms of medical intervention is not clear. It is well known that medical science is imperfect and that there are some adverse consequences from tests, surgeries, or anything else. The question is whether the expected value is positive; and I see no reason why the expected value of tests should be negative when the expected value we assume for all other forms of health care is positive.

Willis Goldbeck's Paper

Seidman

I have two brief comments: one for Diana and one for Willis. I agree with Diana that cost sharing that is unrelated to income would be inequitable. The whole point of the tax credit was to scale the cost sharing to a patient's ability to pay, so I hope she would recognize this new possibility. Second, the poor as well as the affluent suffer from the alternative, which is a system of rationing under regulation. As a matter of fact, I think you could argue that when you have limited supplies under a rationing system, the poor are likely to suffer more than the affluent because they don't have the means to get to the head of the queue.

Willis cited evidence that when people are given the choice, they choose the more comprehensive insurance. I would re-emphasize that this occurs only under the current, very substantial tax subsidy. There is no evidence of what would happen if the latter were removed.

Phelps

I want to make a general comment on Willis's paper. Something he said in these talks carries over into what Diana has said about Patricia's paper, (to which I think Pat adequately responded). It was, in some sense, a rejection of scientific methods as being useful. Willis said that there was a reduction in hospital days that was attainable, although there were no statistical tests to verify it, and that every employer could achieve this reduction. I would like to argue here that it is not necessarily good to leap before you look. I can cite several examples of things intuitively desirable at first glance that turned out to be otherwise. I'm also relating back to my discussion of Larry Seidman's paper. It was intuitively obvious to everyone for years, decades in fact, that if you increase the coverage for ambulatory care, expenditure on hospital utilization would fall, because it would save unnecessary hospitalization. Everyone believed that premise, until it was actually studied in the Blue Cross–Blue Shield Plan in Kansas and turned out not to be true.

Everybody also intuitively believed that preventive medical care was desirable in reducing medical expenses. That is a very explicit assumption made by Diana in her discussion of limited access of the poor to preventive care and in some of the tables she presented. That assumption also turns out to be empirically testable, and Proctor at the University of Utah tested that. The results of Proctor's test showed that when people were enrolled in a comprehensive, preventive screening program, that program did not change their medical expenditures, their number of hospitalizations, their number of hospital days, or their sick days off work. I would like to urge that we stop relying on intuition and start relying on data, when we can. I believe that we will make better-informed decisions when we do that.

On Rationing

Pierce

I would like to comment on rationing, as it has been brought up yesterday and just now—rationing via queues. As an epidemiologist, I know of very little evidence that many medical or surgical procedures have any major effect on health outcome. Queues do not exist when there is indication that the promptness of the medical service has an effect on the health outcome. So queuing is a very effective rationing system in cases where there is no such indication, and the fact that the rich can jump the queue doesn't really matter in terms of the health outcome to the patient.

Seidman

It depends on whose perception you seek. To the person who is waiting on queue, thinking immediate care might well make a difference, the fact that ultimately you could prove that in a particular case it didn't matter is not the central issue. The central issue is that there is a worried individual who might be willing to bear at least a good part of the cost to get that service. If a person wanted to buy a luxury refrigerator, we wouldn't regulate and say: no, you have to wait. But we are moving with our health care system to a point where we will say to the person: never mind the fact that you're worrying for three months; the data show that in 80 percent of the cases immediate care really doesn't make any difference. The individual's subjective feelings are being ignored because somebody is saying that the system knows better. We should be sensitive to the individual patient, not simply look at what is supposedly best for the system in a majority of cases.

Phelps

When we exchange money for a service, that exchange itself does not consume real resources. When we use queuing as a rationing device, the value of that time is in fact a deadweight loss to society. Exactly the same argument applies to gasoline lines in this country.

Ricardo-Campbell

I would just like to comment a little further. There are different types of time costs, and waiting for a hospital bed is slightly less costly sometimes than physically waiting in line. Sometimes, while you wait for a hospital bed you can still work—less efficiently, presumably, but you can function. The time you spend waiting in a physician's office, unless you are able to do work while you are waiting, is a complete dead-weight loss. There is also the structuring or lessening of the demand for care via waiting. An example is the Health Insurance Plan, the largest prepaid group medical plan in Washington, D.C., whose director was quoted in the *AMA News,* and by others, as saying that the average wait for an appointment to see a specialist was about twelve weeks, including an appointment with an OB/GYN physician. This is a form of waiting that creates anxiety costs to the consumer.

Diana Dutton's Comment

Anderson

I was fascinated by table 15.1, which Diana Dutton presented. If I read the table correctly, it means that poor families with incomes of less than $3,000 will pay more than 25 percent of their income in out-of-pocket expenses when they go to the hospital. I assume that this is in addition to whatever payments they get from insurance and Medicare. I wonder if you could tell me what the source of that table is and if you would comment on the validity of the table.

Dutton

The total out-of-pocket expenses paid by poor families (incomes under $3,000) averages 17 percent of their annual income. The source of these data is the National Center for Health Statistics (NCHS). Dorothy Rice, the Director of the Center, is probably in the best position to comment on the validity of the data.

Rice

The data are valid.

Anderson

With Medicaid and other public funding programs, how is it possible that the poor have such high levels of out-of-pocket expenses? Where do families with annual incomes of only $3,000 get the money to pay $714 for hospitalization expenses during the year?

Dutton

You are assuming that all of the poor have Medicaid. Actually, only about half of the poor are on Medicaid at any one time. (Davis and Schoen 1978, p. 54).

Anderson

In table 15.1 of your paper (Dutton's), how can the average annual expense for all types of expenses be lower than the figure for the hospitalization component alone?

Dutton

The average annual expense for all types of expenses is based on all people who had any health expense at all during the year, and this includes many people who had only minor expenses, such as dental care or drugs. Thus, the average expenditure level is lower than that of people who had hospitalization expenses, which were generally much higher. In other words, the average for all types of expenses is lower but applies to more people, while the average for hospitalization expenses is higher and applies to fewer people.

Phelps

Many people with incomes of $3,000 or less who are hospitalized are retired people. They are on Medicare, which could very well pay for hospital and medical bills, as we know.

The second point I want to make about table 15.1 (of Dutton's paper) is that the column labeled "All types of expense including insurance premiums," is misleading. It does not include the premium payment made by families or by employers on behalf of families, which is a substitute for income. In fact, the effect of the employer paying the premium is that a worker's income in the table is lowered by the cost of the premium paid by the employer. To use these figures to suggest that these levels of out-of-pocket expenses are declining by income is completely misstating the facts.

Rice

We are well aware of the limitations of the information that came through the National Health Statistics Survey, but we did make up a National Medical Care Expenditure Survey, which will indeed provide the critical figures. We're just now beginning to analyze this information.

Postscript (Ricardo-Campbell)

Because table 15.1 of Diana Dutton's comments was criticized by several persons at the conference, the chairperson of the session wrote to Dorothy Rice, Director of the National Center for Health Statistics (DHEW), for her official comment. Two excerpts from her letter follow.

> The $714 estimate of personal out-of-pocket expenses for persons with [hospital] expenses among those with an annual family income of under $3,000 has a relative standard error of about 13 percent. This means that the 95 percent confidence interval of the estimate ranges from about $530 to $900.

Moreover,

> given the size of the sampling error, there is no statistically significant difference between the estimates [of personal expenses among those with incomes below $3,000 and $5,000].

To this it probably should be added that the major problem in reading this table is that each column of figures refers to a different group of people, which is unusual in statistical tables. As Diana Dutton explained, "The average for all types of expenses is lower but applies to more people, while the average for hospitalization expense is higher and applies to fewer people." Thus, persons whose health expenses are averaged in the "All types of expense" column may or may not have had any out-of-pocket expenses for hospital care; some may have had only prescription drug expense or dental care expense.

It is important to remember, too, that the lowest income category (less than $3,000) would include persons over 65 on Medicare whose out-of-pocket expenses for hospitalization are higher on the average than those of young adults or children (both because they are hospitalized more frequently and because Medicare pays only 40 percent of their bills).

Chapter 16 References

Davis, Karen, and Schoen, Cathy. 1978. *Health and the War on Poverty: A Ten-Year Appraisal*. Washington, D.C.: Brookings Institution.

Epilog: Can Anything Be Done About Health Care Costs?

*Caspar Weinberger**

Initially, I had thought that the title of my dinner talk should be "Controlling Health Care Costs," but that implied a degree of optimism which, on further reflection, I don't think I have. Mark Twain once said that an optimist is one who thinks that things can't get any worse, and I don't know, under the circumstances, that I feel very optimistic tonight; although, of course, the California Constitution requires all of us native sons to be optimistic, and we try.

I decided instead to title the talk, "Can Anything Be Done About Health Care Costs?" and I think the answer to that is yes. I wish to talk about some of the programs that have been advanced, and some of the ways in which we might consider dealing with health care costs.

One way, of course, is to do nothing, and if this were fifteen years ago, in 1965, that would have been the preferred solution. We wouldn't have health care cost inflation, and we wouldn't have Medicare, and perhaps we wouldn't have a great deal of the problem—maybe not even enough to have a conference about.

Another way is to suggest that government pay all costs for better

---

*Current Secretary of Defense of the United States. Former Secretary of Health, Education, and Welfare in the Ford and Nixon administrations.

health care, and I don't think that topic needs a great deal of discussion tonight.

The third way is to try to reduce, or at least level out, the rate of increase of health care costs by a variety of means, and there are quite a few ways to try to achieve this goal. One could adopt the magnificent dictum of Dr. Lewis Thomas, who said that most things get better by themselves. Most things, in fact, get better by morning, and this he described as the great secret which internists have managed to keep from their patients for generations. But, unfortunately, Dr. Thomas was talking about health care, not health care costs, about which I think we do have to do something.

Let me discuss some of the causes and the culprits in this rather chronic problem that we've all been dealing with for many years; and then some of the cures, none of which perhaps is really new, yet they are being more frequently recommended today. They bear out the precept of Ecclesiastics, that there really is nothing new under the sun. But perhaps it is time to re-examine some cures that have been presented over the years and see if there isn't more merit to them than others have thought.

When I said that fifteen years ago the preferred course of treatment would have been to do nothing, I had in mind of course that we didn't have inflation then, and we didn't have Medicare. And I had in mind also that one of the causes, indeed one of the prime culprits of health care cost inflation, is the faulty design of Medicare. The latter, as you know, injected an enormous demand for health care services into the system by guaranteeing payment by the government for all services available without constraint and to a very large segment of the population, without any regard to questions such as the need for the service, the quality, or the cost of the service. In the euphoria that accompanied the idea of bringing better health to everyone, it was a very difficult concept to get across that there might be some real problems connected with the system. Virtually all the people involved at that time had never before had an opportunity to have unlimited free services; as a matter of fact, very few people have ever had that kind of opportunity before. And there had also been many predictions about Medicare, which I think were roughly as accurate as many other predictions made by people sponsoring programs.

It had been estimated that when the program was fully implemented, it would cost about $200 million. It reached about $43 billion last year, and even allowing for the inflation that may have been partially caused by Medicare, that still is a pretty faulty estimate. The faulty design of the program really came about in a rather interesting way that is not commented on very frequently. It was the result of a very far reaching and, I think, little understood aspect of the whole legislative and governmental process.

In 1965, President Johnson's administration urgently wanted a health care program as a part of what was loosely called the president's vision of a great society; and while we can certainly, at least for the sake of argument, attribute only the best motives to that administration, I think it is fair to say that the tactics employed have caused endless problems. There was, as there had been for many years before, very strong opposition to the whole idea of Medicare and the idea of federal intervention in the health care picture, certainly at the federal level. There have been somewhat similar proposals made to the Congress many times before which had been rejected, or which died by inaction—pretty much the same thing. All the objections that were raised are familiar and need no repetition.

But the administration and President Johnson were committed to securing the passage of some kind of health bill. This is a rather familiar syndrome, and we see quite a bit of it even today. They wanted something that they could point to as a national health care program, and they determined that they would make an offer they felt could not be refused, as a means of defusing the chronic (and thus far successful) opposition to this sort of program. In effect what they tried to do, and I think succeeded in doing, was to eliminate the opposition of the various health care providers by agreeing in advance that the government would not try to regulate or control the health care service to be paid for by the government; and as evidence of their good faith, if that is the word we want, there would be no government challenge to the necessity for the service—no government inquiry into the price of the service or the quality of the service furnished. The opposition crumbled sufficiently so that the necessary votes were secured, and we had Medicare.

For several years the government kept its part of the bargain. They didn't make any inquiry into the need or the cost or the quality, and we were well launched on the road to health care cost inflation. Of course, there are several other causes, and I would not want to say that Medicare was the sole cause, but it suddenly injected this enormous new demand into the system, accompanied by a guaranteed payment for whatever the service. That simply meant that there was now health care available to be used not as needed, but simply because it was there.

In addition, because of the design of the Medicare insurance—a design that is still in effect today—there was a heavy emphasis on the use of the most expensive and, I suppose, sometimes the most unneeded type of care (namely, hospitalization) without sufficient emphasis on other types of care.

And then there is another cause, too, that goes along with it to some extent: American technology, of which quite understandably I am not at all critical. American technology never really rests (nor should it), and as the volume of health care grew, owing to all of these demand factors that I have mentioned, there was also a very substantial increase in the intensity of care as new technologies developed. As they developed in an era of general inflation, and being very expensive new instruments themselves, they, too, added to the expense.

There is another factor that also hasn't been recognized adequately as a major culprit, and that is the explosion of malpractice suits as the old barriers to physicians testifying against other physicians seem to be broken down not only by an increasingly vigorous bar, but also by a general change of standards. In San Francisco there used to be one attorney who specialized in handling malpractice cases. He was the man you went to see if you were a doctor and you were sued. He kept very busy, but there were very few cases, and he could handle them all. That is not the case now. This explosion of malpractice suits brought with it, through a number of verdicts, an obvious increase in the risk which was reflected immediately in the more or less free market of malpractice insurance. The rates rose so steeply that when I was in Washington as Secretary of Health, Education, and Welfare, I became quite alarmed at the number of doctors who were simply going out of practice rather than try to pay those rates. Neurologists and anesthesiologists seemed to be the worst risks from the insurance standpoint, and their rates skyrocketed, some as much as 1200 percent in insurance premiums in a couple of years.

The proliferation of malpractice suits has caused a major increase in the already rapidly rising cost of health care, not just because of the premiums, which of course are passed on to the consumer like everything else, but because it induced a vast number of unnecessary and duplicative procedures, all under the basic title of defensive medicine. Instead of keeping the kind of records that everybody assumed and hoped doctors were keeping before on each patient, now almost from the first day of care doctors must start building a defense against a potential malpractice suit. And this means enormous numbers of unnecessary additional X rays, hospitalization, and other kinds of procedures, done with the idea in mind that, "Well, these things are probably insured for anyway, they are paid for by the government, and if I don't have a record that I've done them, I may lose a malpractice suit."

When I was in Washington, we asked some government estimators for figures as to the cost of defensive medicine, defined as unnecessary hospitalization or other procedures taken as a direct result of the need to protect against malpractice suits. They came up with an estimate of between $3 billion and $8 billion a year. This was in 1973. Because of the lack of precision and the total size of the numbers, I have not questioned the estimate further, but I still think it is a very substantial sum. It is something that one can't blame anyone for but that enormous profusion of suits. A great many things could be done to reduce them, and two of the things I always advocated when I was in Washington, and which made me very unpopular with my own profession, still seem to me like very good ideas. The first is a much shorter statute of limitations for bringing such actions, rather than letting them string out for up to six years, as is the case in some states. The second is disallowing contingent fees for lawyers—a suggestion that brought the wrath of the profession down on my head. When a lawyer in effect finances a case, he really buys an interest in the outcome and then has a double incentive to win the case. In some cases he uses the nominal plaintiff as a virtual pawn, and in some situations, I regret to say, he is not entirely careful about the type and quality of the evidence that he amasses.

Another cause of inflation of health care costs reintroduces the government as the villain, you might say, and this is heavy over-building of hospitals, encouraged and subsidized by the Hill-Burton Act. As is the case with many programs, this one started out right after World

War II with a very necessary and valid purpose: to provide some of the needed additional beds and modernization that had been neglected for many years—and it just kept going, as is the case with most government programs, with a similarity to the Sorcerer's Apprentice. So now we have a surplus of 75,000 or 85,000 hospital beds and a 60 to 65 percent occupancy rate in many hospitals. That ought to be all the evidence we need that the government should no longer continue to subsidize building more hospitals, but it isn't. This still goes on and is one of the causes of inflation, because as a very simple computation will show, it is a great deal more expensive to operate a hospital with empty beds than with full beds, particularly if you are paying off very large construction loans at some rate of interest.

Another major factor is that there is really very little competition in the salutary form known as the free market in the health care system. For instance, it is not in any way practical or possible for a patient to shop around, so to speak, to choose the least expensive or the most efficient hospital. Patients go to hospitals assigned by the doctors, and the doctors use hospitals where they have been admitted to practice. Whether this is good or bad, it means that the opportunities of allowing market factors to help in that particular rather narrow situation are not present, and there are very few situations where any kind of real competition prevails.

There is another factor: the increasing intrusion of government into the system. Like all activities that are regulated or over-regulated, it produces enormous additional nonproductive costs which have to be borne by either the taxpayer or the patient or, as usually happens, both. Other factors to be considered are some very strong lobbies, for instance. I remember the very strong push for a bill in the middle of a small recession in 1973—a bill that would have the government step in and pay the premiums on existing health insurance for anyone who was unemployed. The average time of unemployment at the time was six weeks, and the enormous administrative complexities of trying to get the government into each of these private policies to determine the proper premium to be paid each month during the six-week period when a person was unemployed, didn't seem to bother anyone. And we had to stop and find out who were the people who really wanted this? Well, these were the labor unions, many of which had agreements that they would pay a private form of unemployment compensation to their unemployed members *and* their health premiums; and it was the insurance companies that had carried the insurance and didn't want their premiums to go unpaid.

It reminds me of another enormous humanitarian effort to increase the school lunch program so that it would include all children regardless of need, and the people pushing for that the hardest were not nutritionists or parents, but the Association of American Milk Producers. This is the kind of lobbying activity that is very strong, very effective, not in any sense illegal, but far stronger than opposing factors.

These are some of the factors that have added to the already very high rate of inflation of health care costs, which have run well ahead of the Consumer Price Index for several years, at least in hospitalization costs. I suppose it could be tolerated and you could excuse it if, despite the rising costs and the contribution to the general inflation that this inflation of health care costs produces, it were considered a permissible or necessary cost of society. But the simple fact of the matter is that there seems to be a very tenuous connection between health and costly health care, and we go back to Dr. Thomas again.

We have a number of different studies that indicate that despite the application of a great many modern technologies, more hospitalization, more insurance, and an enormous increase in Medicare expenditures from $200 million to $43 billion and beyond, we don't necessarily observe that degree of improved health to the nation. We seem, on the contrary, to be approaching the point reached by several other governments and countries. It is almost apparent that it is not possible to allocate the resources that seem to be required by these ever-increasing and expanding programs, of which health care is one, and at the same time to maintain any kind of an economy sufficiently strong to enable us to deliver the vastly improved quality and standard of life that people in this country have enjoyed with very few interruptions since the beginning of this century. It is very important to try to preserve this very valuable, rare thing. As the government gets further and further into the process, and as more and more of the gross national product is devoted to governmental costs, we are in danger of weakening, and ultimately destroying, the strength of the economy that has produced that enormously improved quality of life for so many people, not only in this country, but all over the world.

What worries me most is that as more and more resources are devoted to paying for these programs, as we get beyond 40 percent of all government spending for services at all levels, we risk weakening that system to the point that all we can do is get in a constant race for more government grants and government programs to overcome the effects of inflation caused by the increasing costs of government.

I suppose the simplest thing to do is stop right here because I've outlined all the problems and as the cliché goes, there are no easy answers. But I think this may well be one case that defies the cliché; I think there may be some relatively easy answers. Yet with the kind of institutions that we have, the way Congress is structured, and the way it is influenced by special interests, I don't know if we, as a nation, have the courage and the resolution to try any of them.

One of the things we might want to do first is consider rather seriously if we cannot back the government out of its very active role in some health care programs, particularly those of poor design, and reduce some of the extremely unproductive and therefore, by definition, inflationary expenditures.

There are many plans that offer some hope in this area, and some of them would certainly make a vast improvement in the present system. I don't wish to endorse any particular plan tonight except, of course, the one presented to President Ford in 1975, which I consider the best so far, but I'm sure that everybody here with a plan thinks that his or hers is. It is interesting to note how many common features are now shared by most of these plans, such as far more competition, far more aspects of the free market in the area of health care. We have to bear in mind that basically the health of the nation is good. We have had an improving state of health for quite some time by various statistical measures, and I think that they are substantially correct and that we have had some extremely skilled providers of health care, both physicians and hospitals and others. The conclusion from that is that we should be very skeptical, to the point of downright opposition, of any plan to get the government any further into the regulation of health care or of health care suppliers. Rather, we should back the government out of many of the programs it participates in now.

I think, by contrast, that the provision of far more comprehensive, privately furnished health insurance, paid for by employers—bearing in mind that a great many employers do this now for a fairly large section of the employed population—would reduce the demand for hospitalization and increase the utilization of home health care and much less expensive remedies, if the policies were broadly based and covered such things as alcoholism, mental illness, drug abuse, and a number of other things that are all excluded now.

If the entire working population of the United States were covered by privately furnished health insurance with the government's role being primarily to examine the comprehensiveness, the value, and the proper breadth of coverage of health care policies, and perhaps to help pay the premiums of people totally unable to pay, then I think we would have not only a very substantially increased competition among the insurance companies to be the carrier for these programs, but also, because of the enormous breadth of coverage and the base of numbers of covered people, we would have an opportunity to drop the cost. As part of this, the private insurance company should be able to challenge the necessity for the service, the quality of the service, and its cost. I think we would then get a substantial reduction in some of the steadily rising costs, or at least a reduction in the rate of increase. And I'm surprised and pleased to note how many people now come up with one or more variants of this basic idea.

Some tort laws governing malpractice suits in a number of states should be modified, as I have indicated. That has been started in a few states such as Indiana, and I hope will spread to other states and reduce the number and the incidence of malpractice suits.

There ought to be, of course, complete freedom for those who wish to use prepaid health care plans. By the same token, I don't see any reason for the government to continue subsidizing these plans any more than I see any reason for the government to subsidize the fee-for-service insurance or any other form of delivery that the free market might propose.

I would also remove, as I have indicated, any government inducement to more hospital building, and instead give incentives to hospitals to combine and consolidate facilities, so as to eliminate much of the duplication and the waste that necessarily occurs from the natural desire of trustees and the staff of each hospital to be the finest general hospital in the world, even if the finest general hospital in the world is right across the street. Many years ago, long before I went to Washington, I served on a little group in San Francisco called the Health Facilities Planning Committee, and as a result of what we concluded,

I was delegated the task of telling St. Francis Hospital why they didn't really need any more facilities for the care of childhood diseases, that Children's Hospital was fully able to provide these, and that they ought to consolidate those two departments. I have run into a great many fierce opposition nests in the course of long years spent in politics, but I don't recall anything more fierce than the reaction to that simple proposal many years ago. Perhaps now there is some more of this consolidation under way, and this again is something that can reduce duplication and the waste.

I think we are basically a very healthy nation by many if not most of the yardsticks by which health is measured—even though some of those yardsticks may not be all that effective. We have every reason to be very proud, not only of the way in which health services are delivered, but of the enormous research capability that has been developed. A lot of that was developed with government support, and that is one of the things that the federal government has done well over the years. The National Institute of Health is certainly a very great tribute to the kind of support that government can give. It is a little lavish now, and it is a little hard to get it into a somewhat more normal mode, but I think it has done some very remarkable things. I don't think we should tamper with the basic system of health care that we have and its emphasis on the delivery of health services through private sources. But it is very natural for the government to get further and further into it when $42 billion of public money is involved. It is entirely reasonable that the trustees of the $42 billion, the members of Congress, and the executive branch should want to have a very close look at how it is being spent and whether it is being spent in accordance with the statutes, misguided as many of the latter may be. It is natural that if you have heavy government involvement, you are going to get heavy government regulation and, ultimately, control. This is the principal reason why it is so fundamentally wrong—aside from all the fiscal problems involved—to go into a system that involves fully paid, federally furnished national health insurance or nationalized health insurance. We have a very long and unfinished agenda in health care and in health care research, and at the top of that list is the necessity to ensure that people have the opportunity to receive the health care they need in a way they can afford. It seems to me that the basic principles I have tried to outline in very general terms in this talk would help bring that about. If the government limits itself to determining the satisfactory comprehensiveness of the private insurance and its only other role is helping to pay the premiums for the kind of private insurance desired by people who are totally unable to pay for it themselves, then we would have taken several major steps towards introducing competition and backing the government out, and therefore toward controlling health care costs and perhaps maintaining, or even improving, the very high quality of health care that I think we already have.